Cystic Fibrosis in the 20th Century

People, Events, and Progress

Cystic Fibrosis in the 20th Century

People, Events, and Progress

Carl F. Doershuk, M.D.
Editor

Professor of Pediatrics, Emeritus
Case Western Reserve University School of Medicine
Cleveland, Ohio

Carl
Best Wishes
Carl Doershuk

AM Publishing, Ltd.
Cleveland, Ohio

AM Publishing Ltd

Printed in the United States of America

ISBN: 0-9717064-0-9

Proceeds from the sale of this book benefit
the Ronald McDonald House of Cleveland

www.ronaldhousecle.org

This book is dedicated
to every person challenged or touched
by cystic fibrosis,
an enemy not yet unmasked

Contributors

Phyllis S. and Lawson S. Anderson — Past Presidents, Cleveland Chapter, Cystic Fibrosis Foundation, Cleveland, Ohio

Bruce L. Baskin — Member, Board of Trustees, Cystic Fibrosis Foundation, Bethesda, Maryland

Madeline C. and Henry I. Bernbaum — Past President, Cleveland and Rainbow Chapters, Cystic Fibrosis Foundation, Cleveland, Ohio; Past Vice President, Cystic Fibrosis Foundation, Bethesda, Maryland

Richard C. Boucher, M.D. — William R. Kenan Professor of Medicine, University of North Carolina at Chapel Hill, Chapel Hill, North Carolina

Amoz I. Chernoff, M.D. — Past Medical Director, Cystic Fibrosis Foundation, Bethesda, Maryland; Past Director, Division of Blood Disease, National Heart, Lung, and Blood Institute, National Institutes of Health, Bethesda, Maryland

Lourdes R. Laraya-Cuasay, M.D. — Professor of Pediatrics, Robert Wood Johnson Medical School, New Brunswick, New Jersey

Pamela B. Davis, M.D., Ph.D. — Professor of Pediatrics, Medicine, Physiology & Biophysics, and Microbiology & Molecular Biology, Case Western Reserve University School of Medicine, Cleveland, Ohio

Paul A. di Sant'Agnese, M.D., Med. Sc. Dr., Dr. Med. (Hon.) — Past Chief, Pediatric Metabolism Branch, National Institute for Arthritis and Metabolic Diseases, National Institutes of Health, Bethesda, Maryland; Clinical Professor of Pediatrics, Retired, Georgetown University, Washington, D.C.

Jack M. Docter, M.D. — Clinical Professor of Pediatrics, Emeritus, University of Washington School of Medicine, Seattle, Washington

David M. Orenstein, M.D.

Antonio S. and Janet Palumbo Professor of Cystic Fibrosis, Children's Hospital of Pittsburgh; Professor of Pediatrics, School of Medicine; Professor of Health, Physical and Recreation Education, School of Education, University of Pittsburgh, Pittsburgh, Pennsylvania

Barbara L. Palys

Chairperson, International Association of Cystic Fibrosis Adults; Editor, IACFA Newsletter, Harvard, Massachusetts

Paul M. Quinton, Ph.D.

Professor of Biomedical Sciences, University of California, Riverside; Nancy Olmsted Chair in Pediatric Pulmonary Medicine, University of California at San Diego, San Diego, California

Robert C. Stern, M.D.

Professor of Pediatrics, Case Western Reserve University School of Medicine, Cleveland, Ohio

Doris F. Tulcin

Past President, Cystic Fibrosis Foundation, Bethesda, Maryland

William W. Waring, M.D.

Jane B. Aron Professor of Pediatrics, Emeritus, Tulane University School of Medicine, New Orleans, Louisiana

Warren J. Warwick, M.D.

Professor of Pediatrics and Medical Physics, Annilisa Marzotto Professor for Cystic Fibrosis Patient Care, University of Minnesota School of Medicine, Minneapolis, Minnesota

Robert E. Wood, M.D., Ph.D.

Professor of Pediatrics and Otolaryngology, University of Cincinnati School of Medicine, Cincinnati, Ohio

Contents

What is Cystic Fibrosis, Who Has It, What Has Been Done About It?
Clinical Insights and Research Progress

How Has the Community Helped With Care and Research?
Volunteers Organized to Work Together

How Well Have We Done?
Center Directors Remember

Can We Do Even Better?
Looking Ahead

Timeline of Events in Cystic Fibrosis

Event	Year	Approximate Median Age of Survival
Cystic fibrosis of the pancreas described (Andersen)	1938	6 months
Diagnosis by analysis for deficient pancreatic enzymes	1940s	
Pancreatic enzyme replacement	1940s	
Penicillin effective orally and by aerosol	late 1940s	
Sweat salt defect identified (di Sant'Agnese)	1950-53	1 year
Structure of DNA reported (Watson and Crick)	1953	
Broad spectrum antibiotics	1950s	
Founding of National CF Research Foundation	1955	2-4 years
Cleveland CF Chapter incorporated, Ohio	1955	
Diagnostic sweat test reported (Gibson and Cooke)	1959	
Cleveland Comprehensive Treatment Program started (Matthews)	1957	5 years
Start of National Comprehensive CF Care Centers (Landauer and CF Board of Trustees)	1961	
Start of International CF Association (Barrie, di Sant'Agnese, and others)	1965	
Colistin (first anti-pseudomonal agent)	1960	
Semi-synthetic penicillins and aminoglycoside antibiotics	1960s	10 years
"Heparin Lock" intravenous delivery system developed (Stern)	1972	15 years
Completion of "Strategic Plan" (CF Foundation)	1979	18 years
Finding of the chloride ion transport defect (Quinton)	1981	
Research Development Program (RDP) Centers started by National CF Foundation, now 10 Centers	1981	
Increasing CFF/NIH support of CF research		
Identification of CF gene (Tsui, Collins, Riordan)	1989	25 years
Clinical therapy trials begin	1991	
Gene therapy trials begin	1995	
Drug development, drug screening, and other innovative National CF Foundation programs	1999	
Current projected median survival age		32 years

Suggestions to the Reader

The chapters in this book range from very personal essays, to a combination of personal and historical developments in cystic fibrosis (CF), to a virtually straightforward historical approach, or to a blend of the three. Almost all of the lay and professional contributors range from 50 years of age to well into the 80s. Their individual essays, presented in differing ways, cover the CF story from 1938 through the remainder of the 20th Century and serve to make the reading personal and interesting. The "Timeline of Events" will help orient the reader. The chapters vary greatly and some include scientific detail so readers may read only selected sections initially. For a student project report, a great deal of useful information is recorded in many chapters and include relatively detailed science along with the individual personal stories especially in the Quinton, Drumm, and Farrell contributions. The chapter by Stern reviews intravenous therapy from its origins, brings the reader to the current status of home therapy, and provides predictions for future advances.

Historians and those interested in how medical progress came about and the successful interaction of public policy and a voluntary health agency will find many chapters of interest. Events and autobiographical vignettes are found in most chapters. The personal experiences and reports by parents (Graubs, Tulcin, Andersons, and Bernbaums) are especially compelling, as are those by Palys, Baskin and Quinton, each of whom live with the disease.

This enterprise should have been initiated some years ago but now is better than never. As many as possible of the early CF Center Directors who were also involved in the early days of the Medical Advisory Council of the Cystic Fibrosis Foundation were solicited. Sadly, many no longer retained reference information or were unable to contribute. Much of the development and subsequent progress in pediatric pulmonary medicine since the 1960s is the direct result of the action of the Cystic Fibrosis Foundation in initiating its Center Program of treatment and research. The US Center developments are documented in several chapters (di Sant'Agnese, Docter, Lobeck, Waring, Wood, Huang/Laraya-Cuasay, Warwick, Doershuk) and in Canada (Gillespie). The Nova Scotia CF experience, initiated by Dr. William Cochrane, provides database information including improving survival and change in age of diagnosis beginning in the 1950s and documented into the 1990s. Throughout the book there are many references to volunteers in the CF effort and to the impact of the CF Foundation on treatment and research progress that is continuing at an ever increasing rate. Activities initiated in the CF Centers spawned the development of pediatric pulmonary medicine as a specialty, pediatric respiratory therapy, newer airway clearance techniques for pulmonary patients of all ages, long term indwelling intravenous therapy, and, at the least, fostered the development of Child Life programs in children's hospitals.

Review of the Timeline of Events is especially revealing since it demonstrates the Foundation's impressive and accelerating progress. After the description of CF as a disease in 1938, the stimulus to form the National CF Foundation in 1955 followed in 17 years. Five years later in 1961, the essential network of Care Centers was initiated at major medical institutions to improve care and to increase patient numbers and research while the equally essential network of Chapters was developed for education and fund raising.

With the growing success of the Chapters and Centers, by 1975 the need for long range planning was recognized and "The Strategic Plan" was completed 4 years later in 1979 (Tulcin, Chernoff, Doershuk in Medical Program). This creative and pivotal product quickly brought on the innovative Research and Development Program in 1981 (Tulcin, Davis) and, remarkably, discovery of the CF gene followed in just 8 years in 1989 (Drumm). Clinical therapy trials began 2 years later in 1991 followed by gene therapy trials in 1995, the Therapeutic Development Network in 1998 (Davis, Doershuk in Medical Program), and other progressive programs in 1999 (Timeline, Drumm and Knowles/Boucher in Looking Ahead), all with the purpose of more rapidly increasing knowledge, improving therapy, and sustaining productive lives.

The events in the race leading up to the discovery of the CF gene were of interest and exciting even to those observing from the sidelines. To follow the story through the eyes of a research trainee in one of the major genetic laboratories is even more compelling (Drumm). Neonatal Screening and the need for early diagnosis have been discussed for over 25 years and there is increasing interest in this issue now that there is reasonable methodology available (Farrell). In the Looking Ahead section, Drs. Farrell, Drumm, Knowles and Boucher, and Davis graciously offer insight for what to look toward for clinical and research progress over the next few years. We are mindful of the concern expressed by Dr. Davis in the final chapter, Patient Care and Research, (paraphrased) on the necessity for continuance of aggressive, meticulous conventional home care management of the patient, faithfully today, until we have the cures of tomorrow.

The pathologic description of CF, the origin of the CF Foundation dedicated to research and comprehensive treatment, and the stimulus for forming the International Cystic Fibrosis [Mucoviscidosis] Association all originated from the United States. A recounting of these events, of necessity, results in this being a mainly a North American story. However, there are many other important developments and stories about CF to be told and much more recent history to be recorded from the US and from the many other countries where active programs evolved. Further reporting of these activities may be for others to achieve. Meanwhile, readers are free to pick and choose their way through these essays. For those with comments or further anecdotes and stories, I can be reached at cdx5@po.cwru.edu.

Carl F. Doershuk
Cleveland, Ohio

Foreword

In little over half a century, the disease known as cystic fibrosis (CF), has progressed from an unknown entity, to identification as an early-life, almost uniformly fatal disease, to the development of life-prolonging interventions, and more recently to hope for total control or possible cure in the wake of the identification of the gene and its protein product. The history of the many individuals and events that, independently and together, allowed such dramatic progress, even in the absence as yet of detailed understanding the disease, makes a compelling and rewarding story.

Chronic diarrhea and malnutrition were common in infants in the early 20th century. Many of these babies were diagnosed as having "celiac disease" in which normal digestion of food occurs by the pancreatic enzymes, but an abnormal small intestine is the cause of poor absorption of nutrients and subsequent abnormal bowel movements. From autopsy studies, it became evident that some of these celiac diagnosed infants were dying at a very young age, had a normal small intestine, but instead had mucus plugging of the pancreatic ducts resulting in the formation of cysts and scarring (fibrosis). In patients with celiac disease, there had been only a few case reports of fatal associated pneumonia and/or bronchiectasis until 1938 when an American pathologist, Dorothy Andersen, published an extensive autopsy study of infants with the pancreatic abnormalities, and abnormal bowel movements and dying of pneumonia at a very early age. She used, for the first time, the term "cystic fibrosis of the pancreas" (later shortened to cystic fibrosis) to describe the findings in these infants. Additional reports soon confirmed this new entity, almost uniformly fatal early in life. Somewhat later, the indication that this was a generalized exocrine (secreting) gland disease of the body led to the term "mucoviscidosis," which was frequently used in Europe. There was a suspicion that this was an inherited recessive disorder. Thus, a couple who each carried the recessive gene would have a one in four chance of the disease occurring with each subsequent pregnancy. Later this proved to be true in accordance with recessive gene inheritance.

Unfortunately, in the 1940s there was no easy diagnostic test and diagnosis occurred mainly from suspicion. However, physician awareness was minimal as there were no textbook reports, afflicted infants tended to die very young, and the siblings and parents of these infants had no symptoms of the disease that would prompt suspicion. There was some progress in that there was a diagnostic test for intestinal pancreatic enzyme activity (albeit laborious). Pancreatic enzyme extracts from the pancreases of pigs proved helpful in improving digestion of food and nutrition. The *Staphylococcus aureus*, a common bacterium, was recognized as a frequent contributor to the progressive lung infection and damage. The availability of penicillin and other antibiotics provided dramatic early improvement in the pulmonary infection and for the first time effectively demonstrated that it was possible to improve survival in this otherwise devastating disease. Later, another bacterium, *Pseudomonas aeruginosa*, became the more predominant infection agent. It was a greater problem as it proved to be much more resistant to antibiotic therapy.

The surprising discovery of the electrolyte sweat defect (too much salt in the sweat) occurred in New York City in the early 1950s. This led to the development of a diagnostic sweat test which is important to early diagnosis even today. With its ease and accuracy, the sweat test provided rapid confirmation of the disease in any suspected child. Major institutions were located on the East Coast (Boston, New York, and Philadelphia) and using various treatments. Increasing numbers of patients were identified. Parent groups were forming to help each other and to fight the disease. In 1955, the National Cystic Fibrosis Research Foundation (NCFRF) was formed in New York City and, in the same year, a statewide chapter was chartered in Ohio. By 1960, the National Cystic Fibrosis Research Foundation created increasing new chapters and approved a new Regional Center Program concept inspired by the successes of the National Foundation for Infantile Paralysis Foundation (Polio) Center program.

Various treatments for CF were in use and the most promising were assimilated into a "comprehensive treatment plan" in 1957 by a young Cleveland investigator with initial support from a concerned local CF family group known as the "Cousins Club." There was an accompanying evaluation and research program to provide documentation of the clinical treatment success observed. Patient survival improved markedly and provided the nidus for a basic research program. The impressive clinical results led to the incorporation of the comprehensive treatment program into the CF Foundation's Regional Center plan in 1961. The major concept for the Centers was to gather patients, improve care, and increasingly promote research at the major institutions recruited across the country.

Nationally, the result was of increasing success from the collaboration of the lay Chapters in promoting public awareness and fund raising in conjunction with the medical care Centers, which were furthering patient survival and increasing research capabilities. Although national survival improved steadily, the pathophysiology remained a mystery. Various hypotheses were pursued, but despite several interesting - but short lived - observations and scientific reports, there was a lack of real research understanding of the disease. Fund raising gradually increased and the Foundation developed a "Strategic Plan" in 1979 including an effective public policy program to enlist the aid of Congress and the National Institutes of Health in support of CF research. The Foundation increasingly focused on developing the research capabilities of the most qualified Centers. It became increasingly important to identify the CF gene so that research could be better directed on the etiology of this unique and still fatal disease. That focus led to a race to identify the gene. Finally, three Centers collaborated to identify the gene in 1989, another story detailed in the book. This important achievement greatly expanded the research potential, and new therapies and more basic information have followed.

It is almost past the time to relate the many important events that occurred and to acknowledge as many individuals as possible; the volunteers, researchers, physicians and other care providers, families, and, most importantly, CF participants. All these individuals made this a story of lay and medical people working together in support of the CF Foundation and its programs to achieve remarkable treatment and research progress against a formidable and still life short-ening disease.

This book attempts to relate the steps that occurred, wherever possible in the words of those who were involved at the time. Regretfully, too many years have passed and too many are no longer with us or were unable to participate. I am deeply indebted to each of the contributors who have taken the time, patiently endured my requests, and truly have made the effort to join in relating this story of incredible and continuing success. At the same time, it has been a delightful and rewarding experience for me to renew so many old ties and friendships in the course of developing this book.

My medical school and Babies and Children's Hospital/University Hospitals of Cleveland provided the setting for my training and the early opportunity to be exposed to and become involved in the comprehensive treatment program so successfully developed by my mentor, Dr. LeRoy Matthews, who led me and many others not only into CF care and research but also into what became a new discipline, pediatric pulmonary medicine.

I am indebted to Dr. Claire Doerschuk and Dr. Jeffery Wine for insightful reviews and constructive comments. Dr. Frank Primiano, Dr. Robert Stern, and Gayle Meehan were especially helpful with extensive reviews, advice, and editorial comments. Of greatest importance, my deepest thanks and appreciation are for my wife, Emma Lou, for her support and understanding throughout these many years of involvement toward making a difference.

Carl F. Doershuk
Cleveland, Ohio
September 21, 2001

What Is Cystic Fibrosis, Who Has It, What Has Been Done About It? Clinical Insights and Research Progress

1

The Disease and Its Manifestations

David M. Orenstein, M.D.

It seems that we have always known that cystic fibrosis (CF) is the most common life-shortening inherited disease, particularly among Caucasian populations. We now know that it is caused by a "recessive" gene found to be on chromosome number 7 and because it is a recessive gene, both parents have to be carriers of the gene, but have no symptoms of the disease. For CF to occur, both parents must contribute the CF gene so that, with such a couple, with each pregnancy there is a one in four chance of CF occurring. And we have known that somehow CF was caused by the production of abnormally thick mucus in all the affected organs, particularly the lungs and gastrointestinal system. We were a little uneasy about the fact that thick mucus could explain the abnormalities in the lung, pancreas, intestines, liver, and reproductive tract, but the presence of thick mucus could not explain the salty sweat since the sweat glands do not secrete mucus.

Now we know that our assumptions were only roughly correct, in that the basic defect involves the abnormal transport of salt and water across epithelial cells in the affected organs. This transport abnormality then leads through some direct and some indirect pathways to the production of thick mucus in mucous secreting organs, and other abnormalities in organs that don't make mucus, such as the sweat glands. In the lungs, the development of chronic progressive infection leads to destruction and respiratory failure. The lung involvement is the leading cause of death in over 90% of the patients.

Also, CF is not the most common inherited life shortening disease. That dubious honor probably goes to the familial hyperlipidemias, which are as much as 6 to 10 times more common than CF. These hyperlipidemias are not as brutally life shortening as CF though, as they do not begin to evidence heart disease until into the fourth decade of life. With the increasing improvement in survival in CF, the two may be comparable in this regard.

Whatever our early misconceptions about underlying causes and comparative frequencies, we've long known that CF causes clinical disease in many different organs systems (Table 1.1). There are so many organs systems involved that, as a third year medical student, I thought that if I knew everything about CF I'd know most of what there was to know about Medicine. Since I had already decided that I wanted to be a "CF doc" for my career, I applied to take my whole fourth year of

Table 1.1 Organ Systems Involved in Cystic Fibrosis

Respiratory
    Upper
        Nose
        Sinuses
    Lower
        Bronchial tree
        Lungs

Gastrointestinal
    Pancreas
    Intestinal Tract
    Liver

Other Organs
    Sweat glands

Reproductive
    Male
    Female

medical school studying CF. The wiser minds of the Center doctors, Matthews, Doershuk, Stern, and Boat, turned me down and said I should instead study various other disciplines before I entered full time into CF. They were able to delay by a few years my joining them but after my residency training I came back to them as a pulmonary and CF trainee. I think they were right, but I think I was partly right too; it is hard to find an aspect of medicine not touched on by CF at one time or another.

In addition to the listing of organ systems involved in CF, a full accounting of the impact of CF should include the complications seen in these organ systems (Table 1.2).

In this chapter, I'll reminisce about patients I've seen over the years who have represented for me some of the various aspects of CF that occur and mention a few things about my own career.

Upper Respiratory Tract

Nasal Polyps. About 20 percent of CF patients have nasal polyps at one time or another. These polyps may be persistent and relief only comes with surgical removal, but they may also shrink with steroid sprays, or in some cases when they feel like it, without medical intervention, even in a very short time. Unfortunately,

Table 1.2 Complications of Organ System Involvement in Cystic Fibrosis

Respiratory
    Upper
        Nasal polyps
        Sinusitis
    Lower
        Hemoptysis
        Pneumothorax
        Respiratory Failure

Gastrointestinal
    Pancreas
        Pancreatic insufficiency
        Pancreatitis
        CF related diabetes (CFRD)
    Intestinal Tract
        Meconium ileus
        Distal intestinal obstruction syndrome (DIOS)
        Rectal prolapse
    Liver
        Liver cirrhosis and liver failure
        Portal hypertension
            Hypersplenism
            Esophageal varices

Other Organs
    Sweat Glands
        Salt loss syndrome
    Reproductive system
        Male infertility
        Female reduced fertility

they may recur and require repeated treatments in some cases. Polyps can also occur in patients with asthma and allergies. Polyps are not dangerous, but can be a nuisance, mostly by blocking nasal airflow, and requiring mouth breathing, but also in some cases by causing a widening of the nasal bridge or interfering with the ability to smell. In rare cases, they may grow so far forward that they protrude out of the nostril, looking for all the world, as some patients have told me, "like you have a bugger hanging out of your nose all the time." Few patients enjoy this complication. One young girl had this problem many years ago, and I sent her to our ENT (ear, nose, and throat) surgeon, whose offices were some two miles from the hospital. By the time she arrived at the ENT office, the polyp had shrunk out of sight. The surgeon thought that this youngster, her family, and CF physician all had a vivid imagination, since all had described the permanent "bugger" which, during the short trip between hospital and outpatient office, had disappeared back into the recesses of the nose.

Sinusitis. Virtually all patients with CF have pansinusitis (abnormalities of all the sinuses) on sinus x-rays. Some of these patients also have the typical symptoms of sinus infection (headache, stuffiness, posterior nasal drip, etc.), but most do not, and the abnormal x-ray is a problem only for the radiologist. Most CF physicians advise against taking sinus x-rays, because we know that they will show sinuses that are filled up. More recently, CT evaluation of the sinuses can provide better information, especially if recurring or significant headaches are a problem.

A teenager with CF was involved in a car accident a number of years ago and sustained cuts to his face. The emergency room physician in the outlying hospital correctly ordered a skull x-ray to make sure the patient hadn't fractured his skull. He hadn't. But the x-ray was abnormal in a way that anyone who is familiar with CF would have anticipated as the sinuses appeared to be completely filled. The emergency room physician took this as evidence that the sinuses were filled with blood from the accident and the patient was life-flighted to our emergency room. He was fine. I used to tell this story to make the point that all patients with CF have very abnormal sinuses on x-ray. I'd tell anyone who'd listen that my patient was the only one in history to enjoy being life-flighted, since he was perfectly well, except for his minor cuts, and got to enjoy the helicopter flight. I recently made a terrible mistake for a storyteller, however, by checking the story with the original source (the patient), and I can't use the story any more. It turns out that he hated the flight!

Lower Respiratory Tract

Lung Disease. The lung disease of CF begins as obstruction of the smallest bronchi and bronchioles. The earliest chest x-ray abnormality this produces is overinflation of the lungs, an abnormality that can be quite subtle. With progression of the disease over years or decades, this obstruction extends upwards to the larger bronchi, and with continuing bacterial infections and inflammation, it becomes more widespread. In the 1940s, the most common bacterium recovered from the lungs was the *Staphylococcus aureus*, which was then very sensitive to newly available penicillin. Then another bacterium became more common and led to a more persistent, low grade and chronic infection. It was called *Pseudomonas aeruginosa* and, with the *Staphylococcus aureus*, led to the damaging destruction of the lungs. Also it proved harder to treat as it was more persistent and more resistant to many antibiotics, as they became available.

The chest x-ray in more advanced cases can be quite striking, with overinflation, linear markings, cysts, and fibrous (scar) tissue. I remember a young woman who was working as an x-ray technician in a local hospital when her younger brother was diagnosed with CF. She arranged to have a chest x-ray taken of herself. While waiting for the radiologist to give an official interpretation of the film, she put it up on the view box. When she saw her own x-ray, she broke down crying, essentially having diagnosed herself, based on seeing the shadows of her own fairly severely involved lungs staring her in the face. I have another favorite story – and a happier one – of a CF patient staring at – and in this case holding – his own severely involved lungs. For that story, you have to be patient (or cheat, and skip ahead to the section on respiratory failure and lung transplantation).

One of the biggest changes in CF care that has evolved over the two and a half decades since I started my CF fellowship is that we now have the capacity to obtain excellent bacterial cultures of the tracheobronchial tree, even in patients—including newly diagnosed tiny infants—who do not cough out mucus. This information is important in guiding appropriate antibiotic treatment. The tool that enables this to be done safely and in relative comfort is the flexible fiberoptic bronchoscope. The techniques for performing bronchoscopies in infants and children were developed by a doctor who preceded me by one year in fellowship and in joining our mentors on the faculty. That person is Dr. Robert Wood, known internationally as the father of pediatric flexible fiberoptic bronchoscopy. Since we were brother fellow trainees together during one year and faculty colleagues for another four years, I believe this experience makes me the "uncle" of pediatric flexible fiberoptic bronchoscopy. No one else seems to think so.

Hemoptysis. Blood streaking of expectorated mucus is not uncommon in patients with CF, but massive hemoptysis (more than 300 cc in 24 hours) is rare. These episodes result from the infection causing local erosion of the wall of a small bronchial blood vessel. Most of these episodes stop on their own, or with extra vitamin K (to help blood clotting) and treatment of the underlying infection, but some require more aggressive treatment. A few decades ago, the only more aggressive treatment available was lobectomy (surgical removal of a portion of the lung). Lobectomy has in rare cases been lifesaving, but it involves removing healthy lung tissue along with the tiny vessel that is bleeding. There are only five lobes (3 in the right lung; 2 in the left), so loss of a lobe entails loss of a substantial amount of functioning lung tissue, and the current thinking is that this should be avoided in all but the most desperate situations. Nonetheless, I have seen two different teenaged boys who had some bleeding, and underwent removal of not one but two lobes in outlying hospitals, and only when they continued to bleed were they sent into the CF Center. Against these large odds, both young men were able to pull through the acute bleeding. Both went on to have several years of very active life, one employed full-time in a cemetery, and the other a student and part time charming wheeler dealer, always selling this or that to whichever doctor, nurse, or man on the street would listen to his sales pitch.

Today, there is aggressive treatment for hemoptysis that preserves lung tissue. Specially trained radiologists can insert a catheter into a large artery (the aorta) and inject a special chemical that shows up on x-rays, allowing for identification of exactly which small artery(ies) to the lungs is (are) bleeding. They can then inject substances that block those arteries so that blood no longer leaks out. This procedure is called embolization. I have never had a patient who required embolization, but many patients around the country have had lobes (and even lives!) saved by this newer technique.

Pneumothorax. Pneumothorax is the leaking of air out of the lung, into the space surrounding the lung, within the chest. The leak occurs when mucus blocks the bronchi enough to allow air past the obstruction during inspiration, but not out during exhalation. This leads to a "bleb" (a weak part of the lung) which is usually found in an upper lobe. With each breath, more air is trapped behind the obstruction, progressively inflating the bleb, until it bursts. Once this occurs, air leaves the lung and collects outside the lung but within the chest space. This can be dangerous, as eventually enough air collects outside the lung so that the lung is prevented from expanding and can even be compressed. The treatment of pneumothorax used to be relatively straight forward, if not easy. An operation was performed wherein the surgeon would open the patient's chest, identify the blebs, excise them and sew over the holes, and then purposely cause inflammation of the pleura (the membrane covering the lung). The pleural inflammation would heal, with the formation of scar tissue. This scar tissue was quite successful in preventing further leaks. But there was a problem brought about by this medical progress in that the extensive scar tissue surrounding the lung would make removing the lung a difficult and bloody undertaking. In "The Old Days," the only time the lungs needed to come out was literally during undertaking, or more precisely during a post-mortem examination, after a patient had died.

However, science marches on, and lung transplantation has now given some patients a new lease on life. For a patient to undergo transplantation, his or her old lungs need to be removed to make room for the new. The surgical difficulty and bleeding caused by prior pneumothorax surgery made this part exceptionally challenging and precluded transplantation for some patients. We have now developed a new stepwise approach to pneumothorax in patients with CF. The first step is placing a tube into the space between the chest wall and the collapsed lung, allowing the air to escape, and the lung to re-expand. Sometimes this procedure will be enough. If it is not, then more definitive steps may be needed to prevent recurrences of the pneumothorax. These next steps should be taken if the simple chest tube placement has not prevented a recurrence. I have known quite a few patients within the past decade who have developed a pneumothorax and were not able to get the definitive treatment, because of the physicians' or family's fear that this might make future lung transplantation difficult or impossible. Fortunately, modern surgical technique seems to have made transplantation after pneumothorax surgery less risky.

Respiratory failure. Respiratory failure is the term given for failure of the lungs to continue to do their job of bringing oxygen into the bloodstream in adequate amounts and eliminating sufficient carbon dioxide. Respiratory failure is the cause of death in over 90% of patients with CF. Respiratory failure is usually an ominous sign that death is increasingly imminent. However, there are exceptions to the rule of this one-way trip. Today, the success of lung transplantation for some (but still very far from all, or even the majority of) patients has made people aware of the possibility of reversing or halting this downward plunge. I've already mentioned one patient who did very well with his lung transplantation. He wanted to see his old lungs afterwards, so we went to the pathology department. One of my very favorite pictures is of him, with a huge grin on is face, standing there, holding his own badly damaged—and no longer needed—lungs, as if to say, "anybody want these lungs? Only one previous owner!" In years past, well before transplantation was dreamed of, there were exceptions to this rule of "respiratory failure always means imminent death" as well. I remember clearly several patients who were all judged unlikely to survive the night, yet who eked out a few more hours, and then went on to have more good years of life.

The memory of these patients has helped guide me in my belief that there can always be hope. Sometimes there is hope for longer life, even in the face of evidence that seems to point towards death. At other times, when there isn't any more hope of a longer life, there can always be hope for comfort and peace. Most modern CF physicians are guided in their care of patients with respiratory failure by the principle of offering hope: continuing treatment that might allow for longer life if that is to be possible, while not withholding measures that provide comfort whether or not a longer life is possible.

Gastrointestinal Tract

Pancreas. The pancreas is important for its role in digestion, especially of dietary fat and protein. The pancreas makes enzymes that break down (digest) fats and proteins in the duodenum, that portion of the intestine just beyond the stomach. The pancreas seems to be blocked in most (85 – 90% of) patients with CF, preventing these digestive enzymes from reaching the food. In most patients, the pancreas is replaced with scar tissue. The result is the incompletely digested fat and protein failing to be absorbed into the bloodstream, making the stools bulky and smelly, and making it difficult for the patient to gain weight. After CF was recognized as a distinct disease entity in 1938, the only test was for a deficiency of pancreatic enzymes.

The typical child with CF was one who had a large appetite, yet failed to gain weight. In the early years, malnutrition contributed to the cause of death in babies with CF. Then came the introduction of pancreatic enzyme supplements, derived from pigs, and the digestive problems became much more manageable. Still, the powdered enzymes that were available posed new problems. One problem was that the enzymes were easily degraded by stomach acid. So, only a portion of the enzyme doses reached the duodenum where they enzymes are supposed to work in digesting food. Another problem was that these enzymes were designed to digest fat and protein. They did it well, and they did it without discrimination, trying to digest all the fat and protein with which they came into contact. This meant that babies who got enzymes smeared on their lips as they ate in the typical sloppy baby way could get burns on their lips, and breast-feeding mothers could get sore nipples if they were not careful (and quick) to clean up any enzyme transferred from the babies' mouths. Some babies and toddlers hated the bitter taste, and would spit out any food used to deliver (and hide) the enzymes. Derek was just such a toddler, and boy was he ever good at finding which food had been used for the enzymes, and spitting it out!

Then in 1978, a breakthrough occurred that affected most patients with CF: the introduction of enteric coated pancreatic enzymes. This meant that enzymes were packaged in tiny beads, each with a coating protecting the enzyme from stomach acid. The coating also protected lips and nipples from coming in contact with the active enzymes themselves. The coating was designed to dissolve only after it left the acid environment of the stomach. This made a huge difference in the effectiveness of the enzymes, and benefited virtually every patient with CF. And, I thought, at last we can get enzymes into Derek because the new beads have no bitter taste to cause him to reject them. But the little stinker just seemed to have a "thing" for enzymes, and no sooner did he start getting the new enzyme beads in apple sauce than he started sput, sput, sputtering out each little enzyme bead, one after the other, like a machine-gun! Fortunately, he was able to eat enough food to make up for all that he was losing into his diaper by not getting adequate enzymes, and he did quite well. And, eventually, he outgrew his bead-spitting games.

Pancreatitis. Among the 10% or so of patients whose pancreas is relatively spared, and who do not need supplemental enzymes for good digestion of their food, there is still probably some pancreatic duct blockage. This blockage can lead to a backing up of the enzymes that were on their way to the duodenum. When these enzymes back up, they begin to digest the pancreas itself, and then infrequently may cause pancreatic inflammation called "pancreatitis." This condition causes severe abdominal pain, and must be treated by resting the pancreas by causing it not to secrete digestive enzymes. Since the pancreas secretes enzymes automatically in response to a person's eating, this means that people with pancreatitis are made "NPO," which stands for "having nothing by mouth" in Latin. Some patients, including one active 19 year old man and one sassy 3 year old girl whom I remember vividly, can have pancreatitis as the first sign of CF. These two patients were typical of patients who first come to medical attention because of pancreatitis: they have appeared quite healthy and well grown. They might have had what seemed like mild asthma. But since they had not had the typical CF digestive problems, they did not have an earlier diagnosis.

Diabetes. As the pancreas becomes progressively more blocked and replaced with scar tissue, some patients even develop diabetes mellitus (termed CF related diabetes or CFRD). The way this happens is that the special pancreatic cells that make insulin are damaged or destroyed, and less insulin than usual is available to help control the body's glucose (sugar) levels. Rarely does one with CF develop this problem before 10 years of age. Between 10 and 20 years of age, about 10% of CF patients develop diabetes, and then another 10% develop it between 20 and 30 years of age.

In people who don't have CF, diabetes announces itself with fairly sudden loss of energy accompanied by tremendous thirst and very frequent urination, all caused by very high blood sugar levels. Blood glucose levels are regulated with a system somewhat like a dam in a river: if the glucose is below a certain level (180), all of it stays in the bloodstream and can be delivered to the tissues that need it for energy and growth. However, once the level of sugar in the bloodstream exceeds 180, the excess sugar "spills over the dam" in the kidneys, and into the urine. Lots of sugar in the urine pulls extra water into the urine, so one pees a lot. With the loss of all of that water, there is a great thirst and the need to drink a lot.

There are things about CF related diabetes that are different from non-CF diabetes that often make it less dramatic and less life-threatening. Some patients, like Beth, may not have frequent drinking and urination, and may actually think they have pretty good energy, but just have trouble maintaining their weight. Beth was a high school swimmer who swam the 500 yard freestyle in her freshman season. But then in her sophomore year she couldn't last the 500 yards, and she swam the 50 and 100 yard swims instead. She also lost weight – not dramatically, but bit by bit. She and I thought the problem was that her lungs just weren't in as good shape as they should be (even though her pulmonary function tests were not that different from the previous year). Finally, we thought to check her blood glucose level and it was 785 (about seven times normal)! So what seemed like bad news turned out to be not so bad news: we had an explanation for her decreased energy and her difficulty maintaining her weight. And in fact when she started taking insulin shots – something that she adjusted to quite readily—she quickly regained her lost weight and energy. Now she runs long distance with the track team.

Intestinal Tract

Meconium ileus. Somewhere between 10 and 20% of newborns with CF are born with their intestines blocked by thick stool secretions (meconium) or failure of a portion to develop. This blockage needs to be relieved immediately, either by surgery, or—in as many as half of these infants—by special enemas (Gastrografin[R] enemas) performed in the radiology department. This is a way that many patients' families have found out in a sudden and frightening way that their newborn baby had CF. The bad news is that this is a medical emergency within the first day or two of an infant's life. The good news is that once the obstruction has been recognized and treated, most babies do very well, and most begin on a treatment program before they have suffered any lung damage, thus making their long-term outlook very good.

Distal intestinal obstruction syndrome (DIOS). After the newborn period, a number of patients may experience a different kind of intestinal obstruction, for different reasons. Sometimes this happens with "dietary indiscretion," such as lots of ice cream and cake (without adequate enzymes) at a birthday party, as I can remember with one young patient. This obstruction, like meconium ileus, must be relieved, but most of these patients will be able to have this done by enemas, such as with the Gastrografin, but without surgery, while nearly half of newborns with meconium ileus require surgery.

Rectal prolapse. This problem arises when thick intestinal contents "grab" the inside of the rectum and pull it inside out during the passing of a bowel movement. The rectum then is left inside out, outside of the anus. In some cases, it simply goes back inside by itself. In most other cases, if the problem is recognized, the rectum can simply be pushed back inside with gentle pressure. If the problem isn't recognized promptly, there can be swelling that makes it harder to get the rectum pushed back into its proper place. This problem most often happens in very young children. In one of the creepiest "it's-hard-to-think-about-what-almost-happened" scenes etched in my mind, this occurred in a teenager, and the rectum did not go back in immediately. This teenager had not experienced the problem before, and— somewhat logically, I suppose—thought that what was hanging out was just a very large sticky bowel movement. She began shuffling her way across the room to get a large pair of scissors to cut off the offending "stool." By some miracle, the bowel went back inside on its own. Had it not, and had this young patient wielded the scissors as planned, to bisect what was hanging out, the likely consequences are now too horrendous to contemplate. Fortunately, this story had a happy ending, as is true for most people with rectal prolapse. In most cases, simple adjustment of pancreatic enzyme dosing solves the problem. And most patients seem to outgrow the problem.

Liver. Somewhere around 50% of CF patients have liver abnormalities, involving blockage of bile ducts and some scarring, but does not cause symptoms. This is called cirrhosis of the liver. A very small number of patients have liver problems that truly affect their health. These problems result from the back pressure caused by the duct blockage and this is referred to as portal hypertension (see below).

Liver cirrhosis and liver failure. Another change that has occurred in the past few decades related to care of CF patients with liver disease is that in the few cases when the liver completely fails due to extreme progression of the cirrhosis, the patients do not necessarily die, as they would have previously. I remember several patients, some of them with excellent lung function, who died because the liver failed (this has been the fate of some 3 – 5% of CF patients). This is not necessarily the case anymore because of the success of liver transplantation. I was fortunate enough to know the first young man with CF ever to get a liver transplant, as well as to work in the same institution as Dr. Thomas Starzl, the surgeon who performed that transplantation, and in fact single handedly invented liver transplantation. These were two remarkable men. One, the innovative medical scientist, who persisted in his belief that liver transplantation could save people with previously fatal liver disorders despite six years of uniformly fatal outcomes of his transplantation operations. Of course, today, some decades after his first attempts, liver transplantation is an accepted form of therapy for some disorders. It is so widely accepted now that successful claims of malpractice have been brought against physicians for not performing such a procedure! And the other remarkable man was a former high-school football player who was willing to undergo the very first procedure of its kind in someone with CF. He did well, and his twin brother followed him in undergoing the procedure within the following year or two. Since that time, many patients with CF, even some with fairly marked lung disease, have had liver transplants. Many have done well, and have even had improved lung function after the procedure.

Portal hypertension, hypersplenism, and esophageal varices. Much of the body's blood drains from the abdominal organs through the liver to return to the heart. If there is sufficient blockage, blood can back up into the spleen and into the veins in the esophagus. If enough blood backs up into the splenic vein, the spleen enlarges and becomes over active. Since part of its job is to remove some of the red and white blood cells and platelets from the circulation, the patient can become anemic and have a low white blood count and low platelet count. If the situation becomes severe enough some surgical correction becomes necessary.

Also with sufficient blockage, the esophageal veins also can become enlarged (and are then called "varices"). In severe cases, these can rupture causing serious bleeding. In rare cases, life threatening bleeding can even be the first sign that someone has CF. I have no recollection of any patient with this particular dramatic way of announcing the diagnosis of CF, but I have vivid recollection of several patients who had many episodes of serious bleeding that was nearly uncontrollable without major abdominal surgery to relieve the back pressure. And I have been able to see the big change in our ability these days to control esophageal bleeding, without surgery, either through endoscopy performed by the gastroenterologists, or even a special shunting procedure done in the radiology department that relieves the back pressure.

Other Organs

Sweat glands. It is the high salt (sodium chloride) content of sweat that enables the diagnosis of CF to be made using the sweat test. The sweat glands remain normal appearing under the microscope and never develop any pathology or visual changes, but they function abnormally. Patients with CF need to be careful to take in extra salt, especially when they are exercising in the heat. Infants with CF need to be given extra salt to make up for what is lost in the sweat. A few years ago, a young African American baby with CF lost his appetite, and became quite lethargic. It turned out that his blood sodium and chloride levels were very low, despite the fact that his mother had been putting extra salt into his formula. He was suffering from the salt loss syndrome that some people with CF have. This problem seems to be a bit more common among black patients, for reasons that we don't understand. What was especially unusual about this youngster (in addition to his being one of the sweetest children ever) was the fact that he required hospitalization six (!) times for salt loss, including 2 times after he was old enough to select his own food, and salt it. Most patients with CF do fine even if they exercise a lot in hot weather, by just selecting salty foods, without ever being aware that they are making such high-salt selections.

Reproductive system. Most men with CF are sterile because of a blockage or even the absence of their vas deferens, the tubes that carry sperm from each testicle to the penis. These are the tubes that are cut purposely for a vasectomy. In days past, when sexually transmitted diseases were not as prevalent, certain young Lotharios were not averse to advertising this fact to their young lady friends as a reason to enjoy safe sexual indiscretions with them. Most men with CF are aware of their likely infertility, because most CF physicians are careful to educate patients and families about all aspects of the disease. I remember an awkward moment some years ago, when I was taking care of Dr. Doershuk's patients while he was on sabbatical leave. One of his adult patients told me happily that he and his girlfriend were planning to get married, and he was looking forward to fathering many little children. I knew that Dr. Doershuk would not have neglected telling a 23 year old the CF male facts of life long ago, but wondered if perhaps this patient had "forgotten" what might have been a painful bit of information. How could I, a fresh new young CF doc, break the tough news to this happy "father-to-be?" As I stumbled around trying to assess what he did and did not know about his likely ability to father a child, it became clear that he was just having some fun at my expense. He knew full well that if he was to have children, he could do what many others have done, namely, adopt a child, or – less commonly – their wife has in vitro fertilization from a non-CF sperm donor. This young man just wanted to see me squirm in trying to explain to him about the CF birds and bees. Nowadays, in rare cases, it is even possible for some men with CF to have sperm withdrawn from their own testicles and used for in vitro fertilization, so that even with a blocked vas deferens, they can be the biological, as well as the emotional, fathers of their children.

Women with CF usually have a harder than normal time getting pregnant, because of thick cervical mucus, chronic lung disease, under nutrition, or a combination of these factors. Yet, many women with CF have had babies. Unfortunately, if their health has not been ideal, pregnancy can be hard on a woman with CF. I remember all too well a very young woman with CF who became pregnant when her lungs were not in the best shape, and whose health deteriorated dramatically through the pregnancy. She had a healthy baby, but she died within six months after the baby's birth. Fortunately, this is not the typical course of pregnancy in women with CF. If they are healthy prior to the pregnancy, their health does not deteriorate while they carry their pregnancies to term. One of my favorite CF patients, a wonderful nurse, was herself diagnosed only after her own daughter was diagnosed!

My Research Career and Its Roots

Early in my fellowship, Dr. Doershuk took me aside to discuss what field I might choose for my research. We listed many possibilities, but the one that caught my attention was the study of exercise for patients with CF. He was well aware that I was already interested in exercise, especially running. The way he hooked me on embarking on exercise studies was to tell me of a patient who had traveled to Cleveland from another Center. This teenage boy was very active and liked sports, but his mother reported that during one hospitalization the physician had said, "You are not to play baseball again!! And do you know why? Because it will kill you!!" And he then turned to the mother and said to her, "And do you know whose fault it will be? Yours!!" I knew that each of my mentors in patient care had always encouraged their CF patients to be active, and it certainly appeared that those who were more active did better, both medically and psychologically.

But as we thought about how negative this patient's medical advice about physical activity had been, we realized that neither that physician, nor we, had any scientific proof that our way was right. So I was motivated to find the scientific proof that the active lifestyle I saw being encouraged was in fact beneficial (it is). As a result, I happily gained extra training in exercise physiology and began my exercise research studies. Along the way, my colleagues and I have been able to answer a number of questions about exercise and CF, including the responses to exercise in the heat, oxygen levels during exercise, the role of supplemental oxygen, and the benefits of various exercise programs. These initial conversations that sparked my interest have formed the foundation for my whole research career.

After my formative years in Cleveland as a trainee and faculty member, I spent three years in Memphis, Tennessee, some of these as the only trained CF physician in the state. And I began to develop a more acute appreciation of what I had suspected, how special my training had been, including exposure to Dr. Matthew's comprehensive approach to treatment. For I now saw parents from other cities being told to take their newly diagnosed children home to die, because there was no effective treatment for CF. I saw babies from these other cities still being diagnosed using the archaic total body, plastic bag sweat tests. I then had the opportunity to move to Pittsburgh in 1984 and to develop a CF Center and program that had gotten an excellent start under the direction of Dr. Joan Rodnan, who died very young just a few months before I arrived. From that start with one physician, we now have 7 full time CF physicians—including Dr. Glenna Winnie another Cleveland trainee—and an active clinical Center, with 400 patients. We do clinical and basic research, and pass on the principles planted and nurtured in my training.

The three accomplishments of which I'm most proud in my own career stem directly from that Cleveland soil. I saw each of my mentors, and subsequently colleagues, take special interest and time in communicating with their patients and families, teaching them all about CF. In 1989, I wrote the first book aimed at CF patients and families, "Cystic Fibrosis: A Guide for Patient and Family". Actually, it was *published* in 1989, I wrote it from 1986 to 1989. I then updated it with a second edition in 1997, including many of the advances in our knowledge of the cellular and molecular bases of CF[1]. I am told that many patients and families (and medical care professionals) find this a useful tool. I thought that since not every patient/family is lucky enough these days to have a physician with enough time to give all of the details about CF as I had been taught, I would try to give them as many of the tools to understand CF and its treatment[2] that they would have received if they had been so fortunate.

Second, in 1997 I received an honor from the Wellesley Hospital in Toronto in being named their Arthur Squires visiting lecturer. This honor is bestowed on a physician who is judged to practice medicine in the style of Dr. Squires, now in his 80's, who practiced general internal medicine for many years and was revered for his compassion, and for his exemplifying the gentle art of medicine. I remain a bit puzzled as to how I was chosen, but since the gentle art and compassionate care and teaching of patients is what I consider to be the greatest lesson I learned from my teachers and colleagues in my Cleveland "Golden Years," I value the bestowing of this award most highly.

Third, I was honored in 2000 by being installed as the Antonio J. and Janet Palumbo Professor of Cystic Fibrosis at Children's Hospital of Pittsburgh. This professorship recognizes the importance of the kind of CF care that began for me in Cleveland and represents only the second endowed professorship devoted solely to CF. I am grateful that it enables me to continue my work in CF care and research and in writing about them.

From this brief introduction, it is apparent that CF can cause a multitude of problems in various organ systems. Also, CF affects individual patients in different ways, perhaps in part because there are now well over 900 different mutations of the CF gene that have been recognized. I have tried to share my recollections of some of these very special individuals with you as they've illustrated the different manifestations of CF. In the years since I saw some of these patients, we have come a long way. Survival has doubled. Breakthroughs in basic science have given hope for even better progress in the near future.

It is gratifying to think of how much of this improvement can be traced, directly or indirectly, to the Center Program of the Cystic Fibrosis Foundation and the Center where I trained.

References

1. Orenstein, DM. *Cystic Fibrosis: A Guide for Patient and Family.* Second Edition. Lippin-cott-Raven. New York, 1997.
2. Orenstein DM, Rosenstein BJ, Stern RC. *Cystic Fibrosis Medical Care.* Lippincott, Williams & Wilkins, Philadelphia, 2000.

2

Experiences of a Pioneer Researcher: Discovery of the Sweat Electrolyte Defect and the Early Medical History of Cystic Fibrosis

Paul A. di Sant'Agnese, M.D.

I was born in Rome, Italy in 1914 to an obstetrics/gynecology physician father and an accomplished pianist mother. Learning English as a child as my second language would help me a great deal in my future in the United States. A year after graduating with honors from the University of Rome Medical School in 1938, I came to the College of Physicians and Surgeons, the medical school of Columbia University in New York to get a Ph.D. in Biochemistry. Instead, I completed an internship and residency in Pediatrics at the New York Postgraduate Hospital and later received the degree of Medical Science Doctor (MSD) from Columbia. Now 87 years of age and walking with a cane, I have a great many memories of the appearance of cystic fibrosis (CF) on the medical scene and of what I like to call the "heroic age" of medicine, the advent of antibacterial and antibiotic agents which so dramatically changed the outlook and treatment of pediatric and infectious diseases, and of course of CF.

Cystic Fibrosis—The Beginning

From the discovery of the gene for CF and of its 900+ mutations, it has become evident that CF has existed for thousands and probably tens of thousands of years. However, it was not recognized as a separate disease entity until 1938. Patients with CF were thought to have celiac disease because of their gastrointestinal symptoms or chronic bronchopneumonia of which there was so much at that time. We know Guido Fanconi in Switzerland in 1936 published in an Austrian journal the autopsy and clinical findings in three cases a subgroup of patients thought to have "celiac disease," in which he recognized the association between pancreatic deficiency and what he called bronchiectasis. However, it was the extensive pathology study by Dr.

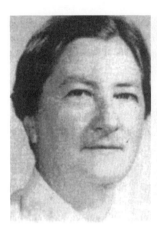

Figure 2.1. *Dr. Dorothy Andersen who gave the first
comprehensive description of cystic fibrosis.*

Dorothy Andersen (Figure 2.1) published in 1938, in which she used the term "cystic fibrosis of the pancreas" in describing the autopsy findings of 38 patients from
the files of the Babies Hospital in New York City, that really put CF on the map as
a distinct disease entity. At the same time in 1938 there were two other smaller
reports which had less impact; one from Blackfan and others in Boston and one
from Australia. However, knowledge and recognition of the disease were almost nil
for several years after 1938.

It was at this time that I came to the CF scene. After the four year residency in Pediatrics at the New York Postgraduate Hospital which was affiliated
with Columbia University, I returned to the Babies Hospital, the Pediatric Unit of
the Columbia Presbyterian Medical Center and of the College of Physicians and
Surgeons Medical School of Columbia University. I was on the Pediatric Faculty of
Columbia University and Chief of the Pediatric Clinics (Figure 2.2). Dorothy
Andersen, who was a pathologist, was looking for a pediatrician for care of her
patients who had been referred with celiac disease and with the new and relatively
unknown disease then called cystic fibrosis of the pancreas. It sounded like a challenging project and I signed up for it, especially as I remembered the several infants
during my residency who had died of a progressive lung disease of mysterious origin. At that time at Babies, there were only a handful of patients with CF. Among
them JD, who was the first patient ever diagnosed in vivo in 1938 at Babies Hospital on the basis of chronic pulmonary disease and a positive duodenal drainage test
showing pancreatic deficiency. Perhaps he was the first living person diagnosed
with cystic fibrosis anywhere in the world.

Most patients died within the first year of life, but occasionally they lived
longer as did JD, who lived until the age of ten or eleven years, despite the lack of
any effective treatment. Sulfa drugs were the only antibacterial agent available at
the time and they were totally ineffective in CF. We were completely helpless

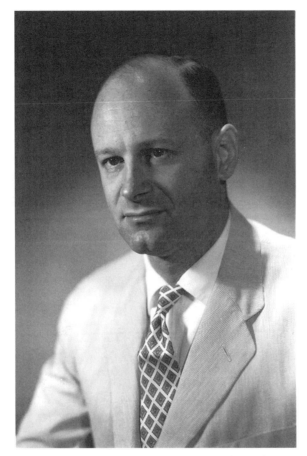

Figure 2.2. *Dr. Paul di Sant'Agnese who identified the elevated salt content in the sweat of cystic fibrosis patients.*

watching patients get progressively worse and eventually die. The first break in treatment came with penicillin about that time. Penicillin was owned by the army and largely reserved for the troops in the field in World War II. However, small amounts were given out for worthy research projects. I remember a Colonel in uniform sitting at a table at Columbia and doling out the drug to the petitioning scientists sitting in front of him. I got a small amount of penicillin for use in CF.

In most patients, the results were dramatic. From death's door, slowly dying from the chronic pulmonary disease while we watched helplessly, patients revived in a few days. The high white blood cell count and the fever decreased, appetite improved, and there was a significant weight gain. For the first time, we had an effective tool to help us control the lung infection as the predominant organism in the bronchi of patients with CF was penicillin sensitive *Staphylococcus aureus*. Penicillin worked whether it was given by injection or by inhalation.[1] Patients who had never had an antibiotic before were very susceptible to penicillin, even though by present standards ridiculously small doses were used. It is interesting that aerosol administration of antibiotics, so effective at the time, later fell in disrepute for decades until it was later reinvented with therapeutic success. I guess we were the first, at least in print, to use the newly available antibiotics in the treatment of the pulmonary disease of CF. The major reason for the success of penicillin was due to the fact that *Staphylococcus aureus* was the predominant organism at that time in contrast to the present flora dominated by the Pseudomonas species.

Antibiotic therapy, of course, was to become the mainstay of therapy of the pulmonary disease of CF. It was quite effective together with physical therapy and other therapeutic methods in improving, although unfortunately not curing, the CF patients. Streptomycin became available in the late 1940s and was remarkably effective despite its side effects, mainly ototoxicity, but there was no choice at the time. As a result, several patients had a hearing loss of various degrees of severity. Also in the late 1940s, tetracycline and chloraphenicol came on the market and were among the first of the broad spectrum oral antibiotics.

At the same time, and while we were spreading the gospel on this largely unknown disease, CF, the number of patients seen at Babies Hospital steadily increased until we were getting 50 to 60 new cases per year. In fact, at that time, CF patients from a large section of the United States were being referred to either the Babies Hospital in New York or to Boston's Children's Hospital, the other institution in which work on CF was being done at that time by Dr. Harry Shwachman.

Sweat Electrolytes and the Sweat Test Story

When a new discovery is reported to the scientific world, they say first, "It is probably not true." Thereafter, when the truth of the new proposition has been demonstrated beyond question, they say, "Yes, it may be true, but it is not important." Finally, when sufficient time has elapsed to fully evidence its importance, they say, "Yes, surely it is important, but it is no longer new."

—Michel de Montaigne
(1533–1592)

At the end of August 1948, there was a very intense heat wave in New York City. It was especially difficult to cope with because there was no air conditioning in most homes or even hospitals at the time. Notably, five of the ten children admitted to Babies Hospital because of heat prostration were known CF patients. All patients had severe dehydration and vasomotor collapse. Only one case had hyperpyrexia, which proved to be fatal. One of the patients without pulmonary disease was not known to have CF which then became suspected on the basis of the heat prostration. Later he proved to have pancreatic deficiency, at that time the test necessary to establish the diagnosis. Parenthetically, he was still alive in Los Angeles at the age of almost 50, not too many years ago.

I took care of these patients as Dorothy Andersen was vacationing in England at the time. However, they were reported in the medical literature by Dr. Kessler, at the time the senior resident, and Andersen in 1952.

In the summers following 1948, we noticed that CF patients appeared to be unusually susceptible to hot weather and heat waves. Reading the textbooks of physiology, it was apparent that the sweat eccrine glands, generally distributed over the body surface, produced aqueous sweat and were responsible for temperature regulation. They were estimated by Professor Kuno in Japan in his book on sweat glands to number about two million and spread all over the body. The apocrine sweat glands were confined to limited areas of the body (armpits, groin, etc.) and had a different and to some extent sexual function, e.g. aroma, etc. Prof. Kuno had not studied the sweat electrolytes (especially the sodium, chloride, and potassium), but there were a few reports in the literature about the normal values of these electrolytes and some information that there was a moderate increase in sweat electrolyte concentration in patients with adrenal insufficiency. A constant temperature room had been used in all of these experiments to induce sweating.

It was at this time in early 1952 that I met up with Bob Darling, who was then Head of the Rehabilitation Department of Columbia Presbyterian Hospital. He had available a constant temperature room and a method to collect sweat was available, although it had to be somewhat modified. I decided, as a "shot in the dark," to see if the sweating function was impaired in CF patients that would lead to a smaller than normal volume of sweat, or whether there was something wrong with the sweat electrolyte concentration, or whether both factors might be present. A sweat problem might have made these patients unusually susceptible to heat and "heat stroke."

Accordingly in April 1952, I selected two patients with CF who were in their early teen age years and two other children of the same age but with other conditions, put them in the constant temperature room, and then collected and analyzed their sweat for the electrolytes, chloride, sodium, and potassium. To my surprise and much excitement, the answer was right there. There was a tremendous difference in the sweat electrolyte concentration between the two groups. In the two patients with CF it was much higher than in the two controls. In contrast, the sweating rate was similar in the two groups.

As quickly as I could in the next few weeks and months, I obtained sweat in the constant temperature room in as many CF patients, normal children, children with a variety of disorders other than CF, and a few adults. I confirmed the great difference in sweat electrolyte concentration with almost complete separation of values for chloride between CF patients and children who were either normal or with almost any other kind of disease.[2] As before, the rate of sweating was similar in the two groups. For sweat sodium there was a little overlap, but some of the results we obtained were too high due to some error that we could never ascertain. At the time, of course, that was thought to be quite the way it was. Sweat potassium was also analyzed and was statistically significantly different in the two groups, but

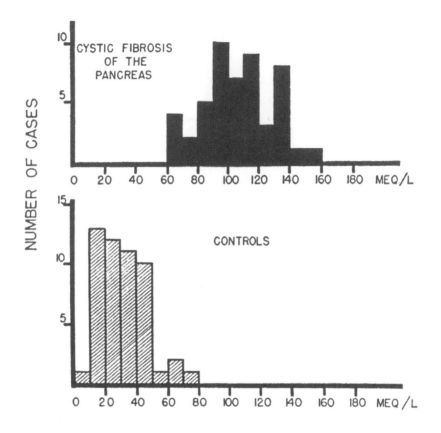

Figure 2.3. *Abdominal sweat chloride in 43 patients with cystic fibrosis of the pancreas (50 determinations) and 50 controls. From Pediatrics 1953;12:549-563 (page 550), with permission of the publisher.*

there was quite a lot of overlap in values. Figure 2.3 describes the results of the chloride concentration in the first 50 CF patients that were ever studied. It is striking that after so many years since the original studies, the results of the sweat chloride concentration have remained essentially the same. Two of the first questions that came to my mind were: Do patients with CF lose salt through their kidneys as well as through the sweat glands? What is their adrenal function?

As previously mentioned, it was known that patients with adrenal insufficiency had a high chloride level in their sweat. Accordingly, I enlisted the help of Dr. George Perera of the Department of Medicine and Head of its Metabolic Unit. A 13 year old male CF patient, CJ, in fairly good condition was tested with the steroids available at that time and was shown to have normal adrenal function. He was then placed on a salt restricted diet and the serum, sweat, urine, and stool electrolytes were determined on metabolic studies. During the period of salt restriction, the kidneys were able to reduce excretion of sodium and chloride amazingly well, so that by the third day the patient was excreting less salt in his stools and urine than he was taking by mouth. Despite this, the patient lost 2 kg of body weight, his serum sodium decreased from 137 to 131 mEq/L and after five days he began to vomit. The experiment was discontinued. Such vomiting is quite characteristic of CF patients in acute salt loss during hot weather when they have lost enough sodium chloride per kilogram of body weight. Similar experiments on a 13 year old male patient with CF, VD, were carried out over a 20 day period with identical results. Indeed, the disassociation between increased electrolytes in the sweat and the low sodium and chloride levels in urine during the periods of low salt diet or heat waves appears to be a unique characteristic of CF.

It is surprising that, with the exception of some limited studies by Dr. Charles Lobeck several years later and our work with Dr. Richard Grand and others in the 1960s with aldosterone and sweat electrolytes, nobody ever repeated these metabolic studies which addressed such fundamental questions of the physio pathology of CF. It must be assumed that these detailed and comprehensive studies answered all questions to everyone's satisfaction.

At that time, at the end of June, there frequently was a heat wave in New York City exacerbated by the lack of air conditioning. This was the case again in 1952 and, of course, I was ready to study the effects of excessive heat on CF patients, already being aware of the sweat electrolyte situation in this group. During this period and later in the summer of 1952, we admitted to the Babies Hospital six "heat casualties" among CF patients ranging in age from 3 to 13 years, and were able to determine the "seven steps" that lead from perspiration to death. High atmospheric temperature, especially sudden heat, causes profuse sweating which, in view of the abnormal composition of sweat and normal sweating rate in CF patients, leads to acute salt loss. As estimated by Marriott in his studies of British soldiers in India in the 1930s, when sufficient salt has been lost per kilogram of body weight, vomiting then ensues leading to dehydration, with vascular collapse following in rapid succession. Then hyperthermia occurs followed by coma and death. The individual may present as an acute medical emergency requiring the most rapid and drastic therapeutic measures, primarily immediate intravenous fluid administration, to restore the depleted extra cellular fluid volumes. None of the six patients observed at Babies Hospital in the summer of 1952 died, although one was admitted in coma and moribund.

This sequence of events, once a relatively frequent problem, has become quite rare now with the advent of widespread air conditioning. However, infants with CF may become salt depleted even in cold weather as they are more susceptible to salt loss than adults, because their inordinate body surface area to body volume makes their water and electrolyte balance more labile.

In the 1950s, we admitted to Babies Hospital five such infants over a period of four years because of hypoelectrolytemia with decreased serum sodium ranging on admission from 132 down to 112 mEq/L. They were thought at first to have adrenal insufficiency, but renal and adrenal function were shown to be normal. All had some vomiting not thought to be sufficient to explain the symptoms. One had slight diarrhea preceding admission, the other four had none. Repeated small excessive losses of electrolytes in sweat and possibly in gastric secretion leading to negative salt balance over a period of time appeared to be factors in the genesis of the clinical picture. CF should be kept in mind in the differential diagnosis of hypoelectrolytemia and dehydration in infancy. This picture was later more precisely described in the studies by Lynn Taussig, and Eliezer Nussbaum.

One of the first dividends of the "sweat test" was the recognition that CF may occur even in the absence of pancreatic involvement.[3] We know now that this is due to the presence of certain mutations of the CF gene. At that time, however, the diagnosis of CF could not be made unless pancreatic insufficiency could be demonstrated. I had a few patients waiting in the wings who had chronic bronchopneumonia and other features of CF, but normal pancreatic trypsin activity and no evidence of pancreatic insufficiency. The first patient with normal pancreatic trypsin enzyme activity that we tested was a three year old girl of normal stature and nutrition, but with chronic bronchopneumonia following whooping cough and a subsequent relapse following measles. Her sister had died at two years of age and was diagnosed with CF at autopsy, while her three year old brother had all of the features of CF, including pancreatic insufficiency (Figure 2.4). The abnormally high sweat test, in addition to the other clinical features, proved that CF could exist without pancreatic involvement. Later I estimated that about 10% of CF patient had normal pancreatic function, which subsequently proved correct.

The sweat test also immediately proved useful in differentiating CF patients on the wards of Babies Hospital from some of the other conditions that mimic this disease; familial dysautonomia, celiac disease, and other syndromes that lead to chronic lung disease (e.g. Kartagener's syndrome, etc.). All of these have a normal sweat test. At the same time, we tested other secretions and demonstrated a statistically significant difference in the salivary electrolyte concentration between CF patients and other individuals. However, there was too much overlap for this to be of practical use.

With the demonstration of the involvement of the eccrine sweat glands (the small sweat glands distributed all over the body surface) and the salivary glands, it became clear that CF in reality was a generalized disease. The name "cystic fibrosis of the pancreas," while descriptive of the pathologic changes in this organ, was a misnomer, and the term "mucoviscidosis," while popular in Europe, was even less justified as at least two non-mucous producing exocrine glands were affected.

Everybody was telling me to hurry up and get the sweat data in print, as they were so easy to reproduce. However, as frequently happens when somebody comes up with a new finding especially with something as unglamorous as sweat, nobody believed these results. Before publication, the data were presented at the May 1953 meeting of the American Pediatric Society in Atlantic City. There was not a single question. Perhaps the most interesting reaction was that of Jas Kuno,

SWEAT ELECTROLYTES IN MEQ./L

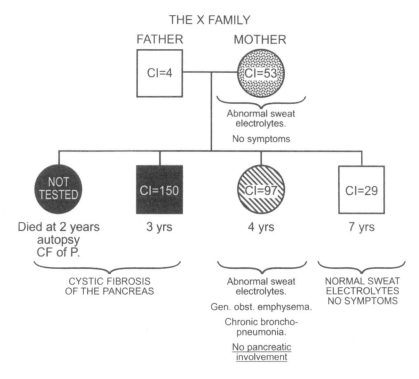

Figure 2.4. *Family tree of X family. The patient is represented by the crosshatched circle. From Pediatrics (modified) 1955;15:683-697 (page 689), with permission of the publisher.*

the famous sweat physiologist. On his visit to Columbia Medical School, I was invited in front of a small audience to present my sweat data to him. Prof. Kuno, a somewhat bullheaded Professor, listened in silence and then uttered one word, "impossible," and stalked out of the room.

It takes time for papers to be published and it finally appeared in Pediatrics in November 1953. The first person to show some interest was Harry Shwachman from the Children's Hospital in Boston, who came to the Babies Hospital in early 1954 to find out more about the sweat test and how it was being done. This was almost two years from the beginning of the investigations of sweat. He soon became convinced of its usefulness and with his usual alacrity and energy quickly went to work and by October, 1954, was able to present a fairly large series of CF patients showing similar results in their sweat and confirming the diagnostic value of the sweat test. I was absolutely delighted to have somebody else confirm my results, as one feels very uncomfortable when one has new data that nobody else has yet confirmed.

Obtaining sweat for analyses with the constant temperature room is a safe and effective method, but not many people have access to such a room. Harry Shwachman introduced the use of plastic bags of various sizes in which patients were enclosed for 45 minutes to one hour and sweat was collected from the back by the usual methods. Plastic bags, although a little unpleasant to the patients, were quite effective and we also used them eventually instead of the constant temperature room. However, there were several reports of deaths from hyperthermia and irreversible brain damage, even in some patients who turned out not to have CF. In a case I was called to see in another hospital in New York City, there was a family history of hyperthermia during anesthesia. This was probably a case of malignant hyperthermia, not realized at the time, and the patient died of irreversible brain damage.

In 1959, Lewis Gibson published his paper on the use of pilocarpine iontophoresis to induce localized sweating by stimulating the sweat glands with a weak electric current in a limited area, usually on the forearm. This simple, safe, and effective method became, and remains to this day, the standard method of performing the sweat test. It is notable that while the methods of inducing sweating have varied, the way of obtaining and analyzing sweat have remained essentially the same.

From the beginning I realized, of course, that the sweat test was a good diagnostic tool, but I never expected it to be as good as it turned out to be. I then thought that five to ten percent of the normal population would have a high sweat electrolyte concentration. As it proved to be, almost all the patients with CF showed this abnormality, and almost no one else. As Beryl Rosenstein said in a recent article, "After 45 years from its description, the sweat test is still the gold standard for the diagnosis of most patients with CF," with genetic studies reserved for the occasional difficult diagnostic case. However, while an abnormal sweat test for many years was a sine qua non of the diagnosis, recent genetic studies have shown that in a tiny fraction of patients it is possible to have an abnormality in the CF gene and some clinical findings, despite a normal sweat test and no apparent involvement of the sweat glands.

It is still strange and unexpected that virtually all investigators have been interested only in the practical diagnostic applications of the sweat defect in CF, and almost no one in the physiopathologic aspects of renal and adrenal function, or in the mechanism and the sequence of events in heat prostration in this disorder.

A final consideration: it was always difficult to reconcile the sweat and salivary defect with the mucus abnormality, which gives rise to most of the symptoms of CF. However, I never imagined that the defect in electrolyte transport would turn out to be the basic defect in CF, as shown by the recent genetic studies of the CF gene and its product, the cystic fibrosis transmembrane conductance regulator (CFTR).

Nature of the Pulmonary Involvement

After a decade of watching most CF patients progress quickly or slowly to their final end, I was convinced that the pulmonary involvement was an almost constant feature of the disease, and that it dominated the clinical picture and determined the fate of the patient. The question at the time was, what was the real nature of the pulmonary involvement?

After review of 211 charts of CF patients, plotting the clinical course, reviewing the chest x-rays, and evaluating the laboratory and pulmonary function tests, I came to the conclusion that bronchial obstruction was the basis of the lung involvement. This appeared to be due to failure to remove secretions and consequent widespread bronchial infection, as described in detail in a series of papers in the early 1950s. Thus, it became clear that bronchial obstruction was the primary and cardinal manifestation of the pulmonary disease component of CF.[4,5]

The cascade of events leading to pulmonary involvement was strikingly uniform in the various patients, except for the degree of severity and the duration of the single phases. Because of failure to remove these secretions, acute respiratory infections usually initiated the cycle by causing increased mucus production. Widespread bronchial obstruction resulted, of which cyanosis, air hunger, and at times atelectasis (collapsed areas of lung) were an expression. After a variable, but usually short period of time, the infection, at first mild and perhaps localized to the main divisions of the bronchi, suddenly became widespread and severe by invasion of the obstructed air passages down to the smaller subdivisions. The infected surface was thus suddenly and enormously increased. In the preantibiotic era, many patients succumbed at this stage because of the spread of the infecting agents to the bloodstream. If the patient survived, this cycle could be repeated again on the occasion of subsequent respiratory infections, thus explaining the characteristic course of these children, punctuated as it was by relatively sudden attacks of markedly increased bronchial obstruction and infection. Any one of these episodes might be fatal.

The main offending organism was consistently *Staphylococcus aureus*, frequently in pure culture in preantibiotic days, although *Pseudomonas aeruginosa*, E. coli, and other organisms were occasionally found in smaller amounts. Collapse of an entire lobe of lung, mediastinal and subcutaneous emphysema, cor pulmonale (heart failure secondary to chronic pulmonary disease), and sudden death from asphxia due to coughing up of large amounts of thick, tenacious bronchial secretions were not uncommon complications.

The advent of effective antibiotics greatly changed this course of events. When the widespread pulmonary infection appears, these agents help the patient to wall off the bacterial invasion and give time for the immune defenses to be activated. Ever since antibiotics have been available, bloodstream infections have essentially disappeared.

The next challenge at this time was the definition and delineation of the pulmonary involvement using specific physiologic measurements. I was very lucky to enlist the help of Dr. John West of the Pulmonary Disease Division of Columbia

Presbyterian Hospital, an outstanding unit that was headed by two 1956 Nobel Prize recipients, Andre Cournand and Dickinson Richards, for their discoveries concerning heart catheterization and pathological changes in the circulatory system. John West studied pulmonary function in just six of our patients who ranged in age from 12 to 14 years.[6] The results of these studies could not be stated better than by quoting the words of Dr. Hans Wessel in the 1983 *Textbook of Cystic Fibrosis* edited by John Lloyd-Still. "…it is remarkable in that West at al clearly identified most of the important features of impaired lung function in CF which have since been verified and expanded on in a large number of subsequent investigations. Notably these authors recognized the wide spectrum of functional impairment of the lungs. They showed that functional impairment correlates well with the clinical assessment of pulmonary involvement. They recognized that an increase of the residual volume and RV/TLC [residual volume to total lung capacity] ratio are manifestations of early pulmonary involvement while a reduced TLC and CO_2 (carbon dioxide) retention are late manifestations of severe chronic disease. They clearly demonstrated that abnormal intrapulmonary gas mixing and increased dead space ventilation were the earliest signs of impaired lung function and concluded correctly that these changes were the result of abnormal ventilation-perfusion relationships primarily due to nonuniform distribution of alveolar ventilation as a result of bronchial obstruction." Unfortunately, John West died of leukemia shortly after completing this study.

Needless to say, strenuous efforts were made incessantly during these years to try to devise the best methods for treatment with the welfare and quality of life of the patients always in mind.

The Unique Liver Involvement in CF

It had been known for several years that the liver was involved in some CF patients. Indeed, in her original paper in 1938, Dorothy Andersen quoted three patients with hepatic cirrhosis (scarring of the liver) from the literature and added one of her own. In the next decade, it was noted by several authors that cirrhosis of the liver was occasionally present in CF patients.

Through the years, I became quite interested in the liver aspects of CF, especially as several patients at Babies Hospital had this liver cirrhosis which can result in portal hypertension (see "The Disease" Chapter) with an enlarged hyperactive spleen and/or gastrointestinal bleeding and massive vomiting of blood due to enlarged esophageal blood vessels, called varices. I was lucky to enlist the interest of William Blanc, who was then the junior pathologist at Babies Hospital. The basic lesion found in virtually all CF patients at autopsy is the so called "focal biliary cirrhosis with concretions" characteristic of CF, at times quite localized and at times more extensive. There are concretions of eosinophilic (pink staining) material, similar to those in the pancreas, which plug the bile ductules and lead to proliferation of the biliary ducts and an inflammatory reaction. If the process spreads, groups of lobules are encircled and trapped by the fibrotic process, while others are spared, resulting macroscopically in deep clefts and excessive lobulation. This is quite different from the usual diffuse liver cirrhosis in which every lobule is surrounded by fibrous tissue. We studied seven such patients, all of whom either at liver biopsy or autopsy had a type of more focal cirrhosis unique to CF, which we named "multilobular biliary cirrhosis with concretions."[7] The presence of biliary concretions on liver biopsy or autopsy establishes the diagnosis of CF, if not already known.

Clinically, because large areas of the liver are normal and spared by the pathologic process in CF, there may be no clinical or laboratory signs of hepatic involvement except the finding of an enlarged liver of various consistency on physical examination. In some patients and in most of those in our study, back pressure in the portal vein developed. In our original patients, there were no cases of liver failure and, of course, it was decades before any liver transplants were performed.

My Stay at Columbia University

First I must state how grateful I am to this country, as nowhere else in the world could one hope to fit so easily into the scheme of things when coming from abroad. Of course, I had some difficulties especially with the language. I knew English quite well when I got here, but I knew the King's English, not the local lingo. My first linguistic experience was the afternoon of the day I landed in New York (no jet lag occurs with ship travel and there were no planes to or from Europe as yet). When I asked directions of a policeman, he informed me I was on, "Toidy Toid Street." Looking at the street sign I realized it was "33rd Street" in New Yorkese! Next I got to Columbia and somebody asked me as to "what neck of the woods" I came from. I was highly insulted and I told the man I didn't come from any "neck of the woods," but from Rome, Italy, the eternal city and the hub of the world.

I must also pay tribute to my wife to whom I owe a great debt of gratitude. Without her help, understanding, and assistance I could not have pursued my career and whatever I achieved, especially after my severe illness and the many permanent physical handicaps that resulted. She was the night nursing supervisor, and I met her the first day I started interning October 1, 1940. We shared many interests including medicine, have been married for 57 years, and our partnership has been and continues to be fruitful and blissful.

After coming to Columbia as previously mentioned, I spent the next four years on the housestaff of a Columbia University Hospital, interrupted by a six month spell at the now defunct Willard Parker Hospital which was the Infectious Disease Hospital for Manhattan and the Bronx. As an intern and resident, I had long hours and lousy board and room, but was otherwise unpaid as the idea at the time was that if you could not afford it, you shouldn't be in medicine in the first place. The work, however, was fascinating and exciting and, as a senior resident in my last year of training, with lots of responsibility. Incidentally, the Chairman of the Department of Pediatrics at the Post Graduate Hospital was named Dr. De Sanctis and people often mixed up our names, much to his discomfort.

When I joined the Babies Hospital at the Columbia Presbyterian Medical Center as Associate in Pediatrics and Chief of the Pediatric Clinics, I also went to work to assist Dorothy Andersen with patients with CF and celiac disease. I have been asked how Dr. Andersen, a pathologist, had patients referred to her? I really do not know the full answer. CF was virtually unknown at that time and patients with celiac disease had to be differentiated from them by duodenal drainage demonstrating the presence or absence of pancreatic enzymes and presumably were referred to her because of her pathology work. Of course, Dorothy had worked with a pediatrician, Dr. Hodges, who I replaced, but she had always had a keen interest in clinical matters. In retrospect, I wonder if she really had wanted to be a clinician, but because of the difficult situation for a woman in medicine when she graduated from Johns Hopkins had to instead be content with a career as a pathologist.

Working with Dorothy was a great and rewarding experience, especially in the first few years. Unbelievably, although she was much better known in the medical world, she was the junior pathologist to Dr. Beryl Paige who was the senior, a relationship which was not always smooth. Dr. Paige retired in the late 1940s and Dr. Andersen became the senior pathologist at Babies Hospital. Dr. William Blanc, with whom I later had a fruitful collaboration, became her junior. Dorothy then was occupied more and more by her duties in the Pathology Department and had less and less time for clinical matters.

With my duties on the wards taking care of CF and celiac patients, running the "Celiac Clinic" (which was primarily CF), serving as attending on the pediatric wards, teaching the students, and fulfilling my duties as Chief of the Pediatric Clinics, my calendar was pretty full. The latter position entailed a fair amount of administrative work and was quite time-consuming. Among other things, every afternoon I had to examine five or six children who had been told to have a tonsillectomy and decide that more than 90% of them did not need this operation.

Then on May 2, 1946, a severe illness called acute disseminated encephalomyelitis, a demyelinating nervous system disease, struck me suddenly with alarming symptoms and changed my life forever. It progressed rapidly and five days after the onset, I was moribund and on the danger list. Most people thought I was going to die and, if I survived, would have to be institutionalized. Instead, surprisingly I rallied and after two months in the hospital I was able to gradually resume my duties at Babies Hospital. However, the acute illness left me with permanent and quite severe physical handicaps.

My main and continued interest in medicine has always been CF. I have been involved in all aspects of the disease; clinical, research, organizational (CF Foundation, International Cystic Fibrosis Association, etc.) and later at the National Institutes of Health (NIH) in the training of promising young investigators. The major part of my 160+ scientific publications, chapters in books and innumerable abstracts, letters to the editors, lectures to medical and lay groups, and presentations at scientific meetings also have been devoted to CF.

However, especially in the 1940s and early 1950s, there were other medical fields to which I was able to make significant contributions. One such opportunity for which the pediatric clinics at Babies Hospital offered an ideal environment was the then relatively new field of immunizations against diptheria, tetanus, and pertussis. My series of comprehensive studies in the 1940s led to important recommendations, which were quickly accepted by the medical community.

Also in the late 1940s, in a clinical, chemical, and pathologic study, I recognized for the first time that glycogen storage disease of the heart was a separate disease entity with different etiology from von Gierke's disease and suggested the name Pompe's disease, which has been generally accepted since.

In the early 1950s, I was finally able to relinquish my duties as Chief of Pediatric Clinics to a successor. The immunization and glycogen storage disease studies were completed and I now had more time for collating, classifying, and investigating my almost decade long experience with CF patients. The next few years were undoubtedly the most productive of my career.

Nowadays, when CF has become a household name, it is difficult to realize that in the 1950s it was still largely an unknown disease entity. As an example, when CJ, a young man with CF and severe pulmonary disease, reached his eighteenth birthday around 1956, he had to register for the draft. I wrote a letter for him explaining his condition so that he could be exempted from military service. The Army authorities looked through their list of diseases, could not find CF, and concluded that CF did not exist. However, they did take an x-ray of the chest and decided that CJ had severe pulmonary tuberculosis and therefore should not serve in the Army.

In 1958, I was asked by Dr. Robert Loeb, the Chairman of the Department of Medicine at Columbia Presbyterian, to write a short chapter of 1,000 words on CF in the *Cecil Textbook of Medicine*. CF was too complicated a disease to be limited to just 1,000 words, but I did manage to condense the chapter to 1,500. As far as I know, this was the first time CF had appeared as a separate entity in a textbook of medicine, although there had been brief information in pediatrics textbooks. Up to this time, if the average non-pediatric practitioner wanted to know something about CF, it could not be found in the non-pediatric literature. Incidentally in 1947, I wrote an article on CF in Italian and translated the name in that language, a literal translation. It was published in an Italian medical journal and apparently it was the first time most physicians in that country had ever heard of CF. Now, Italy is a productive and flourishing area of CF care and research.

In thinking back on my 20 years at Columbia, 1939 to 1960, most of them at Babies Hospital, I realized this was an exciting, exhilarating experience. The environment was pleasant, the other physicians as a whole very cooperative, and the facilities available were adequate. I loved everyone of my assignments whether making rounds on the wards, teaching the medical students, running the pediatrics clinics, and especially the research and the excitement of finding new things, especially in CF, a new disease which needed definition in all of its aspects. In my office at Babies Hospital, I had as many as 250 charts neatly piled on the floor (which would never be allowed these days) trying to analyze the various aspects of the disease in the almost 600 CF patients we had seen by the time I left Babies. I was a clinical investigator and proud of it, as this was the time when not only CF, but also many other disease entities needed definition and recognition of their manifestations. When a foreign geneticist several years ago spoke disparagingly of clinical investigators, I rebutted strongly that if it had not been for the legion of people like me, geneticists and other so called "basic investigators" would not have known what to look for.

The Move to the National Institutes of Health

In October 1958, I received a telephone call from Dr. DeWitt Stetten, a Ph.D. who was the Scientific Director of the National Institute of Arthritis and Metabolic Diseases at the NIH in Bethesda, Maryland. I had known Dr. Stetten since my early days at Columbia when he was my instructor in the biochemistry course and I was one of his first students. Dr. Stetten asked me to come to the NIH and give a lecture on what he called "my favorite disease CF." I complied and went to Bethesda with Dr. Zakarias Dische, Professor of Biochemistry at Columbia and quite a famous person in his field of the biochemistry of mucus secretions, with whom I had a joint NIH grant for the study of CF on which I was the senior investigator. The day started inauspiciously as Dr. Dische, the absent minded professor, forgot and lost all of his slides on the New York subway and had to speak of the biochemistry of complicated mucopolysaccharide structure without the benefit of slides. My presentation, however, went smoothly. In Dr. Stetten's office after my talk, he said, "We really wanted you to come to offer you a job." Dr. Daft, the Director of the Institute, Dr. Bunin, the Clinical Director, and Dr. Stetten proposed to create for me a new branch to be called the Pediatric Metabolism Branch. This would be in tune with the name of the Institute of Arthritis and Metabolic Diseases (CF was under the definition of "metabolic"). I would be the Chief and thus completely independent to do whatever I wanted. Money did not have to be applied for and was available from the NIH budget. I was also promised the close collaboration of the large number of experts at the NIH in various disciplines which made the offer especially attractive; however, this never materialized. I was also anxious to have a university connection and a position as Clinical Professor of Pediatrics was negotiated with Georgetown University through Dr. Frederick Burke, then Chairman of the Department of Pediatrics. In the local jargon, I was a full Professor of Pediatrics, with the term "clinical" indicating that I was not being paid by the University.

I accepted the offer as this afforded several opportunities, most importantly to further the cause of CF, pursue the investigations in the then elusive basic defect, improve the care of patients. In addition, I would have a platform from which to make the public, medical and lay, in this country and abroad recognize the significance and indeed the very existence and importance of this relatively common genetic disease.

However, I was also very interested in glycogen storage diseases, at that time in their infancy regarding general knowledge. The NIH with all its facilities, its expertise, and the fact that patients could be admitted for an indefinite time and have complicated research protocols all without charge, seemed to be the ideal place for such a study. I felt this could not fail and was certain to produce important and novel results. The NIH in theory stood for close collaboration between the clinician and the so called basic investigators, at that time mostly with a Ph.D. degree. Alas, this study was not to be. Although we quickly had the referral of more than 40 patients with undefined glycogen storage diseases, representing a gold mine of certain and important information, the hoped for and expected collaboration did not materialize. There has always been tension between Ph.D.'s and M.D.'s, as the former frequently felt exploited by the latter. The final nail in the coffin of the glycogen storage disease project occurred when one of the well known chemists specializing in glycogen metabolism whose collaboration I had counted on said, "You want me to do the work so that you can write it up." This was a complete misunderstanding of the situation which called for a clinical as well chemical definition, and hardly a reflection of what was supposed to be the NIH spirit. This was my greatest and really the only big disappointment in my career.

Meanwhile, the CF community, the parents, relatives, and patients were elated. This was the dawn of a new day as it represented recognition by the government and indeed the public that CF existed, that it was a major problem, that it deserved to take its rightful place besides the many other diseases that afflicted mankind, and that investigations into its genetic and physiopathologic basis as well as better treatment and perhaps a cure should be pursued.

I started work at the NIH on January 1, 1960 and quickly found that south of Washington, D.C., with the exception of a clinic in New Orleans headed by Dr. William Waring, there were essentially no special facilities for treating or following patients with CF. At the NIH, there was a small program on CF in the Institute of Allergy and Infectious Diseases headed by Dr. Utz, which later merged with our own in the Pediatric Metabolism Branch. Very quickly, we were inundated by more than 200 patients, largely from Washington and points south. This volume was much more than we could care for. With the help of Dr. Robert Parrott, head of the District of Columbia Children's Hospital and who had always been interested in the problem, I started a CF clinic at Children's Hospital where some of our patients could be referred. Later, a number of CF centers were established under the sponsorship of the CF Foundation, meeting this need and greatly improving the care of CF patients.

At the NIH, I was blessed with exceptionally qualified young men and women as clinical associatess, perhaps aided in the early years by the Vietnam War, from which the NIH represented a refuge, as clinical associates were commissioned officers. They all had a superb background, initiative, and dedication to research and care of patients. As Dr. Doershuk from Cleveland once said to me, they are "super people." Almost all of them have remained active in CF, have greatly contributed to this field in the past, and are continuing to do so at present. Almost all have remained in academic medicine and many have achieved national and international stature and outstanding positions, and are leaders in the fight against CF. This is the achievement of which I am most proud.

Together through the years we conducted many investigations, frequently on their initiative; including glycoprotein structure, tissue culture, bacteriology and immunology, recognition of the true nature of so called "Diabetes Mellitus" which occurs in CF, pregnancy in CF, adults with CF, some of the nutritional components of this disorder, including Vitamin E, Vitamin B, fatty acids in the serum, as well as such practical endeavors as evaluation of assisted ventilation in CF, the diagnosis of the syndrome of inappropriate antidiuretic hormone (SIADH) in the disease, and many others.

As I reflect back on my career, I feel very fortunate as a whole. I loved and enjoyed virtually every assignment I was given. I was always keenly interested in all aspects of clinical medicine, the care of patients, the search for a better and more effective treatment, and especially the excitement of research, of finding new explanations and new answers to the riddle presented by the clinical problems and manifestations.

I was very fortunate to be on the ground floor at the very beginning of the recognition of a disease, CF, which needed a description and explanation of all of its many facets. It was only 15 years after its appearance on the medical scene that the sweat electrolyte defect was recognized and a reliable diagnostic test developed, the "sweat test", and many of the pulmonary, hepatic and other manifestations described in detail. The care of patients and the quality of life steadily improved and investigations advanced, culminating in the discovery in 1989 by Lap-Chee Tsui, Francis Collins, and John Riordan of the CF gene and of its product called the cystic fibrosis transmembrane conductance regulator (CFTR), thus opening new vistas in research and treatment.

It is not given to many to be able to watch, as in my case, the unfolding scenario of a new disease in the span of 50 years, a very short time by medical standards and also the length of my medical career. Paraphrasing Winston Churchill from the "beginning to the end of the beginning," or more hopefully to the "beginning of the end," to the dawn of a new day with the ultimate goal within reach; a simple, safe, and effective treatment or even cure of this devastating disease, cystic fibrosis.

References

1. di Sant'Agnese and Andersen D. "Celiac syndrome IV. Chemotherapy in infections of the respiratory tract associated with cystic fibrosis of the pancreas; Observations with penicillin and drugs of the sulfonamide group, with special reference to penicillin aerosol." *Am J Dis Child* 1946;72:17-61.
2. di Sant'Agnese PA, Darling MD, Perera G, and Shea E. "Abnormal electrolyte composition of sweat in cystic fibrosis of the pancreas: Clinical significance and relationship to the disease." *Pediatrics* 1953;12:549-563.
3. di Sant'Agnese PA. "Fibrocystic disease of the pancreas with normal or partial pancreatic function; Current views on pathogenesis and diagnosis." *Pediatrics* 1955;15:683-697.

4. di Sant'Agnese PA. "Bronchial obstruction with lobar atelectasis and emphysema in cystic fibrosis of the pancreas." *Pediatrics*

5. di Sant'Agnese PA. "The pulmonary manifestation of fibrocystic disease of the pancreas." *Diseases of the Chest* 1955;27:654-670.

6. West JR, Levin SM, and di Sant'Agnese PA. "Pulmonary function in cystic fibrosis of the pancreas." *Pediatrics* 1954;13:155-164.

7. di Sant'Agnese PA and Blanc WA. "A distinctive type of biliary cirrhosis of the liver associated with cystic fibrosis of the pancreas." *Pediatrics* 1956;18:387-409.

3

Dueling with Cystic Fibrosis: Finding the Chloride Defect

Paul M. Quinton, Ph.D.

We've both made it to the new millennium and the year 2000. In a manner of speaking, cystic fibrosis (CF) and I were born almost in the same year. CF became genetic in 1946[1] and I unwittingly debuted with the disease in 1944 (personal observation). Together we have been fighting at some level ever since then. In truth, for most of my life I thought that I would not see the millennium and I had hoped that CF would not either. We are not friends, CF and I. In fact, each of us would kill the other. However, we are both still here in our struggle. Now, there is enough distance to look back and wonder, if not marvel, at what has happened in the meantime.

In 1944, only a handful of people had heard, much less pronounced the words "Cystic Fibrosis" and it would be another 19 years before I heard them either. I was 11 months old when my father returned from WW II, the Normandy invasion, and the occupation of Europe. A few months after he returned, my mother complained to my pediatrician that I coughed a lot and couldn't get rid of colds. Dr. Qualtrose diagnosed me as having chronic bronchitis and said that, "I would just have to live with it." Chronic it was; live with it, I have. For the most part, it was a nuisance, sometimes embarrassing to cough so much in public, sometimes feeling lousy when I ran low grade fevers in the winters and had to wait outside in the mornings for school to open. I had a favorite place on the south side of the building in the sun and out of the wind. I still visualize the corrugations in the bricks of the wall. I still wonder how they were made. I wondered a lot as a child; my life was full of curious things. I wondered how hard a crayfish could pinch (we called them "crawdads" in South Texas). I found out -- with my finger. I found that the critter could pinch hard enough to draw a scream, blood, and a fling that instantly converted him into what was probably my first experimental sacrifice. My mother predicted that my curiosity would make me a "Jack of all trades, and master of none." I suspect she was right.

Nonetheless, other than putting up with persistent stomach aches (some of which really hurt) and the fact that I was always "skinny," I did not suffer from overt digestive problems. That is not quite true, because, due to the "skinny" part, I suffered greatly from my mother's body building concoctions of cream rich milk mixed with raw eggs, baker's yeast, malt, and other untold ingredients depending upon the latest rumor or insight from *Reader's Digest*. When I was 11 or 12, I started worrying, too. I ordered a Charles Atlas bodybuilding, stretch rubber from the Johnston & Smith Company, but I remained "wiry" as it was put in polite Texan terms.

Most of my shirts were stained with rust from hanging on wire clothes hangers that corroded from my sweat. My brother's and my dad's shirts didn't stain. And unlike mine, their sweat wetted shirts and pants did not become stiff with white bands of crusted salt after they dried in the humid east Texas heat. These were just curious things that my mother or some family member would occasionally bring up to make conversation more interesting. But it was nothing more than that, not to me, not to them—just curious observations that Paul sure must have a lot of salt in his sweat and why was that? Even now, animals like to give me licks. No one had the slightest idea that it was the mark of a lethal disease. And I hadn't the slightest idea that salt would become a central focus in my life.

Still, my mother had two medications in her medicine cabinet of galactic importance, Watkins salve for everything on the outside and Vicks salve for everything on the inside. When the colds came and my lungs didn't work well, she was fond of dumping a few teaspoons of Vicks salve into a white, electrically heated ceramic cup, which boiled water—and Vicks. She would stuff me and this rumbling geyser, a "vaporizer," under a big white sheet suspended as a tent over the posts of the bedstead, where I breathed the curative vapors. She was also fond of sending me off to school during these occasions, plastered front and back with Vicks salve. I smelled like a eucalyptus tree, although in Texas none of us had ever heard of or seen a eucalyptus tree. Fortunately for me, I was not unique; a few other kids, including my sister and brother, had mothers who also read similar literature and got basted as well.

But no one worried about a fatal disease. "Cystic Fibrosis" was still unspoken and unheard of. At one point my father argued that my cough must be psychological because when we were squirrel hunting and I had to be quiet, I didn't cough. If I was unlucky enough to get CF, I was lucky enough that it spared most of my childhood.

Until I studied inorganic chemistry in high school, salt was the white granular or powdery stuff that messed up my clothes. It was also good on cold watermelon and freshly picked tomatoes. At that time, I was just beginning to recognize that the world could be described with symbols from chemistry, physics, and math. I was completely fascinated by the concept that a molecule, such as salt, could dissolve into water and become two free moving entities (sodium and chloride ions) that could then carry electricity. At the same time, it was upsetting to realize that the things I had previously seen as single units: trees, dogs, horses, people, were complex composites of these little invisible pieces: salts, water, molecules. It troubled me that the trees, the dogs, the horses, and the people could be destroyed, and that only the little pieces were eternal. But the idea that the same pieces that made a rock could also make an animal was completely captivating. Until my awareness of chemistry and physics, the explanations I had were religious in origin.

My chemistry teacher, Mr. Tibbs, set a course for my life. He asked if I would be interested in doing a science fair project. The Dow Chemical Company had given him samples of some ion exchanger resins. He thought that the subject of "ion exchange" might make an interesting chemistry project. I began to read about ionic interactions. I built a shelf in the end of our garage. It was cold and dark, as a laboratory should be, of course. I used an extension cord for light, and a bathroom space heater to cut the damp cold. With a little more ambience, I would have been a real scientist.

I began exploring the electrostatic interactions of the fixed negative site (anions, which are negative charges) with three mobile cations (which are positive charges), nickel (Ni^{++}), copper (Cu^{++}), and iron (Fe^{++}) by pouring them all together onto a column (glass tube) containing the Dowex resin and collecting small volumes (fractions) of the liquid as it drained through the column. Although poured in together, the different cations washed out of the resin in the column in completely separate samples, showing that their chemical association with the negative sites of the resin differed greatly. It was like getting the sugar back into the teaspoon after it was dissolved in a cup of coffee. As miraculous as it was, that was expected and explainable. However, I was confounded by the fact that if I "cleaned" the column by rinsing it with acid, the order of appearance of the different metal ions changed completely during their separation. How could that be? What did acid do to affect the attraction between the metal cations and the negative charges of the resin?

On a senior class visit to the University of Texas at Austin, which was reputed in our parts to be the greatest of all institutions of learning (second only to Rice University in Houston), I asked to talk to someone in chemistry about this puzzle. I greatly regret that I no longer remember his name, but he suggested that the acid might be doing something called "protonating" the negative sites on the resin. I started reading all I could find about protons "protonating," which was not very much, but the idea seemed to make sense with the little I knew. I compiled and presented my data with the notion that protonating with acid might be an economical way to repetitively regenerate resins used to make fresh water from sea water. This project won the school district award and sent me to Houston for the regional science fair. I followed the advice of a previous contestant to give my display a show window effect accenting the beautiful green, orange, yellow, blue and pink solutions on a blue denim backdrop. I learned then that to communicate, the first requirement is to command attention. I also learned that no idea is completely original; all ideas come from other ideas like genes changing with mutations. Even so, my ego was trounced when my name wasn't called, even for an honorable mention. But then it rose like a Phoenix when the last name called for the Grand Prize sounded a lot like mine. It was, and I qualified for my first airplane ride, which incidentally was to the National Science Fair held that year, 1963, in Albuquerque, New Mexico. I still have trouble spelling that name, probably because of a little of the same dyslexia that has always slowed my reading.

I did not want to go to the National event. I was tormented by the possibility that the theory might be wrong, that I had made a mistake, that "protonation" was just a figment of imagination—mainly mine. I went to the school counselor and told her I wanted to give the trophy and award back because I wasn't sure I was right. At the same time, I wanted to ride that airplane. She told me to get on the plane.

I did not win at National, but the experience was exhilarating. I had my first taste of champagne and became a backsliding Baptist. Science was becoming my religion. I had thought that all my relatives were farmers or pipefitters, so I was dismayed by a visitor who came down from Los Alamos to seek me out because he noticed on the list of entries that we had the same last name. He was a half-second cousin, if such a relation can exist. He took me to see work in his lab in which nanosecond photographs were being taken of explosions in progress. I was stupefied by the idea of a "nanosecond," not to mention that, incredibly, his camera could take a photograph almost a billion times faster than a Brownie. It was completely captivating that by "seeing" one could begin to understand how an explosion takes place. Curiosity was appetite; science was food.

The Duel Defined

More practically, however, the Science Fair turned into a full scholarship from Sun Oil Co. in mechanical/petroleum engineering at the great University of Texas in Austin. Early in the second semester of my junior year, I began to look seriously at salt again, and the result was ugly. My thoughts had been more than a little diverted by romance. But the sobering idea of marriage forced me to investigate the source of my chronic cough and also the recent loss of the upper right lobe of my lung that was due to something diagnosed as "bronchiectasis." I needed to know how long people with bronchiectasis could expect to live. I poured through pages of medical textbooks, ignorant of the meaning of words like "atelectasis," "emphysema," "pneumothorax," and "cor pulmonale." Then there was a little added note, "See in connection with *Cystic Fibrosis*." So I looked it up and then the rest of my life began. Cystic fibrosis was "uniquely characterized by elevated concentrations of salt in the sweat ... salt rings and stains on clothing and shoes common ... predominant involvement of upper lobes of the lung (at age 16 years my right upper lobe had been removed) ... stomach pains from digestive complications ... failure to thrive ... incidents of heat prostration (I already had two)." And then the briny conclusion that CF was a "fatal disease; patients do not survive beyond 6–7 years of age."

A cold chill ran down my back. The library reading room with its vaulted ceilings became enormous and distant. Minutes before, I had been reading and learning with intense intrigue and curiosity. Now, I read a death sentence—mine. I would soon die. The fact that I was already more than 12 years older than the then expected age for CF patients had little impact on my conclusion. I read and re-read the descriptions and matched them with mine. I was convinced CF was my disease. I was right, and I soon became the oldest patient Dr. Gunyon Harrison had seen. After 19 years, I knew and pronounced my enemy's name and he had scored the first "touché." The duel was on.

Dr. Harrison was kind and dodged the burning question of how long I would live. Instead, he offered me a summer job in his CF clinic and laboratory. Oblivious again, my career had begun. He asked me to help "count beans" for a patient registry (no desktop computers then) and to help the nurse and therapist in clinic. He even made a major mistake of trying to put me and Dan Seilheimer (a contemporary pre-med and friend at UT) in charge of a CF summer camp. Most fortunately, Ms. Jo Childress, our social worker, graciously recognized that this charge was not even slightly within the realm of my capacities. Her insight of my experience undoubtedly averted the otherwise certain outcome that someone would have gotten killed (most likely me). She took charge and Dan and I helped. It worked and my life was spared again.

More appropriately, Dr. Harrison assigned me to assist a medical student, Jim Passmore, to develop a means of inducing newborns to sweat, so that we could screen for CF with an early sweat test. I was not so fond of "counting beans," but the intrigue of the laboratory with its columns, agar plates, microscopes, electrophoresis gels, and rocket assays had a magnetic draw. Robert Doggett and Stanley Gunsberg were working on isolating a common strain of bacteria, called *Pseudomonas aeruginosa* that seemed to occur uniquely in CF sputum in an unusual form. The slime, a thick gel, that this "bug" produced was composed of a protein called alginate. They speculated that this alginate caused the sputum of CF patients to be so thick and viscous. Finding a way to break it down in the lung might help patients clear the deadly inspissations (plugs) of mucus that gradually blocked the airways and helped destroy the lungs. But I wanted to know why the bug liked to live in the CF patients' lungs so much better than in other lungs. That was 35 years ago; we still do not know, and I believe it is still one of the most crucial questions to understanding the pathogenesis of this disease.

Meanwhile, even though the Passmore sweat project did not fair well, Jim introduced me to voltmeters and Heath Kits. We assembled a heating block made of aluminum and a piece of soldering iron that would heat the surface of the skin in a local area sufficient to make it sweat (if not cook). It produced more tears than sweat from both the babies and us. I would learn later that the sweat glands of newborn babies are very poorly developed and do not function well until several months of age. I learned that great experiments are easily undermined with only a small amount of ignorance.

Learning to Fight

Yet, another kind of experience took place in those two summers. I met Francisco Escamilla and helped give his respiratory therapy. He was four years old and sick. His mother was young, beautiful, and sad. CF was mean. It would kill Francisco for no reason and torture his mother forever. How did it do it? Why did his lungs get infected? Why didn't the antibiotics work? Why did he lose his pancreas? And why was there so much salt in his sweat? And most confounding, what did his lung infections have to do with his failed pancreas and his pancreas to do with his salty sweat? What was the defect common to all these problems? And still why was I alive at 20 and Francisco dying at four? I wanted to know. It became important to do something. It became important to find out. It became important to fight back. Only science offered a weapon but I had no idea how to fight.

My thoughts became caught up between living a short life as fast as a poet, and the alternative of slowly working to get a "union card" to do science. It was already clear that science would demand an advanced degree which would take more years of study. The year before, I had given up my scholarship in mechanical engineering because: 1) I was not normal, 2) I was afraid of being obligated to do something that was not really so important to me, and 3) even before meeting CF, I deeply wanted to understand what life is and why. Then came the movie Doctor Zhivago. My fate seemed sealed. Hollywood imprinted my brain. I would become a poet-doctor. I enrolled in pre-med and was as happy as a compulsive neurotic could ever become.

The first summer after meeting the enemy, I was selected to go with a group of 15 other students from the University of Texas to the University of Pedagogico in Santiago, Chile, as an exchange student. Officially the exchange was for about 30 days, but I was inspired by Dr. Zhivago running around Siberia and by the prospect of dying soon, so I decided to see the world while I could. I reasoned that I would die soon anyway, so I really had little to lose. I arranged to stay in Chile for the rest of the semester on my own. Afterwards, four others decided to stay, too. So instead of going to class, I hitch hiked first to San Pedro de Atacama in the North of Chile with a buddy, Mike Hennen, and then with Mike and Sally Green to the South to Tierra del Fuego; then back up through the pampas of Argentina, and into the dictatorships of Uruguay and Brazil. We lived hard, mostly off the generosity and kindness of missionaries, firemen, and policemen who often gave us food and a place to stay, sometimes in fire stations and jails. I saw poverty for the first time. I learned that to be better off is not to be better than. I remain deeply enchanted with, and committed to, South America.

Perhaps the events were crazy, but not all bad. The two courses that have been most important to me over the years were remedial English and Physical Chemistry, but biology was beautiful, and I was infatuated with evolution because it meant that "life could be explained." Mr. Erwin refused to give me an "A" in English because he said that anyone who had to take remedial English didn't deserve an "A." Instead, he insisted, "Begin by believing nothing. Outline. Support what you think. Defend your conclusions." He was teaching English, but it is clear now that it was the essence of science—logical, analytical thought. For me, a squirrel hunter from Channelview, who came to his course from Sunday school at River Road Baptist Church and who was convinced that, if it was in print, it must be true, this was revolutionary. Since then, I have become monotonous in quoting Benjamin Franklin's axiom, "Believe none of what you hear, and only half of what you see."

Physical chemistry was the most difficult course in my curriculum. But it was also the best for problem solving and understanding life processes. With it, I could conceptually glue sub-atomic particles into molecules, and molecules to cells, cells to organs, and organs to organisms. Most importantly, it gave me a view of how energy flows. Life was a zero sum game. Energy and mass were conserved. Chemistry and electrical forces were interchangeable and conceptually united. The effects of electrical energy on mass were predictable.

Choosing Weapons

In the last semester of my senior year at the University of Texas, I learned that I had been accepted to medical school in Galveston. I was still waiting to hear from Baylor in Houston. I had been open in my interviews about having CF, but I was very worried that it might keep me from being admitted. When I returned to Houston for a visit, I went to tell Gunyon Harrison that I was going to medical school. He really blew a fuse. He started poking his renowned finger into my chest and bellowing "Why the hell did I want to do a thing like that?" Getting myself into the clinic to see all those patients with all those bugs in Ben Taub (the county hospital) was just what I needed. "No, sir", he yelled, "You don't want to be a doctor, you want to be a scientist. Besides he said, look at me. I'm a zookeeper. You don't want to be a zookeeper. You want to be a scientist. You go over there and talk to that guy, Charles Philpott, at Rice and see if you can be a scientist." I went.

Dr. Philpott had two "new" electron microscopes that he used to see the incredible inside components of cells, even the insides of a cell membrane. Suddenly, instead of looking at going into debt for ten thousand dollars a year in medical school, the government was going to pay me six thousand dollars a year to become a scientist. Not a bad deal, I reasoned. Besides with a Ph.D., I could go to med school later and become that most revered of academic species, the M.D., Ph.D. I never did. I withdrew my pending application from Baylor and notified UT Galveston that I was going to graduate school at Rice, instead.

I went on the fast route to my union card, directly to a Ph.D. in Cell Biology in four years, skipping the Masters (besides the government was not very interested in spending any more money on me). The lab was a wonderful place in the late sixties, filled with neurotic people. Philpott knew I had CF, but I had resolved not to tell anyone I didn't absolutely have to about it. Why? I had at least two reasons. First, for all of us death is a hard thing to deal with. A lethal disease is a constant reminder of death and a person with a lethal disease is likewise a constant reminder. I did not like being reminded that I would die, and I was sure that other people didn't like it either. So I decided to try to avoid making myself any more unpleasant than I already was, by not telling everyone that knew me that I had CF and reminding them of our mortality. Indeed, my fundamentalist protestant training endowed me with great guilt for this deceit, but I rationalized it as justified. Second, also because of my Protestant training, I had to be sure that whatever I got, I earned. I had a deep seated fear that if people knew that I had this disease, I might be treated differentially or favorably for reasons beyond what I was. So only in moments of weakness and after building great trust did I cautiously tell only my very closest friends about my enemy, and I always made them swear, despite my own hypocrisy in telling them, not to tell anyone else. Most people, who did not know, were satisfied with the explanation that I had had "rotten lungs since infancy" to explain the constant cough. That subtly informed them that it was not contagious and that I was not dying of tuberculosis. Now, over the years, I guess I have become almost famous for having CF. I regard this as profound evidence that Mark Twain was right. "Two people can keep a secret if one of them is dead."

At home I took my antibiotics and puffed on my Mist-O-Gen nebulizer. At parties I "got stupid" and puffed other stuff. (I did "inhale"). And I conducted experiments at home as well as in the lab. The sixties were experimental. The miracle is that I (and we) survived them. I also puffed all kinds of "ideas" in my nebulizer: mixtures of antibiotics, alcohol, acetic acid, $NaHCO_3$, etc. Some of the results were definite. The lungs do not like Tequila, even if it is an antiseptic and they resent acid even more. $NaHCO_3$ is OK. Chloromycetin didn't nebulize well, but taken orally is a wonderful bug killer, but after a while it made me feel as sick as the dying bugs it killed. Tetracycline caused terrible abdominal pain. We now know that some CF patients who have pancreatic function develop pancreatitis on this drug. We don't know why. But no matter what, the cough remained. The colds and infections came—sometimes short, sometimes long, sometimes mild, sometimes tough. They took away a little lung function with them each time, but a great loss occurred when I had to give up walking on my hands because it caused hemoptysis. "Touché," again.

My biggest problem in graduate school was that I was not a cell biologist. I was too mechanically oriented. I was a physiologist and didn't know it. The process of fixing and imbedding dead, static tissues, and sectioning and examining them for microscopy, even electron microscopy, was boring in comparison to Dr. John Palka's animal physiology course. It was exciting to see the moving traces on the oscilloscope or chart recorder when a live contracting muscle, firing nerve, or ion-transporting frog skin was connected. To see an immediate response to an electrical pulse or to an applied drug was mesmerizing, and in and of itself, a self-perpetuating motivation to do just one more manipulation. But I had signed on to Cell Biology as my Ph.D. major, and to finish up and get my union card, I must continue. But I worked out a compromise. For my thesis, I decided to study the structural effects of large positively charged molecules (polymeric cations) on cell membranes and on the "movement" of salt transport across them. I was lucky in that these molecules caused both morphologic as well as physiologic changes in cells.

Aside from inadvertently being drawn into salt again, two things happened which shaped another phase of my life. One, at that time there was a great to do about results published in *Science*, that a factor in the serum from CF patients could stop normal cilia from beating [2] and that CF sweat could stop salt transport in normal saliva and sweat glands.[3] The test for the latter was hideously complicated, so I decided to use the lessons of my physiology course and added sweat from normal subjects and CF patients to a frog skin in a Ussing chamber, which is a device used to measure salt transport electrically. These experiments did not have a good outcome. First, one of my normal volunteer subjects was my Department Chairman's son. To collect sweat, I placed him in a portable, plastic tent type sauna and turned on the heat. After I had enough sweat, I opened the tent and allowed him to go shower. He, the Chairman's son, stood up, took one step, and then wilted like an old lily. I grabbed for him, but his heavy, wet body slipped through my arms like a hot fish and he collapsed into a putty of protoplasm on the floor. I was sure we were both dead—he, then, and me as soon as his father found out. My career and life had been ended by Cystic Fibrosis in the cruelest way. Then after three seconds, the putty moved, my eyes bulged, and the putty began to gather itself up and stood. The putty asked, "What happened?" I prayed, "Thank you, Lord" and sat down. I learned a lot about heat, vasodilatation of the blood vessels, cerebral circulation, and consciousness.

The other event at least started on a positive note. When I placed my own CF sweat on the frog skin, the salt movement was much slower than when I put the Chairman's son's normal sweat on it. I was ecstatic. I ran off and told Gunyon Harrison of these stupendous results. He telephoned Dr. John Herndon, the Medical-Scientific Director of the National Cystic Fibrosis Research Foundation in New York, and told him. I enthusiastically returned to the lab to do more experiments, but then I realized that they were not reproducible. There was no difference between my sweat and anyone else's. I learned that one experiment does not a conclusion make. "Believe none of what you hear and only half of what you see," and don't announce it until you are very sure. But I had found my weapon. It would be the physiology of salt transport.

More important, however, in 1969 my interest in salt transport led my Ph.D. advisor to suggest that I go to Los Angeles to the lab of Dr. John Tormey to learn the technique of preparing gallbladders to study salt transport. In two weeks, I fell in love with the West Coast. Terry Machen, Jared Diamond's graduate student at the time, showed me how to prepare rabbit gallbladders. I returned to Houston and two years later I defended my thesis on the "Effects of Polymeric Cations on the Mucosal Epithelium of Rabbit Gallbladder." I'm glad Jesse Helms never noticed what I was doing with the government's money. Science may never recover, but it did secure my Ph.D. union card. The prior introduction to John Tormey set me up for a postdoctoral fellowship with him in the Department of Physiology at UCLA. I applied for and received my first grant to continue training at UCLA. It came from the National Cystic Fibrosis Foundation and had greater implications than anyone suspected.

Most post-docs did not have their own funding but since I did, John Tormey was more inclined to let me follow my own nose and work on subjects of my choosing. At first, I tried to duplicate the studies of CF sweat factors which had gotten me into trouble with the data on frog skin that I had announced too prematurely. I initiated several projects, but eventually decided that the basic defect in CF would most likely be accessible for study in the human sweat gland. I managed to get enough preliminary data to have a stab at applying to the CF Foundation for a "new investigator" program being initiated to help young investigators interested in CF get established. I needed little encouragement, as I needed money. I was learning that research is expensive. The award was for the unheard of sum of $50,000 a year for three years. I later learned that the Medical Advisory Council of the CF Foundation decided at the last minute to fund, not one, but three of the Research Scientist applications. I was the third. The awards were made to William "Bill" Shearer (who later received acclaim as the physician in charge of the "bubble boy"), Dr. Ricardo Martinez (now Director of Dental Research at the National Institutes of Health [NIH]), and me -- in that order. Years later I learned that the grand old physician, Dr. Harry Shwachman, who, along with Dr. Paul A. di Sant'Agnese, probably contributed more to understanding the clinical picture of CF than any living bcing, had opposed my application because I was a CF patient and he felt patients should not study their own disease. If he was correct, it is clear that the best thing was that I did not go into psychiatry. Later, this award led to a Research Career Development Award from the NIH. Ultimately, it was these awards and John Tormey's tolerance that gave me the time and space to develop the techniques needed to study the human sweat gland in CF and subsequently define the basic defect in chloride transport.

By now, I was in the career stream, moving from Post Doctoral Fellow, to Research Physiologist, to Assistant Professor of Physiology and Medicine in Residence at UCLA. My lab was actually in the Department of Medicine by the good graces and wonderful generosity of Dr. Charles Kleeman, Chief of Nephrology, who also displayed incredible tolerance of my tinkering with sweat glands. Chuck Kleeman was a wonderful example for and influence on me. He asked me to write a chapter with him that he had been invited to write on Water Metabolism (his area). The chapter requested was to be entitled "Water Metabolism: Protozoa to Man." [4] I eagerly, and naively, said yes to my first invitation to write a book chapter. I worked my fanny off for about six months. When I finished the editor said that, in this case, it was a good thing the chapter was so long because he needed the filler to thicken the book. But when I presented the manuscript to Dr. Kleeman to review and co-author, he refused to put his name on it saying that I had put too much work into it to share authorship. He knew that his name on the paper would completely overshadow mine. I learned a lot about water and grace from that experience.

A short Visiting Assistant Professorship at Harvard University with Claude Lechenne, where I worked on x-ray analysis and experienced the "coldest winter ever," cooled my enthusiasm for the Northeast forever and I kept one foot in the Department of Medicine and the other in the Department of Physiology at UCLA. Wilfried Mommaerts was chair of Physiology and had arranged for my position in Medicine. He also recommended me for a tenure track position that had become available at the University of California, Riverside (UCR), about 60 miles east of LA—and still in Southern California. Tenure track positions were scarcer than hen's teeth. I was resolved to stay in California and I was more than delighted to join the faculty and move my laboratory to Riverside.

En Garde

Another match with CF was about to begin. In January 1982, shortly after moving my lab to Riverside, the idea that the basic physiological defect in CF was an impermeability to chloride leaped at me from the pages of the New England Journal of Medicine (NEJM). I was sitting at my desk at UCR where I had just received tenure largely on the basis of my work in x-ray microanalysis, not physiology. I thought that x-ray analysis, with its ability to quantitatively analyze incredibly small samples of fluids, would be essential to understanding the abnormal functions of salt transport in CF. I had just talked with Ricardo Martinez at the University of Missouri, to discuss plans for a Guidance, Action and Projection (GAP) Conference that I had asked the CF Foundation to sponsor and let us organize with Ulrich Hopfer. It was to be the first such conference, specifically dedicated to electrolyte transport in CF. Ricardo had told me that I should look at a recent paper by Knowles, et al, [5] because they had found something abnormal about Na^+ (sodium) transport in CF airways. I have always been atrocious about staying up with the literature. I dutifully subscribed to several journals with every intention of reading them, but somehow they always managed to pile up and I usually have to learn what is in them from someone else.

It was the same in this case. I requested a copy of the NEJM article from the library and began to read about increased electrical potential differences across respiratory epithelia in CF. My immediate reaction was a cold chill followed by a fury that came with the sudden realization of being "scooped." "Scooped" means that someone else publishes your work or conclusions before you do. In science, the pay is not the salary, but academic credit or acknowledgement. It is like any other competition and the credit goes to he who publishes first. Getting scooped means working for no pay. It is among the worst things that can happen to a scientist. And as I read, I felt myself slipping in to a very big scoop.

I had already invested several years work in the hope of defining a "basic defect." Very simply, I reasoned that before we could begin to fix it, we needed to know what was wrong in the affected cells. I had chosen to try to find it in pieces of isolated human sweat glands. It seemed clear to me that the duct of the sweat gland was probably the best system to explore the basic defect. Why? Because a high salt content in the sweat was almost diagnostic for the disease. Indeed a positive sweat test was considered virtually essential to confirm the diagnosis. We needed to know the defect that causes salt, sodium (Na^+) and chloride (Cl^-), to be more concentrated in the sweat of CF patients. I thought it very likely that definition of that defect would lead us to understand similar defects in the lungs, pancreas and other affected organs that were much more significant to health than the abnormality in sweat. Thaysen and Schwartz [6] had presented good evidence that fluid emerged from salivary glands in two steps. They proposed that the fluid was secreted first in an early part of the gland and had about the same composition as an ultrafiltrate of plasma, and then, second, the fluid was modified as it passed through subsequent tubules and then ducts on its way out of the gland. Reasoning that the process was the same in sweat glands, Cage et al [7] and Slegers[8] independently made regression plots of sweat composition versus sweat rate and showed that the composition of sweat from both normal subjects and CF patients approached that of plasma when extrapolated to "infinitely" high secretory rates. Importantly, these conclusions dictated that the problem with CF sweat was in the second step, a modification of the initial fluid after it was secreted into the duct, and not due to a more concentrated primary secretion in CF, as some had speculated. Therefore, I decided to go after the isolated sweat duct as the target tissue to investigate for the basic defect.

The decision to work on isolated sweat ducts was naive. My inexperience led me to think the tissue was perfect. It always expressed the defect clearly; skin was the only human tissue that could be obtained without major surgery, and the sweat gland was not destroyed by secondary complications such as occurred with lung and pancreas tissues.

But the practical, devastating problem was that I couldn't find sweat glands in the skin when I tried to isolate them. They were too small and Mother Nature didn't color them to make them stand out. A single sweat gland is a tiny ball about as thick as a sheet of paper. Methylene blue had been used by others to locate the glands in the native skin but methylene blue killed the glands, rather counter productive for studying living functions. Luckily, I discovered that neutral red, a vital stain, accumulated vividly in the lumen (the inside opening of a tubule) of the sweat duct if the skin was bathed in a solution containing a small amount of the stain. It was beautiful. Tiny little red ribbons formed in the duct lumens and ran from the epidermis to the gland. My dissection nightmare turned into a sweet dream. After adding the stain, I could watch through the microscope, like a hunter waiting for prey. As the red thread slowly appeared and betrayed the hidden duct, I attacked the glands with my tiny spears and sharpened tweezers and dragged them into the light. As I learned the hunt, I learned to recognize the glands without stain. Now, it is almost easy to find them, but then, due to partial color blindness, I doubt if I could have ever seen them without the aid of neutral red.

Finding a sweat gland was just the first problem. What to do with it was an even bigger problem. The little beasts had to be kept alive and constrained without harming them. The abnormal salt concentration demanded that I determine the concentration of salt in the fluid from the lumen of the duct. A careful dissection would yield a 1/32 inch length of duct, but its diameter was only about 0.001 inch and the diameter of its opening was only about half that. Thus sampling the fluid from the lumen was not trivial. Fortunately, much of the problem had already been solved by Burg, Grantham, Abramow, and Orloff [9] who, while touring the Public Health Service instead of Vietnam, developed a method to perfuse single renal tubules isolated from rabbit kidneys. Tubules from the kidney are about the same size as sweat ducts, so that I only needed to adapt their design to the duct. At the request of John Tormey, Jared Grantham kindly allowed me to visit his lab to see the technique of microperfusing renal tubules. I sketched a drawing of his micropipette holders and presented them to Don Curtis, our department machinist in Physiology at UCLA. Don turned the sketches into precision pieces of metal and plastic. I will remain deeply indebted to him for his sincere interest and incredible skills in fabricating these beautiful tools. He often worked with a jeweler's loop because of limited eyesight. I loved the smell of machine oil and fresh cut steel in his shop. He taught me much about patience, precision, and machining. Without the infrastructure support for machining and electronics available in the UCLA Physiology Department at that time, my intentions would have been doomed.

Of course, the sweat duct was not eager to be microperfused. Even with Don's precision micropipette holders, I spent more than three years poking on the ends of isolated sweat ducts trying to get a tiny glass pipette tip into the lumen of a duct. The anatomy of the duct was no help since its epithelium is composed of two concentric layers of cells so that the lumen diameter is very small compared to the overall duct diameter. But even worse, its inherent ability to absorb fluid kept the duct lumen tightly closed. In other words, like a child refusing to eat, it kept its mouth shut. Thus, getting the micropipette into the lumen was like finding a hole in the dark and then forcing it open. I accidentally managed to do it a few times— just enough to keep me convinced that it could be done and to keep me from giving up. I found that by placing a small mirrored prism in the bath beside the duct, I could see it from two dimensions. With the prism, I could move the microscope and view the alignment of the duct and pipettes from the side as well as from below. I could then align the pipette to any position with any crevice or fold that might indicate the position of the mouth of the lumen. Cannulating and microperfusion of a duct never became a foregone conclusion, but successes became more frequent than accidental, making it possible to think about conducting experiments.

The next major problem of analyzing the micro samples of fluid perfused through the lumen was potentially solvable by using a helium glow-photometer, which could vaporize a sample of about 10^{-9} (10 nanoliters [nL]) and accurately quantitate the amount of Na^+ and K^+ or Ca^{++} present in the sample. The prototype from NIH was at Harbor, UCLA. I expended many hours and innumerable expletives on this cantankerous instrument. At last, John Tormey, my postdoctoral mentor, saved me from the abyss of never publishing by pointing out a new technology called "Energy Dispersive X-ray Analysis." It theoretically provided the possibility to non-destructively analyze a fluid sample of much less than 1×10^{-12} L for all elements of atomic weight of Na^+ or greater. Sweat glands can secrete about 10 to 20 x 10^{-9} L/min when maximally stimulated and even can be perfused at much higher rates. Thus, a single micro sample of sweat was an abundant volume for analysis, but then there was another hang-up. We would need pipettes tiny enough to accurately pipette such miniscule volumes. I found that with the aid of an old DeFonbrune microforge, I could forge a small ampoule of glass to contain a volume of less than 10^{-10} L or 0.1 nL. Annealed to a larger pipette, the ampoule self-filled by capillary action, and then its contents could be expelled by positive pressure. Under oil, the contents formed a tiny drop of fluid at the tip of the ampoule. Even though extremely small, the samples transferred were all of the same exact volume so that the ion concentrations of unknown samples could be calculated from samples of known standards.

I hedged my career adventures with this technique, because I knew that if I could not perfuse a sweat duct, I could apply the x-ray analysis technique to the sweat I could collect directly from single sweat glands from skin, both *in vivo* and *in vitro*. I also found that collecting single drops of sweat under oil on the skin surface was infinitely easier than perfusing the sweat duct. This ability presented the attractive advantage of producing publishable data, without which my career was certain to end ignominiously. In retrospect, it is ironic that, after the years spent in developing this analysis, it ultimately was peripheral to the actual experiments which would reveal the basic defect in chloride impermeability. However, it did produce data that helped focus my attention on Cl^-. The most significant advantage was that is was the basis of my securing tenure with the University of California so that I could continue to do research. These concerns probably seem trivial to people not in academics, but at the heart of our system, scientists who do not publish are asked to do something else. Without publishing on something, my life in research would probably be shorter than my actual life. And I wanted to continue doing research in CF.

"Je Touché" to CF

As I read the Knowles paper, my studies of electrolyte concentrations in sweat from single glands crystallized in my mind the concept for chloride (Cl^-) impermeability in CF. Previously, I had examined the data on the concentrations of electrolytes in the sweat from single sweat glands from CF patients and normal subjects. I knew that in normal sweat the sodium (Na^+) concentration was always higher than that of Cl^-, while in CF sweat the opposite was the case. In CF, the Cl^- concentration was usually higher than that of Na^+. Slegers[8] had reported similar differences with studies of concentrations of whole sweat and had suggested that, as a rule, the ratio of Na^+ to Cl^- concentrations in normal sweat was greater than 1.0 and in CF sweat it was less than 1.0. This information suggested that rather than an inhibition of transport of the cation, Na^+, as was thought then, perhaps it was the transport of the anion (Cl^-) that was inhibited in CF. The rule of Occam's razor, which insists that the simplest explanation is likely to be the correct explanation and which would have immediately suggested Cl^- impermeability (the inability of an ion or molecule to pass through a barrier such as the cell membrane), I, of course, had to begin with the most complicated explanation, as follows.

I also knew that in normal sweat there was usually an "anion gap." That is, in all fluids the number of negative charges exactly equals the number of positive charges, a phenomenon affectionately known to physiologists as "electroneutrality." I could measure Na^+, K^+, and Cl^- with the x-ray analysis technique. In sweat, most of the positive charges are Na^+ and K^+, and most of the negative charges are Cl^- and a few other small anions. Thus, the sum of the Na^+ plus K^+ should equal the sum of the Cl^-, but in normal sweat there was an "anion gap." The difference between Na^+ plus K^+ minus Cl^- (the anion gap) was a measure of the other anions which were most likely bicarbonate (HCO_3^-) and/or lactate, neither of which were measured by x-ray analysis. It seemed important that the anion gap in CF sweat was always small or missing as compared to normal sweat.

At the time, much attention had turned to the role of a $Cl-/HCO_3^-$ exchange in the red cell, so that it was fashionable to think of anion exchangers in epithelial transport physiology. Anion exchangers move different ions of the same charge in opposite directions across a cell membrane simultaneously. I naively jumped to the conclusion that this could be the problem in CF. Not only would a defect in a $Cl-/HCO_3^-$ exchange in the sweat explain the observed differences in the anion gap, but also it was consistent with the less than 1.0 Na^+/Cl^- ratios in CF. Moreover, it was well known that the pancreas in CF was also a primary target organ. After all, Dorothy Andersen had named the disease "Cystic Fibrosis of the Pancreas." Even better, we knew that the pancreas normally secretes great quantities of HCO_3^-, but Beat Hadorn[10] had shown HCO_3^- secretion was defective in CF patients. Thus my conclusion was that the basic defect in CF must be in an abnormal anion exchanger. I was elated with my insight. I hurriedly wrote my first paper on CF and unfortunately it was published.[11] Those were clearly days when one could publish almost anything on CF. Nonetheless, I am still convinced that abnormal HCO_3^- transport is central to much of the pathology of the disease.

But as I read the paper from Knowles, et al., which reported that the electrical potentials across the CF airway (nasal epithelium in this case) was significantly more negative in CF than in control subjects, it became increasingly evident that I had been more than stupid. Of course, I was being scooped. I deserved it. Clearly, it was not a problem with an exchanger at all; it was a problem with the cell's ability to let Cl^- go through it; i.e., Cl^- impermeability. If Cl^- could not cross the membrane when the driving force was on Na^+, then surely, the negative charge on Cl^- would be kept behind, in a manner of speaking, and the electrical potential in the lumen would become much more negative in CF than in normal cells. If Cl^- could not cross the membrane, other anions should be absorbed preferentially and my anion gap would disappear preferentially in CF sweat. This simple phenomenon of a blocked Cl^- movement could also explain the less than 1.0 ratio of Na^+/Cl^- in CF sweat if another cation (K^+ or H^+) could not exchange for much of the absorbed Na^+ in sweat. Occam's razor was consistent.

I was dejected and embarrassed as I continued to read, but as I reached the end of the article, I began to realize that maybe I really was not completely scooped after all. Knowles, et al had concluded that Na^+ absorption was increased, not that Cl^- was impermeable. That is, for whatever reason, in the CF airway, the driving force on Na^+ appeared abnormally enhanced. Therefore, relatively more positive Na^+ charge would be absorbed across the CF epithelium into the blood side, making the lumen side electrically more negative.

I had trouble with this idea because it was a foregone conclusion for me that Na^+ absorption from the CF sweat duct was inhibited, not enhanced, as compared to that in normal ducts. Indeed, the poor absorption of Na^+ and Cl^- (salt) was the basis of the cardinal diagnostic test for CF, the "sweat test." Inhibition of Cl^- absorption would explain the higher salt in CF sweat because in salt transport, both the anion and cation must move in the same direction at the same time in order to maintain electroneutrality. Thus, if either Cl^- or Na^+ absorption were inhibited, salt transport would be blocked. Now it was just as clear that a Cl^-/HCO_3^- exchange could not be the problem because this mechanism does not separate charge (Cl^- goes in one direction while HCO_3^- goes in the other). It simultaneously exchanges, but does not separate charges, so it cannot generate an electrical potential. It is "electroneutral." Thus, a defective exchange could not explain the increased separation of charge, the electrical potential Knowles, et al had observed in CF. And my paper had to be wrong, because to explain both the greater negative potential in the airway and the decreased salt absorption in the sweat duct, the problem had to be inhibited movement of Cl^- alone. But how could one prove it? Was the CF sweat duct, like the airways, also more electrically negative?

The approach to measuring the electrical potentials in the CF duct was more obvious than proving that the duct was impermeable to Cl^-. I needed to put electrodes inside my microperfusion pipettes and measure the electrical potential across the duct tubule. Jan Bijman, who had joined me from the University of Nijmegen, in the Netherlands, on a post doctoral fellowship, and I were perfusing ducts and trying to collect the perfusate for analysis. We were trying to analyze samples of fluid perfused through isolated ducts to show that its composition had changed and thus prove that the ducts were alive and functioning as *in vivo*. To measure the potential, I needed an electrometer with a very high input impedance. I had such an instrument, which I had purchased second hand from the renowned physiologist, ornithologist, and philosopher—Jared Diamond. Actually, I had measured the potential of the normal duct previously and had concluded that it was so low that changes in composition were more likely to be better evidence of function. I connected the two electrodes of the electrometer to the solution bathing the outside of the isolated, microperfused sweat duct and to the pipette perfusing the inside of the duct. The voltage between the two electrodes measured the electrical potential across the sweat duct epithelial cells through which Na^+ and Cl^- had to pass to be absorbed. The results would be easy to interpret. If Cl^- could move as easily as Na^+ through the duct cells, there would be little or no separation of their charges and the voltage would be low. If Cl^- were inhibited and could not move easily, compared to Na^+, the negative charges on the Cl^- would be held back, the two charges would be relatively separated, and the resulting voltage would be increased. The magnitude of the voltage would be a function of how poorly Cl^- crossed the membrane relative to Na^+.

When I measured the potential in normal ducts, it was small, but when I measured it in the CF duct, although I expected it to be larger, I could not believe my eyes. The meter needle was instantly off scale, indicating a very large difference. As I increased the scale three fold, the needle was on scale, but rising. It pegged off scale again. I switched the scale to 10 fold higher, and it nearly pegged again at 100 mV. As corny as it was and despite my experience with the frog skin at Rice, I couldn't contain myself and literally ran out of the room yelling "Eureka." It was stupid, but it is these few ecstatic moments that drive scientists. Usually these come very seldom and slowly, but the experience of seeing or realizing something for the first time—something that has never been seen or thought before (even if it has and one just thinks it hasn't)—is perhaps the greatest joy reserved for humans. It may even be better than sex.

Of course, I was still some distance from "direct proof" that Cl⁻ was impermeable in the CF sweat duct. The idea for the proof came from a suggestion from Maurice Burg, who had helped develop the microperfusion system for kidney tubules that I was using to perfuse sweat ducts. Maurice was giving a plenary lecture at the European Working Group for Cystic Fibrosis in Belgium and came by the poster display of my sweat gland results. I explained my problem and that I didn't think that I could show the Cl⁻ impermeability with the classical approach of radioisotope tracer fluxes for Cl⁻ because the specific activity of its isotope was too low to be measured accurately in the tiny volumes I could collect from the perfused duct. He suggested that it might be done indirectly with diffusion potentials. Diffusion potentials are voltages that result from the unequal mobility of ions diffusing across barriers. Thus, for example, if Na⁺ and Cl⁻ at equal concentrations are caused to diffuse down a concentration gradient across a membrane, the ion that moves faster contributes more of its charges to the other side of the membrane. For example, if Na⁺ moved faster across the sweat duct than Cl⁻ from the inside (lumen), the outside bath would become positively charged, the lumen inside would become negatively charged. Thus, the measured electrical potential across the duct wall of cells would become more negative in the lumen relative to the bath. But since this measure depends on a completely passive system (no biological energy can be expressed into the system), to use this approach, I had to eliminate the influences of active transport (salt movements caused by expending biological energy). So I poisoned the Na⁺ pump, which drives all active salt transport, with ouabain, a well-known transport inhibitor. When I created a diffusion gradient for NaCl across normal duct cells by diluting the luminal NaCl solution, the electrical potential inside the ducts became very negative, indicating that Cl- could move much faster than Na⁺ into the lumen. On the other hand, when I did the same experimental maneuvers in CF ducts, the potential in the lumen always became positive, indicating that Cl⁻ could not move as fast as Na⁺ across the luminal membrane of CF ducts.

Moreover, when I did not block the active transport machinery with ouabain and simply replaced Cl⁻ with another anion known to be impermeable, the normal duct behaved almost exactly like the CF duct. The same manipulation hardly had any effect on the CF duct. This result showed that the normal duct could be "converted" to a CF duct by making the anion of the salt in its lumen impermeable. While this is complicated information, these two results, the diffusion potential data and the substituted anion data, do not absolutely prove that Cl⁻ is impermeable in the CF sweat duct. However, they do give very strong evidence that is very difficult to explain in any other way. Occam's Razor cuts well for the simple idea of Cl⁻ impermeability. Our results were published shortly thereafter.[12,13]

The Running Duel

These events occurred nearly twenty years ago. Since then, Cl⁻ impermeability has been demonstrated in every tissue examined that is affected in CF. I had thought that with a basic cellular defect in hand, we would rapidly strike the long desired mortal jab into the heart of CF and vanquish my enemy. It was not to be so. First, I was surprised at the length of time it required for these findings to be accepted. It was more than five years before it was generally acknowledged that Cl⁻ impermeability is a characteristic defect of CF. We have since defined many of the physiological and biochemical properties defining Cl⁻ and Na⁺ transport in CF, but we have not been able link this basic defect to the cause of the pathology in the lung or the pancreas. Meanwhile, a genetic marker was found placing the CF gene on chromosome 7. Then shortly thereafter, in 1989, the gene and its most common mutation were identified.[14,15] In addition, mutations in the gene were shown to characteristically result in Cl⁻ impermeability in cells and tissues expressing the gene, thus establishing with certainty that Cl⁻ impermeability is a basic defect in CF. With this new found knowledge, the promise of gene therapy was quickly seized upon and it seemed we would quickly seal the fate of the disease, CF, without ever needing to understand the link of Cl⁻ impermeability to the pathology. Each new finding was a hit, a strike, a "touché," but not a quick mortal wound to CF. Each blow gave a hope, filled with optimism, but not yet realized. We are now into a new millennium and CF still brandishes its sword almost as perilously as ever. CF is a relentless adversary and it continues only because we are still learning to fight.

But, just as surely as we learn, we will put an end to CF. Our resolve to end the disease has not faded, but doubled and redoubled. When I began to try to research CF, it was easy to read every article that was published. That was nearly 30 years ago. Now it is almost impossible to follow the progress in my own field alone. The number of investigators dedicated to solving CF problems has soared from "CF Club," a meeting of fewer than 100 physicians and scientists, to the annual North American Cystic Fibrosis Conference attended by nearly 3,000 scientists, physicians, and allied health professionals from all over the world. In order to help key investigators keep pace with the rapid and vast increases in knowledge, the CF Foundation also annually sponsors the Williamsburg Meeting. This is by invitation for over 100 highly active international investigators who are dedicated to defining the still imposing unknowns that will eventually reveal the solution to the defeat of CF. These meetings serve the vital function of bringing ideas, which might otherwise take years to be appreciated, to this most important and knowledgeable audience.

It is these meetings and the inspiring dedication and intelligence of the participants that I have met there that leave me with the conviction that we will find an answer. It is taking longer than I thought. The challenge has been more formidable than I ever imagined, but the size of the force we have mounted to meet it has also defied my imagination. We are still diluted by the fact that we do not know exactly what we need to know, but I suspect that soon, someone, in some laboratory somewhere, will say, "This is it. This is what we need to know." Then our forces will focus, our efforts will concentrate, and CF, as a disease, will cease to exist.

CF and I have both managed to make it into the 21st century. We both continue to struggle. Of course, I am very intrigued to know who will last the longer. If I win, life will have been worthwhile because of the struggle. If I do not win, life will have been worthwhile because of the struggle. Kazantzakis in Zorba the Greek captured it well, "Life is trouble, only death is not." Despite the trouble CF has given me, it has also resulted in much meaning and reason to live. It has provided colleagues, who have also become life long friends of the highest caliber and commanded my highest respect and affection. M.M. Reddy, Jan Bijman, Jeff Wine, Mike Welsh, Pam Davis, Mike Knowles, Ray Frizzell, Rick Boucher, Jonathan Widdicombe, Hinda Kopelman, Ricardo Martinez, Maynard Case, Ricardo Pinero, Carl Doershuk, Tom Boat, Barry Argent, Jack Riordan, Caroline McPherson, Peter Durie, Doris Tulcin, Lap-Chee Tsui, Birgitta Standvik, John Dodge, Bob Dresing, Omar Pivetta, Manny Buchwald and Bob Beall, have all counted immeasurably in the quality of my life. They have been dedicated allies whom I would not have been privileged to know had it not been for this disease. As a young and beginning scientist, I was extremely fortunate to have known and been able to take inspiration from the forerunners of physicians and scientists who shaped this disease into a known entity. These included Gunyon Harrison, Paul di Sant'Agnese, Giulio Barbero, Harry Shwachman, Pete Gibson, LeRoy Matthews, Dick Dooley, Charlotte Anderson, Gordon Gibbs, Giani Mastella, Dick Talamo, Alex Spock, J.G.F. Slegers, Jean Feigleson, and Dick Dobson who were all monuments of knowledge that taught me much about using the weapons of science.

But the relentless beacons of courage were those compatriots, some fallen, who were genetically conscripted into the duel with CF including Pancho Escamilla, Faye Smith, Barbara Palys, Paul Downs, Ies Fride, and Steve Alamo. And most special among all is my wife, Liesbet, who has not only generated a wealth of medical insights, but who also had the incredible courage to marry me. These are some of those who have provided a lifetime of inspiration throughout the struggle and to whom my gratitude will never be appropriately expressed.

References

1. Andersen DH and Hodges RG. "Celiac syndrome V. genetics of cystic fibrosis of the pancreas with a consideration of the etiology." *American Journal of Diseases of Children* 1946;72:62-80.
2. Spock A. "Abnormal serum factor in patients with cystic fibrosis of the pancreas." *Pediatric Research* 1967;1:173-177.
3. Mangos JA and McSherry N. "Sodium transport: inhibitory factor in sweat of patients with cystic fibrosis." *Science* 1967;158:135-136.
4. Quinton PM. "Water Metabolism: Protozoa to man"; in Rechigl M (ed): *Comparative Animal Nutrition*. Basel, S. Karger AG, 1979, pp 100-231.
5. Knowles M, Gatzy J, Boucher RC. "Increased bioelectric potential difference across respiratory epithelia in cystic fibrosis." *N Engl J Med* 1981;305:1489-1495.
6. Schwartz IL and Thaysen JH." Excretion of sodium and potassium in human sweat." *J Clin Invest* 1956;35:114.
7. Cage GW and Dobson RL. "Sodium secretion and absorption in normal subjects and patients with cystic fibrosis." In di Sant'Agnese PA (ed): *Research on Pathogenesis of Cystic Fibrosis*. Bethesda, National Institutes of Health, 1964, pp 67-79.

8. Slegers JFG. "A mathematical approach to the two-step reabsorption hypothesis." In Rossi E, Stoll E (eds): *Modern Problems in Pediatrics*, Vol. 10. Basel, S Karger AG, 1967, pp 74-88.

9. Burg MB, Grantham J, Abramow M, et al. "Preparation and study of fragments of single rabbit nephrons." *Am J Physiol* 1966;210:1293-1298.

10. Hadorn B, Johansen PG, Anderson CM. "Pancreozymin secretin test of exocrine pancreatic function in cystic fibrosis and the significance of the result for the pathogenesis of the disease." *Can Med Assoc J* 1968;98:377-385.

11. Quinton PM. "Suggestion of an abnormal anion exchange mechanism in sweat glands of cystic fibrosis patients." *Pediatric Research* 1982;16:533-537.

12. Quinton PM. "Chloride impermeability in cystic fibrosis." *Nature* 1983;301:421-422.

13. Quinton PM and Bijman J. "Higher bioelectric potentials due to decreased chloride absorption in the sweat glands of patients with cystic fibrosis." *N Engl J Med* 1983;308:1185-1189.

14. Riordan JR, Rommens JM, Kerem BS, et al. "Identification of the cystic fibrosis gene: cloning and characterization of complementary DNA." *Science* 1989;245:1066-1072.

15. Rommens JM, Iannuzzi MC, Kerem BS, et al. "Identification of the cystic fibrosis gene: chromosome walking and jumping." *Science* 1989;245:1059-1065.4

4

A New Era in Diagnosis: The Sweat Test

Lewis E. Gibson, M.D.

When I went to medical school at Johns Hopkins University (1949-53) we had summer vacations. I spent my vacations at my home in Atlanta working as an extern at the Henrettia Eggleston Hospital. The Chief of Staff at Eggleston was Dr. M. Hines Roberts. I still consider him one of the most outstanding physicians I have known. He had a busy private practice, but still did an excellent job of keeping up with the literature. Included in his reading were the early papers of pathologist Dr. Dorothy Andersen at Columbia University in New York City about a disease she discovered named cystic fibrosis of the pancreas.

Dr. Andersen discovered this disease from autopsy material, where she noted numerous cysts and fibrotic changes in the pancreas in infants dying of pneumonia and bronchiectasis. She found enough cases to say that the disease was not uncommon and correctly postulated that the malabsorption seen in these patients was due to a failure of the pancreas to produce digestive enzymes. She found that the disease could be diagnosed during life by demonstrating a lack of enzymes in pancreatic secretions. Pancreatic secretion was obtained by placing a rubber tube in the duodenum. A fluoroscope was used to insure proper placement of the tube. The lack of enzymes, specifically trypsin, was demonstrated by the failure of the secretion to liquefy gelatin. This was all before the CF sweat abnormality had been discovered by Dr. Paul di Sant'Agnese, who worked with Dr. Andersen.

Dr. Roberts thought it would be good for the enterprising extern to set up the gelatin liquefaction test Dr. Andersen had described. I did this with success, as our laboratory technician knew how to mix Knox gelatin. We then proceeded to ask patients, who we (mostly Dr. Roberts) had seen and had suspected the diagnosis, to return for the test. We diagnosed a number of cases. I well remember one attending physician, not Dr. Roberts, who asked me what was of current interest in the hospital. I replied we had two cases of this cystic fibrosis of the pancreas. He said, "Don't be silly. That is a very rare disease."

During these early experiences, I was greatly impressed by the kindness of Dr. Andersen. I wrote her a letter signed as *Mr.* Lewis Gibson saying that we had set up the gelatin liquefaction test, but that I sometimes encountered considerable difficulty getting a tube through the pylorus and into the duodenum. She replied to my letter and included a drawing of a small brass dumbbell, about the size of two

BB shot, which she tied to the end of the duodenal tube. This would pass through the nose and make the tube easier to manipulate. She had filed the dumbbell to size and shape herself. I also filed a brass dumbbell and found that it was quite helpful.

My internship and junior assistant residency (note the old titles) were at Boston Children's Hospital. I cannot say that Dr. Charles Janeway, the Chairman of the Department, increased my interest in CF greatly. He did, however inspire me by being an outstanding person. During his rounds he had a patient way of leading us through a differential diagnosis that was an excellent learning experience. One night about 9 PM, I was looking at patients when I noticed Dr. Janeway sitting at the nurses desk. I quickly walked over and asked if I could help him. He replied, "No Peter, I am just looking." Since then I haven't noticed many Chairmen "just looking" at 9 PM (even including me). But as a Chairman somewhat later on, I did sometimes snoop around in the early morning hours.

While in Boston, my interest in CF was increased when I had the opportunity of working with Dr. Harry Shwachman, who was seeing as increasing number of CF patients in his Nutrition Clinic. I told Dr. Shwachman about the weight on the end of the duodenal tube, which he tried and liked. He was also trying an apparatus that used an iron weight on the end of the tube and a magnet over the abdomen. This approach turned out to be a disappointment.

In 1955 I joined the U.S. Public Health Service and went to the National Institutes of Health (NIH) in Washington, D.C. I was in the Institute of Microbiology (now Allergy and Infectious Diseases), which had the distinction of being the only Institute which hired pediatricians. Things were a bit loose at the NIH at that time, and my immediate boss, Dr. Robert Parrott, asked me what research I would like to do. The CF sweat abnormality had been found and reported by Dr. di Sant'Agnese by that time, and I suggested that I would like to ascertain why CF sweat had such a high concentration of salt. Though it may not be immediately apparent what sweat has to do with microbiology Bob (Robert) said O.K. But he did exact a price for this approval. In return, I had to accept the transfer of his CF patients to my service and care. He was following a few CF patients because they had lots of bacteria in their sputum and therefore might be subjects for microbiological research, in case we thought of a suitable research project. The patients could get free drugs from the NIH, which probably influenced Bob's thinking.

The NIH had a wonderful library and I assigned myself the task of reading everything ever written about sweat. I think I actually did this. Sweat was not one of the primary subjects of medical research. Curiously enough the Japanese wrote much of this literature. Thank goodness they published in English! I am still not sure why they did this research. It may have been related to the fact that most Japanese lack apocrine sweat glands which are mostly in the armpits. Before deodorants became available, the Japanese immediately noticed and did not welcome the proximity of a Westerner. Occasionally a Japanese girl was born with apocrine sweat glands. With them, she was completely unmarriable. Surgery was devised, before anesthetics, to remove these glands. Many young ladies committed suicide to avoid this procedure. Possibly this aroused medical interest.

Sweating is produced by the so called autonomic nervous system. These nerves control the things our bodies do automatically such as digestion, respiration, and, as mentioned, sweating. This part of the nervous system is divided into two types of nerves, the adrenergic with adrenaline as the chemical transmitter and the cholinergic, which uses acetylcholine.

From my reading I learned that the process of sweating is unusual in that both adrenaline and acetylcholine are involved. I suspected that CF was a disease of the autonomic nervous system involving an imbalance between adrenergic and cholinergic stimulation and I wanted to produce sweat with both types of drugs to ascertain the effect on the salt concentration. Systemic administration of either type drug however could be quite dangerous.

Then I remembered seeing my physiology teacher in medical school produce a hive on his arm by the iontophoresis of histamine. Iontophoresis is the introduction of a drug into the skin with an electric current. The process is similar to electroplating. If a solution of an ionized drug with a positive charge is placed on gauze under a positively charged electrode and a negatively charged electrode is placed elsewhere on the body, the positively charged drug will enter the skin. The dose can be calculated using Faraday's law. But the only medical application of iontophoresis that I had read of was to stimulate vasodilatation of the lower legs by putting them into a bucket of priscoline.

Iontophoresis seemed to be the way to go, and I was soon iontophoresing the autonomically active drugs pilocarpine, acetylcholine, adrenalin, and norepinephrine. Unfortunately there was no dramatic effect on the electrolyte composition of the sweat that was produced. At that time, I was really out to cure CF and was not too interested in diagnosis. Friendly Dr. Parrott, however, was interested in finding if CF carriers had abnormal sweat and suggested (strongly) that I sweat test some parents. To produce sweating we routinely placed the patient's body, not including the head, in a plastic bag. The only known carriers then were the parents of CF children. Fathers mostly worked, so the volunteer for the sweat test was usually the mother. One of our nurses would supervise undressing the frequently chubby subject, usually not removing some of the fairly formidable underwear fashionable at that time. Less athletic females, incidentally, tend to sweat slowly. The nurse started the test, but I had to come into the room to hear the complaints. These adventures made me think that iontophoresis might be a great advance for the diagnosis of CF.

In order to iontophorese pilocarpine, I initially looked up what I could about the dosage of this drug. The effective oral or injected dose was said to be 5 to 10 milligrams. The toxic dose was unknown. I knew that iontophoresis was not 100% effective, but that by using Faraday's law of electrolyte equivalents, I could calculate the maximum possible dose. I used 2 to 4 milligrams. Initially I controlled the dose by the amount of drug put on the gauze. Later I noted that the only unpleasant side effect was from the electric current, which could produce small burns, so I put excess pilocarpine on the gauze and controlled the dose with the current. The results did not vary particularly with these machinations. As most of the CF subjects had had previous sweat test using sweat bags, I found that the results were almost identical by both methods.

After two years at the NIH I returned to Johns Hopkins to complete residency training. Dr. Robert E. Cooke was then Chairman of Pediatrics. Dr. Cooke was excellent as a Chairman. He seemed to have a fresh way of looking at everything. In rounds he would bring up exotic diagnostic possibilities we had never considered. We learned by defending our initial diagnosis. He was also very enthusiastic about new research ideas, either ours or his own. He had an unfortunate desire for political power which led to later difficulties. As a Department Chairman though he was great.

Dr. Cooke had worked with CF at Yale and told me that he also had used iontophoresis. We thought it would be a good idea to write a paper about this since it certainly made the procedure easier. A few babies had died in the sweat bags, which further made us think we should publish the technique. We set up the appropriate studies and wrote a paper which described the method and demonstrated its accuracy.[1] This paper has been widely quoted and was found to be a *Current Contents* classic. Since then I have been involved in various ways as an authority on the sweat test. I helped to show that a number of "simplified" methods of performing the test were unsatisfactory.

One used a gelatin plate containing silver nitrate and did turn more white (silver chloride) when the palm of a CF patient was placed upon it than when a control was used, provided that they both sweated at the same rate. Since the sweat rate on the palm is very dependent upon emotions, the test was very inaccurate. Another test using local heat to stimulate sweating did not work well, mostly because local heat does not cause sweating. The fact, that a person sweats only when the blood entering the brain becomes warmer, is well shown in the literature. In heaven, possibly people will read before they write!

The fact that our method required collecting sweat on a gauze pad, which was weighed on a chemical balance before and after the collection, upset many people. This procedure takes some time, a little skill, and total accuracy. Instead, after iontophoresis, sweat was collected under a cup and then scraped up for analysis. Since the cup was at room temperature and the skin at body temperature, distilled water condensed at the top of the cup and a more concentrated salt solution remained on the skin. There was no way to get proper mixing so the results by this technique were fairly erratic.

Another method of doing a sweat test was by using the Orion electrode that measures chloride concentration. This approach sounds good until one tries to think how to control evaporation at variable sweat rates. I had the dubious pleasure of directing a combined study of three methods of doing the sweat test. We tested the Orion, the cup method described above, and my original method. The results showed that the old method was the only sufficiently reliable one. One Orion enthusiast had better results with it than any other investigator and was fairly hard to persuade.

Finally the weighing problem was eliminated with a device named the Macroduct®. A shallow cup fits tightly over the skin. After iontophoresis, pure sweat is forced into a small plastic tube. The sweat's conductivity and/or its chloride concentration can then be measured. Since there is more data to support the chloride concentration than the conductivity as being diagnostic, most people want the chloride measurement for the definitive diagnosis.

At Hopkins, I also became interested in 'a possible relationship between CF and allergy. There had been a paper saying that asthmatic patients had an abnormally high sweat test. We found that this is not true.

In 1960 after a brief episode of private practice, I went back to the NIH to work as a clinical associate with Dr. di Sant' Agnese. Again I primarily worked with sweat. Among other things, I devised a method of simultaneously measuring sweat rate and conductivity. I found that the CF patient, like the normal control, has a diminution of salt concentration with decreasing sweat rate. From these data I tried to calculate the concentration of the sweat precursor solution from the slope (first derivative) of the salt excretion versus the sweat rate curve. I did not achieve sufficiently rapid sweat rates to obtain accurate slopes. Later Dr. Sol Brusilow at Hopkins used the melting point of frozen skin biopsies to find that the precursor solution in CF patients' sweat is, like that of normals, slightly hypertonic.

We also wondered if there is anything abnormal about the number of sweat glands in CF patients. To count the number of sweat glands per unit area, we iontophoresed pilocarpine and then placed graph paper over the stimulated area. The paper was then stained with ninhydrin. The protein in sweat formed a dark spot. We found that CF patients have the same number of sweat glands as others, so I don't think we published this. It is interesting that one is born with all of his/ her sweat glands. The number of glands per unit area is inversely proportional to the total surface area of the body.

I was very lucky to be able to work with Dr. di Sant'Agnese at the NIH. We all know that both he and his many clinical associate trainees have made excellent contributions to research, both in CF specifically and in medicine generally. He took a great interest in his fellows and gave us all very sound career advice.

In 1966 I became the CF Center Director at Yale University in New Haven, Connecticut. Here the Departmental Chairman was Dr. Dave Cook. I seem to work for Cooks or Cookes. Both were inspiring leaders, though very different. Dave was a great critic. His nihilistic approach to many treatments inspired me to have frequent doubts and to make a few useful discoveries. He taught his junior faculty a great deal about writing papers. The process was painful, but when a paper finally pleased Dave, journal editors rarely changed the style or grammar. He could smell a split infinitive a mile away!

Things I remember from the Yale days include the first CF Club meeting I attended as a Center Director. I had been at these meetings before, but not as a Director. Someone gave a paper about the bacteria *Hemophilus influenza* and I was inspired to comment that, "I don't know how to give antibiotics to CF patients."

The audience sort of gasped. A Center Director doesn't know that! I went on to say that there might be some benefit from a daily therapeutic dose of an antibiotic as a prophylactic, but there also might be some difficulties. I stated that I did not have enough patients to have a controlled study of this, but that we might consider a combined study. This was greeted with a prolonged silence, until the CF Club President said that it was time for coffee. In the coffee line, two outstanding, but here nameless, Center Directors separately conferred with me. Director A said, "Peter (my nickname), the children have to have the prophylactic antibiotics. Your study would kill people!" After he moved on Director B addressed me, "Peter, it is not just that prophylactic antibiotics are useless. They are actually harmful. Your study would kill people!"

This experience led me to one accurate conclusion. The study would not be done for some time. Ultimately, when a variant of it was finally done, the result was inconclusive.

In 1968 or there about, the CF Foundation had a so-called GAP Conference on sweat. As I mentioned, the big authorities then came from Japan. Professor Jas Kuno, who had written a book on sweat, was there. It was an enjoyable conference, though we did not figure out why CF sweat contained so much salt. One of the Japanese participants visited my house in New Haven. He was charming. I remember that his wife did impressionistic paintings. This conference occurred before the Japanese invented the Toyota and the Japanese scientists all returned to Japan with a desire to study CF and bring NIH money home in wheelbarrows. Unfortunately they could not find one CF patient in all of Japan!

At Yale Dr. Thomas Dolan worked in the CF clinic. Tom is an outstanding clinician and is really responsible for our work on iodine. My predecessor as Center Director had believed what she read. She read that iodine liquefied mucus and therefore gave all the patients SSKI (saturated solution of potassium iodide). Tom and I weren't convinced it did much, but we did not want to change things too rapidly. A number of patients did not grow very well, but we attributed this to their CF. Then one patient's hair began to fall out. This woke Tom up. In the differential diagnosis of hair loss, he recalled hypothyroidism. We tested and she had it. We tested the whole clinic and reported the highest incidence of hypothyroidism due to iodine ever recorded.

This inspired the Academy of Pediatrics to look into iodine therapy generally. They found no convincing proof it ever did anything good for anybody. On the other hand there were a few charming side effects such as newborns dying from goiters produced when their mothers took iodine. Dave Cook inspired doubts scored again!

A few years ago I was unhappy to see a paper again promoting the benefits of iodine. It was given to adults with chronic lung disease. No improvement in pulmonary function or other objective benefit was found, but in a supposedly "blind" (neither patient nor researcher aware of the test treatment) study, it was reported that the patients thought they felt better with iodine than with placebo. Iodine is secreted in saliva and tastes bad. That study could not have been blind!

It is impossible to say when early adventures stop. Possibly it occurs when one is put on more than two committees and actually tries to attend all the meetings. CF related adventures continued for me, but patient care, administration, and teaching took more and more time. Some people can continue useful research throughout their careers, but they are exceptional.

I spend a good deal of my retirement time training my Labrador retrievers. When I watch a young lab leap into water trying to make the world's most rapid retrieve, I am reminded of the youthful researcher. He should be more careful. He should take more time. But boy is he eager!

References

1. Gibson LE and Cooke RE. "Test for concentration of electrolytes in sweat in cystic fibrosis of the pancreas utilizing pilocarpine by iontophoresis." *Pediatr* 1959;23:545-49.

5

The Matthews Comprehensive Treatment Program: A Ray of Hope

Carl F. Doershuk, M.D.

When I returned to Cleveland for pediatric training at City Hospital, now Metro-Health Medical Center, I first learned of a relatively new cystic fibrosis (CF) program. It was located at what was then Babies and Children's Hospital (B&C Hospital), now Rainbow Babies and Children's Hospital, where I had two months of pediatric training as a medical student but had not seen a CF patient. Although the medical school's innovative "New Curriculum" was entirely revised in 1952 when my class started, we had no lectures about this serious disease. The CF treatment program was started in 1957 and was reported to be providing impressive results by the time my clinical rotation returned me to B&C Hospital as a senior resident in July 1960. I had developed a strong interest in asthma, pulmonary diseases, pulmonary function and physiology, and care of chronic disease. As a result, I wanted to know more about the pulmonary involvement and overall treatment of CF and about this new program.

Before long I was learning how the program was initiated in 1955 by a dedicated small family group, known as the "Cousins Club." The family members were determined to start, and then provide ongoing financial support for, a new research program for children with CF. Their effort was initiated out of concern for one of the Cousins Club families who had already lost one young child to CF and had another who was becoming progressively more ill due to the disease. Their first act was to found the Cleveland CF Chapter in the State of Ohio in 1955. Next they approached Dr. William Wallace, then Chairman of the Department of Pediatrics at the hospital, about establishing a CF research oriented treatment program at B&C Hospital.

Dr. LeRoy Matthews, a young 29 year old faculty member (born in 1925), was the one Dr. Wallace recommended to plan and initiate a comprehensive treatment and research program for CF patients. He also recommended that a Medical Advisory Board be formed to advise the family group on projects worthy of their support. The program was just starting its third year when I arrived in July 1960.

Leroy Matthews was a good storyteller and was especially good at relating the past history and telling of his experiences that led to the comprehensive treatment program he developed. He termed it "**the comprehensive and prophylactic (preventive) treatment program**" for the treatment of CF patients.[1] With his keen insight in defining issues, he developed the treatment program in conjunction with clinical and basic research planning (Table 5.1). This arrangement provided data for frequent progress reports to other physicians then active in CF.

LeRoy had been involved in diabetes and metabolism research and had two excellent mentors in Drs. Samuel Spector and Walter Heymann. Because of his biochemistry expertise, Dr. Wallace had requested him to develop what was probably the first micro blood sample laboratory in the country for routine blood chemistry determinations in children. Reducing the volume of blood needed for analysis was an important contribution in improving the care and management of small ill infants and subsequently proved important for the care of CF infants as well. It was years later before a commercial automated microanalysis system would become available.

The CF assignment for this young faculty member was truly unique because it offered not only the opportunity to plan and develop a research and treatment program from the outset but also provided a commitment of continuing financial support, assuring further growth. It was also a daunting undertaking against a serious and life threatening disease entity for which there was no cohesive treatment plan or recognized successful intervention up to that time. As a result of his training and previous experience, he was well positioned to initiate a CF research program, which he initially devoted to study of the biochemistry of mucus secretions. These studies resulted in a number of seminal publications over the years. On the clinical side however, he needed to learn as much as possible about current practices in CF care and evaluation. There were several fairly large groups of patients in Boston, New York, and Philadelphia where there were various approaches to the care of these children and multiple years of experience.

Dr. Matthews was a 1948 graduate of Harvard Medical School and had studied under eminent faculty there including gastroenterologist, Dr. Harry Shwachman, and Dr. Sidney Farber, who were both very much interested in CF. On a return visit to Harvard, LeRoy learned about the segmental postural drainage positions with clapping and vibration techniques from Dr. Shwachman, who had a large CF population in his Nutrition Clinic at Boston Children's Hospital. Dr. Shwachman had been in England where there was a great deal of chronic pulmonary disease and had observed the use of the postural drainage technique, which was reported to be effective for many types of pulmonary patients. He later reported that "the methods employed are in constant use in chest clinics in England." [2] He had been using this therapy in the treatment of his CF patients and felt it was beneficial in helping mobilize and clear lung secretions.

Later, my review of the literature revealed a bit of the evolution of this therapy stemming from the early 1900s when *intermittent* postural draining was being used for chronic pulmonary conditions. Gradually it was recognized that this brief positioning (tipping) alone was not very effective in moving secretions, even

Table 5.1 Components of the Comprehensive Treatment and Clinical Research Program

Problem: A complex, time consuming, expensive, life-long treatment program and an early, but correct, diagnosis are essential.

Action: Sweat test repeated to confirm diagnosis. Sweat test of siblings
Assure correct diagnosis
Public and medical education for early recognition of the disease

Problem: CF is a chronic insidious disease, often with slow progression to irreversible lung damage before notable symptoms are evident.

Action: Comprehensive program to deal with all recognized aspects of the disease
Prophylactic and preventive wherever possible, starting at diagnosis
Initial hospital intensive treatment to achieve the best possible control
Initial hospitalization for complete evaluation, family and patient education, and institution of home treatment plan
Daily aerosols and airway clearance treatments, nightly mist tent therapy
Adequate diet and calories, pancreatic enzyme replacement, fat soluble vitamin supplements
Antibiotic therapy as indicated by respiratory symptoms and cultures
Regularly scheduled outpatient visits for every patient
Annual influenza vaccine and routine immunizations
Continuing education
Social and psychological support
Prompt rehospitalization for uncontrolled symptoms or problems
Continuity of care provided at specialized Center

Problem: Data collection is required to validate the impact of treatment on morbidity and survival.

Action: Accurate records
Standardized information collection at each outpatient visit
     Interval well being and clinical history
     Change in respiratory symptoms
     Complete physical examination
     Growth measurements
     Bacterial culture of respiratory tract and antibiotic sensitivity test
Chest x-ray evaluation at least yearly
Pulmonary function test regularly after age 5-6 years
Continuing database update
Clinical score (Shwachman-Kulczycki) assigned every 6 months
Initiation of clinical studies and research projects
Later, combined Center studies

when accompanied by coughing. As a result, *continuous* (2-3 hour or even overnight) postural draining was then recommended.

The Superintendent Physiotherapist at the Brompton Hospital, Jocelyn M. W. Reed, was perhaps the first to report that "clapping and pressure-vibrations, during long expirations, are the most effective forms of mechanical stimulus to elimination of secretions," in the treatment of lung abscess, collapsed lobes, and bronchiectasis (dilatation and destruction of the bronchi).[3] She advised that clapping was not allowed in cases in which severe hemoptysis (bleeding from the lungs) complicated bronchiectasis. Since bronchiectasis does result from the progressive lung infection in CF, it would be reasonable for clapping to be discouraged in this condition. Such experience may account her not including CF as a condition for postural drainage and clapping, or in another British report as late as 1959.[4]

Dr. Shwachman was typically at the forefront of seeking out potentially useful diagnostic or treatment measures for CF. He found that positioning along with clapping and vibrations to selected areas of the lungs was beneficial and encouraged one of his British trained visiting physiotherapists to publish the description of "the methods used at the Hospital for Sick Children at Great Ormond Street and adapted to CF patients at the Children's Medical Center in Boston"[5] so that others could benefit. To my knowledge, this was the first published description of this treatment for patients with CF. In follow up, our publication in 1964 was the first in the pediatric literature to further describe and emphasize with words and pictures, this therapy for *all* areas of the lungs and for every CF patient from the time of diagnosis,[1] unless significant bleeding was present. Subsequently, Drs. Bettina Hilman and William Waring at the Tulane University Center in New Orleans produced an excellent pictorial and written set of teaching aids promoting this therapy for distribution to the growing number of CF Centers.

Twelve positions, including those in the head down position, were used. The goal that evolved for CF patients was to drain any excess or retained mucus from smaller airways where the obstruction, infection, and inflammation were felt to have their origin. Hopefully, this treatment could be started before irreversible damage, such as bronchiectasis, had occurred. It was not unreasonable that at least a few observers felt it unlikely that clapping and vibration of the chest wall could reach these small airways deep in the lungs, however, the treatments did seem to be effective, as confirmed by Dr. Shwachman.[2] The Nutrition Clinic was the base for Dr. Shwachman's CF program. There, LeRoy also learned about the current rationale for and use of diet and vitamins, enzymes for aiding digestion, and the intensive, extended treatment course, full dosage, often double-drug and even triple-drug antibiotic therapy that Dr. Shwachman found useful for the effective treatment of the lung infection.

Since most CF children were dying of irreversible and progressive lung damage, pulmonary function testing would be important in the evaluation of pulmonary status and the impact of therapy in individual patients and groups of patients over periods of time. Dr. Charles D. Cook, at the Harvard School of Pub-

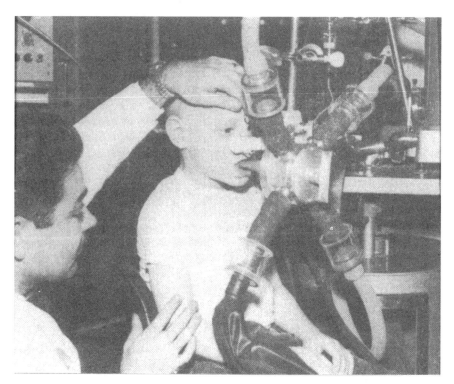

Figure 5.1. *Dr. LeRoy Matthews encouraging a young child during a pulmonary function test. The equipment was very complicated for a child in the early days. Courtesy of Dr. Carl Doershuk.*

lic Health, was a respected leader in pulmonary physiology doing pioneering studies in pediatric pulmonary function and establishing normal values for children. Lee essentially took a pulmonary function and physiology course with Dr. Cook and followed his recommendations completely in equipping a new pulmonary function laboratory at B&C Hospital.

In 1958, Dr. Melvin Wise from Montreal and the first CF trainee in the treatment program at B&C Hospital, soon established a "state of the art" pulmonary function laboratory so that patient and therapy evaluations could be started. The recommendations made by Dr. Cook included basic spirometry using a Collins water-seal spirometer for measurement of the vital capacity and its subdivisions. One could also determine the rate of airflow during a forced exhalation. This unit was ideal for children about age six years on and was also large enough that older patients could be studied as well. Included were the complicated equipment, valves, and tubing needed for the helium dilution test method used to determine the resting volume of the lungs. (Figure 5.1) Both procedures had been set up and standardized and routine tests and research studies had been initiated with the support of the Cleveland Chapter and the Medical Advisory Board. Dr. George Eddy followed Mel. Each had come from Canada as a pediatric resident and remained for an additional year of pulmonary experience and returned home to be involved in CF care and research. Dr. Wise continues to be an active participant and teacher at Montreal Children's Hospital.

At Babies Hospital in New York City, LeRoy met with Drs. Dorothy Andersen and Paul di Sant'Agnese to learn about their approaches to treatment. Of considerable importance to his plan for evaluation, he was impressed with the newest microbiology techniques relevant to CF patients as described and used by Dr. William Blanc, the pathologist in charge of laboratories. Included were the special techniques that had been developed to deal specifically with CF respiratory tract cultures including rapid and accurate detection of the various microbial pathogens encountered and the best method for antibiotic sensitivity testing.

In Philadelphia, Dr. Robert Denton and his pediatrician wife, Dr. Wynne Sharples, were the parents of two CF children. Dr. Denton was studying mucus rheology and investigating ways to thin respiratory mucus. He was nebulizing a 3% saline solution or a dilute (10%) propylene glycol solution to make a mist for inhalation,[6] and felt the latter was helping their children when they slept in mist tents at night. Dr. Shwachman had already been using this mist tent treatment and later reported, "We are impressed with the effectiveness of the use of mist in the management of a number of patients who have moderately severe impairment due to thickened bronchial secretions ... many small patients find such a tent comfortable, as it may reduce or eliminate coughing and permit them to sleep through the night."[2]

The potential for this form of treatment further intrigued LeRoy because of his experience as a Navy Radiation Safety Officer monitoring several atom bomb tests in the South Pacific in the early 1950s. Radiation follow up studies revealed that small radioactive salt particles could be detected as deposits even in the smaller airways of the lungs of individuals who had been exposed. Since glycerine had been noted to prevent rapid evaporation of water from mist droplets,[6] it was reasonable that the use of salt or propylene glycol would also prevent total evaporation of water droplets, might well help moisten or thin the airway mucus layer, and thus make it easier to clear any retained secretions. Leroy's past experience, coupled with the reports of Drs. Denton and Shwachman, led to the use of a 10% propylene glycol (to prevent total evaporation) and water solution nebulized into a tent at night as a part of the comprehensive treatment program. However, as patients grew older their compliance with the program, as expected, became more difficult and this was especially true for the tent therapy. The ultrasonic nebulizer, developed later, produced a more dense mist. However, heat from the transducer made the solution a growth medium for the *Pseudomonas* organism and maintaining sterility became a problem. These and other events led to discontinuation of tent therapy.

There were three additional important contributions to the overall success of the comprehensive treatment program. The first, and one that especially interested me, was the daily use of medicated aerosol inhalations. For the CF patients beyond two to three years of age, the use of aerosol treatments with dilute phenylephrine (for mild decongestant effect at 1/8% dilution) [6] delivered by a compressor driven nebulizer was new to me. These aerosol treatments were in comparison to use of the relatively expensive positive pressure machine used for adult aerosol treatments in which the idea was to force medicated aerosol into obstructed or narrowed airways. In addition to the extra expense, the positive pressure machine was more complicated to use and, of even greater importance, infants and children tended to fight it. It was readily apparent to me that, with the addition of a bronchodilator to the compressor driven aerosol solution, this treatment would easily be adaptable for home treatment of children with asthma and other lung diseases. The other way to deliver inhaled medication to the airways, at that time, was by a hand-held inhaler, which required a significant degree of hand and breathing coordination that most children could not accomplish effectively. The use of the compressor nebulizations could be adapted easily to relatively inexpensive home therapy for continuing treatments out of the hospital for other pulmonary conditions, especially asthma, which was a common enough and significant problem even then. For the CF patients, an antibiotic also could be nebulized as needed, as others had previously noted.

The second contribution was the inclusion of the microbiology information as provided by Dr. Blanc that led to LeRoy's decision to incorporate respiratory tract culture and antibiotic sensitivity testing to the monthly out patient visits for each patient. This enabled whatever bacterial pathogens were present to be identified and their susceptibility to antibiotics determined. Then the antibiotic treatment could be specifically tailored for each patient's bacteria to better maximize effectiveness.

The third contribution, the sweat test, was a less apparent contribution but the fact that it was made available from the beginning of the program was very contributory to the overall success of the plan. From then on, relatively simple, rapid, and accurate diagnosis was available. The sweat electrolyte defect in CF individuals was first observed and accurately described by Dr. di Sant'Agnese in the early 1950s. For a long time, sufficient sweat could only be collected by placing the subject in a very warm room or even in a body sized plastic bag for a sufficient period of time for enough sweat to be produced. The sweat was collected in pipette quantities in order to have enough for analysis and determination of the amount of salt (sodium and chloride). Sweating forced in this way proved dangerous for a few patients and was even life threatening.

Drs. Lewis (better known to all as "Peter") Gibson and Robert Cooke provided further progress in sweat testing.[7] They devised a method of safely driving a chemical, pilocarpine, into a local area of the skin over the forearm by a small electrical current that stimulated sufficient sweat from this small area for accurate salt (usually the chloride part) analysis. Drs. Gibson and Cooke's publication of the pilocarpine iontophoresis sweat test method with quantitative analysis for salt (chloride and sodium) represents the single greatest diagnostic advance for the diagnosis of CF. Their basic method has remained essentially unchanged. For some years a number of children around the country were "undiagnosed" thanks to the simplicity and accuracy of the sweat test when performed by experienced personnel. Fortunately, we did not have the experience of misdiagnosed individuals.

By as early as 1953, a modified form of the test was used at B&C Hospital on a research basis that was facilitated because a clinical research unit with a warm room was available. Because he knew of Dr. Gibson's work, by 1957, well before the sweat test methodology was published, LeRoy had established the pilocarpine method at B&C Hospital and it was routinely available. It was essential for technicians to have skill and experience in applying the pilocarpine, in handling the sweat sample, and in the laboratory analysis using a machine called a chloridometer. Because of the potential expense there was little stimulus for institutions to set up the pilocarpine sweat test. Even after the establishment of Centers by the National CF Foundation, the approved sweat testing method gained only slow acceptance. The locations that used it extensively from early on, chiefly New York, Boston (Dr. di Sant'Agnese related that Dr. Shwachman was an early visitor to learn about it), and Cleveland were provided with the opportunity to make an earlier diagnosis that put them well ahead of other areas in getting treatment started. This was important to the patient, not only with an earlier age of diagnosis, but also a diagnosis at a time when there was only suspicion of the disease and hopefully well before significant pulmonary symptoms, recurrent pneumonia, or irreversible lung damage (bronchiectasis) had occurred. Thus the sweat test provided a less visible but very important advance in the care of CF patients and afforded the patients enrolled in the comprehensive treatment program devised by Dr. Matthews the best opportunity for early diagnosis and for long term survival benefit.

The sweat test permitted the testing of a growing number of children referred because of a suspicion of CF. Ultimately up to 400 children a year were tested in Cleveland. For the small number who tested positive for CF, it represented a great advance in the ease and rapidity of diagnostic testing and permitted diagnosis at a much earlier age. It replaced the previous standard duodenal pancreatic function test, which was time consuming, uncomfortable for the patient, and involved having a tube pushed through the nose and into the stomach, as described in several other chapters. While an abnormal test was consistent with CF, it only later became apparent that some 10 to 15% of CF patients do not have the pancreatic involvement at least early on. Before the sweat test, this normal pancreas variation was not recognized and led to delayed diagnosis in many cases. Fortunately for the great majority of patients referred for a sweat test, the diagnosis of CF was efficiently and effectively ruled out and indicated that other tests were needed for the diagnosis of their problem.

In the early 1950s, CF was usually a disease of acute lung infection and malnutrition in infants and the average age at death was about one year. However, it was apparent that there was some variability in severity and onset of symptoms of the disease and some older children were being recognized as evidenced by a copy of an article from TIME magazine provided by Doris Tulcin. Pathologist Dr. Andersen was featured as the one who "defined cystic fibrosis." This one page summary was undoubtedly the best public relations achievement for CF up to that time and provided a detailed description of the disease along with the current treatment (low fat and high protein diet, vitamins, pancreatin to replace the missing pancreatic enzymes, and tetracycline for antibiotic therapy). It stated in part:

In the wards of Children's Medical Center in Boston last week, or making regular visits to the outpatient clinic, were 200 young-sters suffering from a mysterious disease with a forbidding name: cystic fibrosis of the pancreas. At Babies Hospital in Manhattan there were seven in beds and 80 outpatients; attending Los Angeles' Childrens Hospital were 150 known or suspected cases. Across the country are thousands of other victims, most of them probably unrecognized. For to most doctors, pancreatic fibrosis (also known as mucoviscidosis) is a "new" disease.

TIME , March 1, 1954

Use of the Hospital

In many parts of the country in the mid 1950s, the treatment for CF (if the diagnosis was indeed recognized) was to hospitalize the patient when pneumonia or severe respiratory symptoms developed and only then to treat the infection intensively. As Dr. di Sant'Agnese published in 1946, penicillin worked wonders (even when given as an aerosol) for these ill infants and later oral antibiotics became available and were also effective. However, after discharge from the hospital and usually all too soon, the pulmonary symptoms would recur and the opportunity for further lung damage, now possibly already irreversible, could result. On returning from the East Coast and reflecting on what he had learned and discussed, LeRoy wanted to make the most of his unique opportunity: to plan an ideal program of treatment and research. The result became his concept of what he termed a "**comprehensive and prophylactic (preventive) treatment program.**" He incorporated the variously applied effective measures of evaluation and treatment of the many aspects to the disease into an ongoing treatment program. From that time forward, admission to the hospital was the essential first care step in his plan for every new patient diagnosed or referred.

Initial hospitalization was to accomplish two goals:

Goal 1 was to treat intensively to achieve as much pulmonary and nutritional improvement as possible.

Goal 2 was multiple and was to allow sufficient time to thoroughly educate the family about CF, to promote a positive attitude, and to prepare the family to be able to effectively continue the previous hospital-only treatments in the home. This included training in postural drainage with clapping and vibration (termed PD&C treatments by the house staff). Since almost every patient had some degree of pulmonary disease at diagnosis, the PD&C therapy then was continued at home after discharge.

Furthermore, there was a **long-term outpatient goal** which was to prevent or delay the occurrence or recurrence of the lung injuring bacterial infections as much as possible and to maintain good nutrition. This included continuance of the therapy at home (aerosols and PD&C) several times each day (at first 3 to 4 times a day for the youngest children), and follow up visits initially every four weeks. Oral antibiotics were prescribed in the full treatment dosages and time periods as recommended by Dr. Shwachman (as opposed to the continuous, so called "prophylactic," low dosage approach used by some). As previously noted, the antibiotic therapy was guided by the results of the culture and antibiotic sensitivity testing on a sample from the respiratory tract taken at each visit.

This comprehensive treatment program was the highly visible part to everyone. Less visible was LeRoy's emphasis on the clinical evaluation research projects central to his concept of learning as much as possible about the effect of treatment. Additionally, the concomitant development of laboratory based research would hopefully uncover the fundamental abnormality posed by CF.

The intensity of continuing care at home coupled with the effort to anticipate and/or prevent complications, as much as possible, signified a marked change in the philosophy of CF patient care. One manifestation of change was the training of the parents in administering aerosols and carrying out the drainage procedures at home. Some professionals objected as they felt that only they could (or should) do the postural drainage treatments. In particular, they felt that these treatment procedures were too complicated for parents to learn and do unsupervised in the home. Next there was the need for suppliers of nebulization equipment at reasonable cost. Some kind of tilt board was needed to facilitate the drainage treatments when children became too big for a parent's lap. The monthly out patient visits were scheduled on a regular basis to permit more timely medical evaluation, collection of the respiratory culture for antibiotic sensitivity test, periodic chest x-ray and pulmonary function tests in the older children, and especially for additional education as needed for the families. The organized collection of information from these studies provided the results necessary to evaluate the treatment program and to provide survival results for presentation to others involved in CF care.

The effect on survival was soon apparent, as well as the improved well being of the children. There were many known deaths in Cleveland in the year prior to 1957. After the program was started, there were only 3 deaths among the patients enrolled to mid 1961. This dramatic reduction in annual mortality to less than 2 percent per year after the treatment program was started was met with considerable skepticism elsewhere for a long time. It just did not seem possible that this approach could be that effective for such a serious condition.

Initially, LeRoy personally did the inpatient aerosol and postural drainage treatments, but soon the nurses were so impressed with the results that they volunteered and took over. He and his fellow did all of the education and instruction, as hospital staff was not available for this purpose. Only later did trained physical and respiratory therapists and other support staff become available.

Building the Program

The new Regional Cystic Fibrosis Research and Teaching Centers concept was announced by the National Cystic Fibrosis Research Foundation (NCFRF) in 1960 and funding initiated. The first meeting was held in Cleveland the following year, in part to present to the potential Center Directors the various components needed to make a comprehensive care program successful. This included providing the information from Boston's Dr. Cook about age appropriate pediatric pulmonary function testing equipment; the specialized bacterial culture, identification, and antibiotic testing methods required for CF respiratory cultures; and information about the aerosol and specialized postural drainage therapies.

As one of the earliest Centers in the national Center program (later termed CTR Centers for Care, Teaching, and Research), the Cleveland patient volume and education aspects grew rapidly. Meanwhile, LeRoy worked hard to improve the local research focus beyond that of individual projects. Local support for these projects had grown to about $62,000 per year by 1962. Additional support for research funding at the hospital and medical school would result if he could put together a successful application for a Program Project Grant in CF to the National Institutes of Health (NIH). Rather than support just a single investigator, the Program Project Grant was designed to support the collaboration of several investigators around a common theme. Drs. Sam Spector, Bernard Boxerbaum, Sam Gross, Jerome Liebman, Leroy, myself, and others beyond my recall were involved. The usual panel of experts was assembled and visited the institution, reviewed the planned projects, and subsequently approved the grant, to start in 1964 for a seven year period. It was reported to be the first Program Project Grant in CF to be awarded by the NIH. Old notes indicate that the NIH research support grew to $105,200 per year in 1965 and to $417,100 by 1976.

The widely acclaimed "New Medical Curriculum" at Western Reserve University School of Medicine, initiated with my medical school class in 1952, resulted in an ideal research setting for the CF program. As a result of collaborating closely to develop the new integrated curriculum, the basic science faculty, who were based in the medical school, and the clinical faculty, who were based in the adjacent University Hospitals of Cleveland, were very familiar with one another and accustomed to working together. This experience established a high degree of faculty collaboration, greatly facilitated the growth of the Program Project, and added significantly to the CF related research development.

Leroy's next goal was to develop an application to the NIH for a training grant that would provide financial support of trainees in pediatric pulmonary disease and CF. Such a multiple- year grant would eliminate the need to make an individual application for each potential trainee and would greatly facilitate recruitment for both the program and the applicants. Based on his positive relationship with the medical school and hospital based faculties, he developed an unusual training proposal. His plan was for a program not only for clinical research trainees who would be hospital based, but also included both pre and postdoctoral research trainees, each to be supervised by a basic scientist in the field of interest of the trainee. This would permit the opportunity for cross-training of the fellows and provide research and clinical exposures that could occur for every trainee. Just as with the Program Grant, this training concept also fit readily into the Western Reserve medical campus setting. The site visitors assigned by NIH to review this new proposal were necessarily of mixed academic background to enable them to appropriately review all aspects of the plan, the instructors and their extent of prior collaboration, and the strengths of the Institution. During the morning session, the plan seemed too revolutionary and several site visitors expressed dissatisfaction with the concept. Things did not look promising for approval, despite excellent presentations by the mix of significantly qualified clinical and basic scientists, who expressed their enthusiasm, full support, and cooperation.

Fortunately, the informality and collegiality that can occur during lunch break conversations served to change the perceptions of the review group and they recommended an award of five years by the NIH beginning in 1969. LeRoy, then myself through 1984, and subsequently Dr. Pamela Davis successfully competed for each five year renewal to the present time. The training grant has been an integral part of and very beneficial to the development of the CF research program and has provided an excellent means for the clinical and basic science trainees to have this combined exposure within the same training setting.

During all this time, LeRoy was very active in the Medical Advisory Council of the Foundation. He was the first chairman of the Center Committee and he spent a great deal of time in successfully organizing the Center program and designing the annual reports from each Center to the National CF organization. He also traveled a great deal, especially with Dr. Gunyon Harrison from Houston, to help recruit new Center Directors. His next role was as Vice Chairman of the Medical Advisory Council and he then served as the Chairman for a two year period. Back home and around the same time, he was selected as the new Director of the Department of Pediatrics in 1969, after the untimely and unexpected death of Dr. Wallace. A new hospital was in the planning stage and he had the major staff responsibility for the design and overseeing of construction of this new building which opened in 1971. While he continued to lead the Program Project Grant, he turned the direction of the CF Center to me. Due to the growing number of pulmonary patients, he established a new Pulmonary Division to include the CF Center, and I became the first Division Chief.

The program continued to grow. We were fortunate to recruit Dr. Don Carlson, who had a Ph.D. in biochemistry, from the University of Michigan. He headed the Biochemistry Research Laboratory and further developed the research program in 1964. Don was a highly regarded researcher and an excellent choice. The 1969 availability of the training grant facilitated the recruitment of trainees, especially excellent new physician trainees to the program including Drs. Robert Stern, Thomas Boat, Robert Wood, and David Orenstein. (Figure 5.2) These four trainee additions marked significant support and new growth for the program as each of them subsequently joined the faculty as members of the Pulmonary Division and CF Center. The timing to be able to retain them as new Division mem-

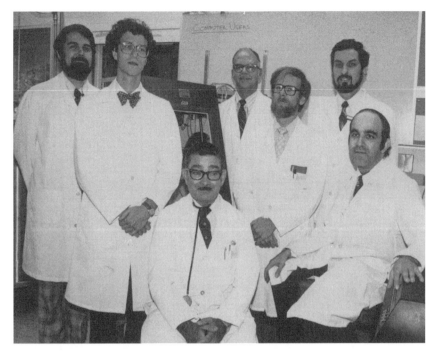

Figure 5.2. *The Rainbow Babies and Children's Hospital Pulmonary Division Faculty in 1980. In the front center, Dr. LeRoy Matthews. From the left, Drs. Robert Wood, David Orenstein, Carl Doershuk, Dorr Dearborn, Thomas Boat, and Robert Stern. Courtesy of Dr. Carl Doershuk.*

bers was excellent as their arrival followed completion of the new Rainbow Babies and Children's Hospital in 1971. This new structure provided the necessary laboratory space needed and each of them went on to become well known and established in their own special area of expertise:

> Bob Stern for intravenous therapy innovations (including the "heparin lock" and long term indwelling so called "Stern" intravenous lines) and prolific writing.

> Tom Boat for mucus biochemistry research and regulation of secretion studies.

> Bob Wood for the pioneering of pediatric fiberoptic bronchoscopy and being its guru.

> David Orenstein for early innovative studies of the pathophysiology of exercise in CF and continuing exercise studies.

These four were, and are, a stellar and talented group who kept the program on the cutting edge in their areas of interest, but they also were wonderful and much appreciated compatriots. They are outstanding and caring clinicians as well.

In addition to these four, Carolyn Kercsmar, Michael Konstan, John Carl, Paul Smith, Tom Ferkol, Mike Infeld, Jim Chmiel, Laura Milgram, and Dan Craven were trainees who became welcome additions to our faculty. Many of our other pulmonary fellows have gone on to successful and productive careers at other CF Centers and Pulmonary Divisions. Hopefully without overlooking anyone, these include Mel Wise, George Eddy, Sue Miller, Sue Pittman, Terry Gillespie, Ed Charnock, Barry Fisher, Pierre Vauthy, Bob Fink, Ricardo Pinero, Eli Nussbaum, Jim Sherman, Glenna Winnie, Chris Green, Greg Legris, Bob Cohn, Youngran Chung, Mike Fiedler, Jim Stark, David Birnkrant, Girish Sharma, Ann Chetty, Juan Martinez, and Starla Glick.

After Don Carlson became Chairman of the Department of Biochemistry at Purdue University, biochemist Dorr Dearborn, Ph.D., M.D., was recruited from the NIH and continued the excellent leadership of the Biochemistry Laboratory. He and Dr. Margaret Bruce, a trainee and then faculty member, were probably the first to observe and report on high levels of uninhibited elastase activity in CF pulmonary secretions and the presence of elevated elastin degradation products in the urine.[8] Elastase products from the neutrophils (the white blood cells that enter the lungs to fight the infection) have subsequently been recognized as a major source of airway damage in CF and have been the target of several treatment measures.

Other Ph.D. staff in that era included Tom Gerken (awarded the first Kathy Graub Fellowship from the Foundation) in mucin biochemistry, Mary Jane Thomassen and Jeff Klinger in microbiology, Cathy Klinger in genetics, Carol Liedtke in biochemistry and cell physiology, Frank Primiano in biomedical engineering, and Jay Horowitz in physics. The latter two individuals taught the pulmonary trainees about medical instrumentation, developed pulmonary function tests for children and adults, computerized data collection and analysis, and studied ventilatory mechanics and water transport in the airways. They also served as faculty advisors for graduate students in biomedical engineering among whom was Jim Ligas who graduated from the MD/PhD program. Tony Bacevice, who also worked in Dr. Herman Hellerstein's cardiovascular research laboratory, was our machine language programmer in the pulmonary lab prior to entering medical school. Kathy Germann Henke, before she went on for her Ph.D., worked with David Orenstein in the study of exercise in CF. Fred Montague provided technical support, and Rob Chatburn worked with Marv Lough in studying and developing infant ventilator systems. The collaborative efforts of this entire group contributed to the extensive publications generated from our Pulmonary Division.

Non-pulmonary division faculty who have provided important leadership and have been strong contributors to the research program include Melvin Berger, Jeffrey Blumer, Dennis Drotar, Richard Hanson, Robert Harvey, Ulrich Hopfer, Charles Hoppel, Jianjie Ma, Michael Reed, Mark Schluchter, John Schreiber, and Alan Tartakoff

As time went on, it was apparent that Lee's history of diabetes mellitus from the mid 1940s was taking a serious toll on his health. Blood sugar control was difficult and episodes of low blood sugar, his heavy schedule, and long and strenuous workdays did not help. Those were very busy times for all of us. To ease his load, I developed the grant renewal application for the Program Project that was awarded another 5 years by the NIH in 1979. Subsequently, the NIH announced funding for a Core Center Grant for CF whose concept was to provide additional laboratory or other needed support for an established and focused group of projects around a central theme, such as CF. As our Program Project was well established with a productive program, our application resulted in the award of the first Core Grant in 1983 for $1.8 million over a 3 year period. I was proud to be the Principle Investigator responsible for that proposal in support of continuing growth of the program. At the same time, we were all saddened that Lee's health was failing following a heart attack and stroke, but he fully appreciated the successes of the program and the continued growth provided by the leadership of Dr. Pam Davis. Sadly, he died in 1988 at the all too young age of 62 years. His legacy lives on, in part, as the LeRoy Matthews Cystic Fibrosis Center, LeRoy Matthews scholarships awarded by the National Cystic Fibrosis Foundation to promising, academically-oriented young physician trainees, and the fine family he raised with the love and support of his wife, "Rock."

In view of the poor long-term prognosis for CF patients in 1955, it was far from evident that LeRoy Matthews' insight, strategic planning, and determination would lead to the impressive and significant improvements in survival for those with CF. It took the combined efforts and long-term support of many dedicated people working selflessly, as well. The Comprehensive Treatment Program he designed and promoted by 1957 was key to the improving survival. The introduction of the program served to decrease the previous year after year after year mortality rate from 10 percent (or greater) per year in the 1950s to 2 percent or less per year by 1960. When his program concept spread nationwide through the Foundation's Centers Program starting in 1961, the annual mortality rate began to fall elsewhere as well. There are now over 19,000 patients under care at the 114 CF Centers in the US. Over 9,000 are adults and there is at least one active international adult CF organization providing a regular publication. While LeRoy Matthews' treatment and research program and his story are but one of the many important contributions made by many others over the years, his accomplishments do stand out as exceptional. The history of the many other contributors to advances in treatment, in research, and in the vital areas of public policy, fund raising, and program development are detailed in other chapters.

References

1. Matthews LW, Doershuk CF, Wise M, Eddy G, Nudelman H, and Spector S. "A therapeutic regimen for patients with cystic fibrosis." *J Pediatr* 1964;65:558-75.
2. Shwachman H. "Therapy of cystic fibrosis of the pancreas." *Pediatr* 1960;25:155-63.

3. Reed JMW. "Physiotherapy for chest diseases," in *Diseases of the Chest*, G Marshall, KMA Perry, Eds. Butterworth & Company, St. Louis, 1952, volume 2 pp. 395-413.

4. Thacker EW. *Postural drainage and respiratory control.* London, 1959, Lloyd-Luke, Ltd.

5. Doyle B. "Physical therapy in treatment of cystic fibrosis." *Physiotherapy Rev.* 1959;39:24-27.

6. Denton R. "The clinical use of continuous nebulization in bronchopulmonary disease." *Dis Chest* 1955;28:123-40.

7. Gibson LE and Cooke RE." Test for concentration of electrolytes in sweat in cystic fibrosis of the pancreas utilizing pilocarpine by iontophoresis." *Pediatr* 1959;23:545-49.

8. Bruce MC, Poncz L, Klinger JD, Stern RC, Tomashefski J, and Dearborn DG. "Biochemical and pathologic evidence for proteolytic destruction of lung connective tissue in the cystic fibrosis patient." *Am Rev Resp Dis* 1985;132:529-35.

6

The Race to Find the Cystic Fibrosis Gene: A Trainee's Inside View

Mitchell L. Drumm, Ph.D.

I always had an interest in genetics and that became my major at Ohio State University. After graduating in 1984, I entered the Department of Human Genetics graduate program at the University of Michigan in Ann Arbor. Part of the inauguration into the Department was a cookout for the new students and the opportunity to meet the more senior students and the faculty. One of the recreational activities was volleyball, which most of the students and a few of the faculty were playing. I found myself on the opposite side of the net from a tall lanky guy who had just joined the faculty the week before my return to Ann Arbor. Despite his good-natured appearance and demeanor, he proceeded to send volleyball missiles at me from above. I asked one of the other students who this guy was and he told me he thought the name was Collins. Over the next few weeks, I got to know this Dr. Collins a little better and seeing as he seemed to be a pleasant sort of person, I asked him if I could do one of the compulsory research rotations in his laboratory. To my great fortune, he assented to my request.

In the meantime, I was in the midst of my first of three basic rotations. Laboratory rotations were a requirement of the Department in order for students to make informed decisions about the type of research they would like to carry out and with whom. One evening during this rotation, my parents called me to tell me the family across the street had just received the news that their infant son was diagnosed with a disorder called cystic fibrosis (CF). This was the second time I had heard of CF in my small home community, but this was the first time it had hit so close to me. This was a family for whom I had watched the first two sons grow from 3 and 5 year olds to young adults, watched the boys when their mom and dad went out, and with whom I wrestled and showed how to play football. They were just about family to me. The kind of people that you could just walk into each other's house without knocking. Needless to say, I was interested in this CF disease. Up to this point CF was just something used as an example in my genetics textbooks for an autosomal recessive inherited disease. I asked around about this CF disease that I knew nothing about and read up on it. I was devastated by what I learned of its severity and ultimate life ending outcome.

The following year, in 1985, I was finished with my rotations and had officially joined the lab of Dr. Francis Collins. This was the same Dr. Collins who went on to head the Human Genome Project. That initiative evolved into an Institute at the NIH, called the National Institute for Human Genome Research, and is directed by Dr. Collins. About 1985, a report came out summarizing a large collaborative study that the gene causing CF was found linked to a genetic marker. As I was to later appreciate, this was a monumental finding for the time, as it used a technique called linkage analysis to make this discovery. A new, young investigator, named Lap-Chee Tsui, at the Hospital for Sick Children in Toronto headed the report. Dr. Tsui and his colleagues had taken a large number of pieces of DNA (deoxyribonucleic acid) that represented various positions on the different chromosomes and looked to see how those segments were inherited in families where CF occurs. The way it works is that between individuals there are subtle variations at numerous positions throughout the chromosomes. The genetic information on the chromosomes is contained in the DNA, a long polymer consisting of 4 different chemical bases. It is the order of the bases adenosine (A), cytidine (C), guanosine (G) and thymidine (T) that dictate the information. While the DNA sequence between two individuals is greater than 99.99% identical throughout the 3 billion or so As, Cs, Gs and Ts that they carry on their chromosomes, there are some differences between any two people who are not identical twins. When these variants can be detected, the ability to do so allows one to label, or mark, the segment of the chromosome in which the variation resides. If the parents of a CF child and at least one other of their children are typed for their array of these markers, one can follow the inheritance of these markers and see how it follows the disease. If the marker is close to the CF gene on the chromosome, most or all children with CF in a particular family should have the same complement of markers. This strategy is outlined in Figure 8.1. The non-CF siblings should have only one or zero chromosomal markers in common with their CF brother or sister. After analyzing dozens of markers from 39 families, the study found one marker, DOCRI-917, that was inherited with CF more often than chance alone would predict.

To this point, the genetic markers used were at random; that is, they represented different chromosomal regions, but it was not known what the regions were. Once a marker of interest was found, the next step was to figure out which segment of which of the 23 chromosomes it represented. By various manipulations, the identified marker was found to be on chromosome number 7. Subsequently, just about every other DNA marker for chromosome 7 was analyzed to see if one might be even closer to CF, and several were found that, in fact, were closer.

One of the closely linked markers found was not in the form of a DNA fragment, but rather a liver enzyme gene with two variants. The variants of this enzyme, paraoxonase, were assessed by examining the enzyme's activity found in an individual's serum, rather than by the simpler DNA assays used for other markers. This was necessary as the gene for paraoxonase had not yet been cloned (identified and isolated) and so no DNA probes existed. A probe is a small piece of DNA that has been isolated and can be used to detect related pieces of DNA from a complex mixture of fragments. As it turned out, two other DNA markers were identified

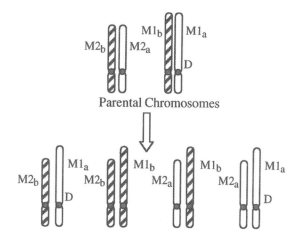

Parental Chromosomes

Likely combinations of chromosomes

Figure 6.1. *Determining the location of a disease gene. During the production of the parental egg and sperm, their chromosomal segments recombine an average of one exchange per chromosome. The result is that two points that are close together on a chromosome will be inherited together while those far apart or on different chromosomes will only be inherited together about 50% of the time. Molecular markers (shown as M1 and M2) with detectable different forms (a and b) can track the chromosomal regions to see if the disease gene (D) in question segregates with one region more than others. In the example shown here, the disease gene tracks with the M1a marker.*

that looked to be even closer to the CF gene than DOCRI-917. One of the two markers was a gene called *met* that was found because of its role in certain cancers, while the other marker, J3.11 was a DNA fragment of unknown function but which existed in two different, detectable forms and could be used as a genetic marker.

Met and J3.11 were tested against a large number of CF families for linkage, and appeared to be quite close together, about 1-2 centimorgans (cM) in genetic distance, or probably about 1-4 millions basepairs in physical distance by best estimates. Most important, it appeared that the CF gene resided between *met* and J3.11. The order of the three sites, or loci as they are referred to genetically, was extremely important. But the existing technology, by which one could move from one genetic position to the next, would not readily allow us to know whether we were going in the right direction. As there are only two directions from any point on a chromosome, having flanking markers meant that you could go both directions from both markers until two of the searches collided. Those two markers then would determine the interval in which the CF gene should reside.

The distance between *met* and J3.11 is quite large, but in a genome of 3 x 10^9 basepairs, The important thing was that the 1-4 x 10^6 basepairs meant that 99.9% of the genome had been excluded from containing the CF gene. Nonetheless, such a region could contain dozens of genes in addition to the CF gene.

The Collins Laboratory Gets into CF Research

Upon entering Dr. Collins' lab, he and I decided that my graduate project would be to work on a technique called "chromosome jumping," a process Dr. Collins, or Francis as he was more commonly called, dreamed up while he was a postdoctoral fellow at Yale University. Chromosome jumping, originally called hopping, was a method to move along a chromosome more quickly than the existing technology allowed. The purpose was to more expeditiously find genes of interest, such as those involved in disease. With the rough localization of the CF gene, it seemed to me that perhaps I could apply my graduate project in the lab to the CF problem. Francis agreed to my using CF as a prototype for chromosome jumping. The first step required obtaining DNA fragments in the CF region of chromosome 7, so Francis contacted Drs. Michael Dean and George VandeWoude at the National Cancer Institute to inquire about obtaining fragments of a gene called *met*. *Met* was a gene they had identified earlier and was important because it was the closest known gene to the CF gene, at that time. Drs. Dean and VandeWoude were very helpful and soon provided us with the DNA fragments. Then we commenced our trek along the chromosome.

Chromosome Jumping and Mapping

The conventional process of moving from point A to point B on a chromosome is called "chromosome walking". The walking process involves breaking the chromosomes up into very small pieces so they can be manipulated, and then analyzing them one at a time. Since the pieces come from the chromosomes of many cells, there are multiple copies so some of the pieces will overlap with other pieces. Without the overlaps, it is impossible to know how two pieces relate to each other. The process can be thought of, by analogy, to taking several hundred copies of a book written in a foreign language, cutting up the pages into pieces and throwing them into a pile. One then pulls out pieces of pages, analyzes the text without knowing what it says, and looks for stretches of text that are in common between different pieces. By pulling out enough of these overlapping pieces of pages, one can eventually re-construct the entire text. As one might imagine, the process is slow and inefficient. In the case of a chromosome, one does not even know whether the overlapping pieces are heading toward the center of the chromosome or to the ends.

The idea that Dr. Collins had was to speed the process a bit by not needing all the overlapping pieces in between two points. Going back to the book analogy, his idea was to glue every hundredth page of each book together, with the first page used in each book being different. In this way, if one found a page with some text in common to some starting page, one would know the adjoining page came from 100 pages away without having to read through the intervening 99 pages. One would gladly sacrifice those 99 pages to get to the part of the book that was of interest. However, the deficiency was that one would not know if the adjoining page came from a point 100 pages closer to the beginning of the book or the end. A schematic comparison of the walking and jumping techniques is shown in Figure 8.2.

With technician Jeffery Cole, I constructed what is referred to as a library of these adjoining "pages," or pieces, of chromosomal fragments. As the *met* gene was the closest one available to the CF gene, we used a piece of it as our starting point. The DNA sequence of *met* (its text) allowed us to fish from the library a piece of DNA we called CF63. CF63 looked as if it originated between 50,000 and 100,000 basepairs from the *met* sequences we had started with. This was an overwhelming success for us, unequivocally showing that the jumping process could, indeed, work.

However, for the process to be useful for CF, we had to know if we were jumping toward or away from the gene. We were able to establish, fairly rapidly, that we were moving away from the far end of the *met* gene, and we felt that was the most likely direction for the CF gene to be, but it was by no means certain. Therefore, the next job at hand was to find a way to make a map of the region so one could be certain of the direction of travel.

Thus, mapping the region on chromosome 7 had to be the next step. Another marker from chromosome 7 was identified as being closely linked to CF. This marker was a random piece of DNA that was different in that it was not known to be from a gene. Called J3.11, it statistically appeared to be on the opposite side of the CF gene from the *met* gene. With these two markers apparently flanking the CF gene, we invoked a new technology called pulsed-field gel electrophoresis (PFGE) to develop a map of this region of chromosome 7. PFGE allows the separation of very large DNA molecules, on the order of hundreds of thousands of base pairs, whereas conventional technology would only allow resolution of up to about 20,000. The biotech business was not quite in full swing at this point, so we home designed our apparatus for the PFGE work. That was part of the fun of being in Francis' lab; he was right up on the cutting edge technology, and that meant the stuff we worked on was not yet available commercially. I like to tinker and make things, so this kind of environment was good for me.

The result of the PFGE work was that we were able to build a sort of map of the region between the *met* and J3.11 markers. Two immediate pieces of information were derived from this map. The first was that we could approximate the size of the interval between *met* and J3.11 to be between 1,300,000 and 1,700,000 bases. The second bit of information was that CF63 did indeed jump in the direction of the CF gene. These two bits of information together provided a major victory for us, as they suggested that by jumping from both ends we could close the gap in 6 to 8 jumps. Few things are as simple as they seem, and subsequent events were reminders that we were not the only ones interested in this gene.

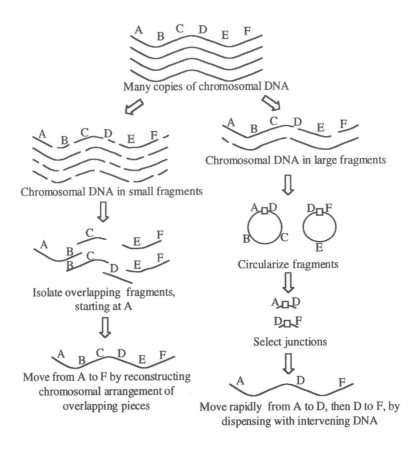

Figure 6.2. *Chromosome walking and jumping. The purpose of both procedures is to move along a chromosome from some marker position (A) toward a target (F) such as a disease-causing gene. To do this, chromosomal DNA from millions of cells is purified and cleaved into fragments. For walking (left), the fragments are relatively small and one begins by identifying fragments that have sequences in common with the marker. These fragments will also have sequences (B) that extend past the marker, which can then be used to identify another set of fragments that extend even a little farther, such as to C, and so on. Since each of these steps can take weeks to complete, traversing the stretch from A to F is a time consuming process. In jumping (right), the DNA is cleaved into large fragments which are enzymatically converted into circles in such a way as to allow identification of the point where the two ends came together (shown as a square). The circles are cleaved into small fragments just as in the walking technique and pieces with sequences in common to marker A are selected. Unlike the walking technique, sequences extending past the marker originate from a point much farther from marker A, thus bypassing sequences not of interest. In this way, one or two jumps replace five to ten walking steps to expedite the process.*

Support from the Cystic Fibrosis Foundation

The CF Foundation was the most obvious group to be interested in the quest for the gene. We had not had any involvement with them, in fact I did not know of its existence, but as it became apparent that we were serious about CF gene research, the Foundation became very interested in what we were doing. One day, Francis asked us to get all of our data in a presentable form because two of the head honchos from the CF Foundation were coming and he wanted to show them what we had been doing and what we intended to do. Shortly thereafter, Bob Dresing and Bob Beall, then the CEO and Scientific Director respectively of the Foundation, came to see us. After Francis gave them one of his typically moving presentations, the Bobs, as they became affectionately referred to by the lab and everyone else, said, "What do you need, our checkbook is with us." I was too naive to understand all the ramifications of the visit until that critical point.

There were other groups interested in the gene as well. In London, Robert Williamson's lab published an article describing the identification of a gene between *met* and J3.11, and reported that this gene was a candidate for the CF gene. Up to this point, a number of high powered labs were involved in the search, but the news that Williamson had found the CF gene, or was at least much closer than anyone else, seemed to quench the desire for a number of these investigators to continue in the search. It also stimulated an alliance between two labs, and shortly a third lab, to forge ahead.

While we were trying to jump along the chromosome, Lap-Chee Tsui and his lab members, were continuing to screen pieces of chromosome 7 by genetic analyses to see if other, closer markers could be found. Two such markers were found that mapped genetically between *met* and J3.11. Francis and Lap-Chee realized that the obvious way to conquer the problem more quickly was for us to band together. We could see where his new markers were actually located and potentially use them for new launch points for our jumps. Our collaboration with Lap-Chee thus began.

The Race for and Discovery of the Gene

The Williamson lab published another paper shortly after the first, indicating the gene they had identified could not be the CF gene based on genetic evidence. They were, nonetheless, much closer to the actual CF gene and had narrowed the gap to 500,000-600,00 bases. When we mapped the new markers from Lap-Chee's lab we found that they were substantially closer to the CF gene than CF63, but not quite as close as the gene reported by Williamson. But, Lap-Chee's markers were not that far away, either. Unexpectedly, these new markers were almost on top of each other. Although we had hoped they would give us two new points from which to search, they really only provided one point, but this position was substantially closer than we had been.

Lap-Chee had been working with Dr. John Riordan on the CF problem, and both were situated at the Hospital for Sick Children. The Riordan lab was collecting CF tissues and constructing what are known as cDNA libraries, resources for identifying genes active in a tissue of interest. As each of the labs seemed to have different expertise to offer to the project, we developed a three-way collaboration. Many telephone conversations ensued between the various researchers from each lab, but for some issues the telephone just cannot accomplish what is really necessary to carry on a project as complicated as this. We needed to know each other, see each other's data in detail, and get a feel for how things worked in each other's labs. Fortuitously, Ann Arbor, Michigan is only about a 5 hour drive from Toronto, Canada, so we ended up having meetings at a point about halfway between, in London, Ontario, Canada.

The most recent work from the Williamson lab showed that the CF gene had not been found and Lap-Chee's new markers put us much closer to the CF gene than we had been. So, the jumping and mapping got back into full swing, now that we knew we were not out of the gene chase race. We knew we were closer with each jump, and were now at risk of jumping right past the gene without even knowing it. We soon started isolating all of the DNA between our jumps, as any fragment might actually contain the gene. We were now faced with a problem. We knew it would come up eventually, but had not really figured out how to deal with. The problem was, how would we know when we actually had the gene? It can be very simple to exclude a gene if it is not the one in which you are interested, but finding a gene amidst all of the other sequences in the DNA and then proving it is the gene you want, is not a trivial task.

One of the ways we went about trying to accomplish this identification was to use a functional read-out test. It was pretty clear that a fundamental problem in CF was the reduced ability for chloride transport across the cells lining the airway, intestine and several other tissues. Francis had a good friend from medical school days at the University of North Carolina, Dr. Richard Boucher, who worked on ion transport in organs like the lung as one of his major research interests. Dr. Boucher used some techniques to monitor chloride movement from cells and came up with a scheme to put those assays to use in identifying the CF gene. The idea was that as we isolated the small pieces of chromosome 7, he would inject them into cells they had isolated from a CF patient. If the piece of DNA contained the normal version of the CF gene, it should restore normal chloride movement to the cells. The assay certainly looked promising, but did not help. As we now know in retrospect, the CF gene was much too large to fit on any one piece of DNA that we could isolate with the existing technology.

The trek across the CF region continued, and as each piece of DNA was pulled out, we looked for any sign that it might contain a gene. This was particularly difficult, but very important to the CF gene search, because there were no clear signs as to where the gene should be. Genes responsible for any other genetic disorder, up to that time, had been identified because of some clear chromosomal abnormality, or because the protein encoded by the gene had been identified first. For CF, there were no chromosomal abnormalities found in any patients, nor did anyone know what the protein product from the gene would be. Therefore, it was necessary to rely on more suggestive evidence.

One of the tricks that helped to identify the gene for Duchenne muscular dystrophy was to look for regions of DNA that were very similar between different species. The idea is that through the course of evolution, genes need to maintain their function and so diverge less than regions not containing genes. Another observation that had been made as more and more genes were being cloned was that the ends of many genes had lots of Cs and Gs, whereas most regions more randomly mix up the four bases of DNA, A, C, G and T. We scanned all the pieces of DNA we found for species conservation as well as CG-containing regions. After a number of false leads, including pieces of DNA that either looked like genes but weren't, or were genes but not the right one, we found a fragment of about 40,000 that contained a CG stretch. We whittled that piece down to about 4,300 basepairs that still contained the CG region and sent it to Toronto. Johanna Rommens, a postdoctoral fellow in Lap-Chee's lab found that this piece, which we referred to as E4.3, also had sequences with very close relatives in mice and cattle. This was all enticing, but we'd been down similar roads before, and it was too early to get too excited.

John Riordan's lab took the next step. His lab had generated what are called cDNA libraries from a number of tissues affected in CF, such as sweat glands, intestines, and airways. cDNA libraries are a collection of DNA fragments, all of which are from genes active in the tissue from which they are derived. It is estimated that of the 40,000 different genes found on our chromosomes, only about 10,000 are active in any given cell or tissue type. Therefore, finding evidence that the gene we were investigating was active in tissues affected in CF would be significant evidence toward it being the right gene.

After screening several million DNA fragments, a single piece of DNA called 10–1 was isolated from a sweat gland library. This piece was sequenced and by a variety of analyses was found to be only a small segment of the gene from which it originated. It did provide a means to determine in which tissues the gene is active and clearly tissues containing a specific cell type, epithelial cells, had this gene turned on. Now we were excited.

10–1 was used as a starting point to find more of the gene and eventually the whole thing was isolated in a series of overlapping pieces. Still, what was missing was a way to know if this was the right gene. Even though only a fraction of genes are active in any given cell, the epithelial specific feature was not proof since many other genes would certainly show the same trait. Then, just before Christmas 1988, the Toronto group found that when they compared cDNA derived from CF epithelia to those derived from non-CF epithelia, there was a difference. Some of the CF genes were missing three fragments, which would be predicted to make a very subtle change in the protein encoded by the gene. I think we were all expecting a more striking change in the gene if it were truly a mutation that caused CF, but any change had to be pursued.

Lap-Chee and his group then screened the large bank of DNAs he had collected from CF patients and their families for this 3 base pair deletion. Because of all the markers on chromosome 7 that Lap-Chee had characterized, he could determine which copy a parent passed on to their CF child and which copy wasn't passed on. In that way it was possible to separate the CF chromosomes from the non-CF chromosomes. Each chromosome 7 was analyzed, and of the several hundred CF chromosomes looked at, about two-thirds carried the deletion, but not a single non-CF chromosome had it. This was the evidence we were looking for.

While the population study was being carried out, there was still the task of trying to figure out what this gene was. The entire DNA sequence was determined and, by computer analysis, we could deduce the type of protein this gene would make. By looking at the amino acids the protein would contain, one could predict with some degree of reliability whether a segment of the protein was likely to be contained in the lipids of a cell membrane, or exposed to the cytoplasm or outside of the cell. It was also possible to compare the sequence of the protein to that of other known proteins and see if any similarities existed. Several features showed up. First, the protein looked to be something that would reside in the cell plasma membrane. It also had regions that showed strong similarity to other proteins that use ATP as an energy source to carry out some function in the cell. Third, it had sequences that looked like they could be modified by an enzyme called a kinase, and it was known from other studies that the chloride transport defect found in CF is normally activated by kinases in the cell.

At this point, there was no doubt that this was the correct gene, but we still couldn't figure out how it fit into the cell physiology of the disease. All the physiology work indicated that a chloride channel should be the culprit, or at least something that influenced the channel. This protein looked like it would sit in the membrane much like a channel would, and it had the kinase regulatory sites in it, but a channel wouldn't need the ATP that this protein looked like it should. This paradox left not only a biological question, but also a quandary as to what the gene and protein should be named. The consensus was to not over interpret. It was clear that this protein affected the ability of epithelial cells to conduct chloride across their membranes, and even affected sodium conductance as well, at least in CF patients. So the name that resulted was the cystic fibrosis transmembrane conductance regulator, or CFTR. It was also noted that this acronym included the last initials of the three primary investigators, Collins, Tsui and Riordan.

In mid 1989 the work was put together for publication. It was a massive amount of work from a large number of people, and so there was an understandable amount of debate as to who should appear, and in what order, on the authorship of the work. In the medical and biological sciences, credit for who did what is acknowledged by order of authorship on manuscripts. To solve some of the debate, the work was divided into three parts and the three articles describing it were published in the September 8th issue of Science in 1989[1-3]. A personal offshoot of the work was that it allowed me to graduate the following spring.

Since the CFTR Gene was Cloned

With the gene in hand, there were great expectations as to what could be done clinically, as well as furthering our understanding of the basic biology involved in CF. I stayed in the Collins' lab as a postdoctoral fellow and one of the next steps we took was to work with Dr. James Wilson, also at the University of Michigan at the time, to determine if gene replacement therapy could be feasible. Jim's lab was expert with retroviruses, a type of virus that was very efficient at infecting a variety of cell types, as a means to getting desired DNA sequences into cells. We replaced some of the virus' DNA with that of a condensed version of the non-mutant CFTR gene, called a cDNA, and used this virus to introduce the cDNA into some CF cells. The cells we used were from a tumor from the pancreas of a CF patient and were epithelial cells, the type of cells that line the tubular structures of the tissues affected in CF, such as the lungs, pancreas and intestines. Dr. Wilson later moved on to head the Institute for Human Gene Therapy at the University of Pennsylvania to explore gene therapy for a number of different disorders.

From the past several years of work on the physiology of CF it was known that CF epithelial cells did not properly allow certain ions, such as chloride or iodide, to pass through them. In conjunction with Ray Frizzell at the University of Alabama at Birmingham, the CF cells into which we had placed the non-CF version of CFTR were compared to the untreated CF cells and CF cells infected with only virus (no cDNA) for their ability to allow chloride and iodide ions to pass through. We found that the cells with the non-CF version of CFTR had a much greater ability to transport these ions and reported this work in 1990 at the same time another group showed similar resulted in airway CF cells. The implication of these two studies from a scientific standpoint was that they verified functionally that the gene in hand was in fact the CF gene: it restored ion transport to the CF cells. From the clinical and public standpoint, it meant that with some finessing it should be possible to treat patients with CF by some form of gene therapy. While much work has been done to improve the gene transfer technology for use in patients, the therapeutic use of the technology is yet to be realized.

The following year, we began working with Dave Dawson and Dan Wilkinson in the Department of Physiology at the University of Michigan. The Dawson lab's interest was in epithelial ion transport and ours was in finding out how CFTR works. Dan Wilkinson, also a postdoctoral fellow, was using a system based on frog eggs to study how various genes affect ion transport. I used my molecular biology training to create several variations of CFTR, including a number of changes that cause CF, and Dan stuck them into his frog eggs and watched how they changed ion transport. Once again we were surprised at the results. The normal version of CFTR created a very large change in ion transport when the eggs were treated with particular drugs that signal CFTR to open, but surprising to us was that the mutant CFTR also responded. The mutants didn't do as well as the normal CFTR, but important to us was that they did respond and that they showed that increasing the amount of drugs gave greater responses. The implication was that gene therapy may not be the only route to correcting the basic defect in CF, but that there may also be drugs that can be taken advantage of to accomplish a similar task.

After Michigan

In 1992 I left the University of Michigan and joined the CF research group headed by Pamela Davis, M.D., Ph.D. in the Pediatric Pulmonary Division and CF Center at Rainbow Babies and Children's Hospital and at Case Western Reserve University (CWRU). Shortly after that, Francis Collins went to the NIH to head the Human Genome Project and the National Institute for Human Genome Research.

My research at CWRU continues to revolve around CF. Shortly after my arrival, Thomas Kelley, Ph.D., joined my lab as a postdoctoral fellow and we pursued the observations about activating mutant CFTR that were made in the frog eggs. We investigated whether human epithelial cells from a CF patient could be persuaded to allow chloride to pass by using drugs similar to those that worked in the frog eggs. We found that certain related drugs did, and others did not. We were excited by these findings, but realized that many of the important interactions that occur between different tissues in vivo could not be addressed in our experiments, a limitation of experimenting on cells grown in a culture dish. An *in vivo* model was necessary.

Beverly Koller and associates at the University of North Carolina first engineered a mouse model for CF in which they had completely inactivated the mouse Cftr gene so it would make no Cftr. This was a useful first step to having an *in vivo* model on which to investigate new therapies, but our research was aimed at activating the existing channel that didn't work very well. Not long after, Kirk Thomas and Mario Capecchi at the University of Utah engineered a mouse with the F508 mutation found in most CF patients. We used our drugs on these mice and found that we could increase chloride transport across airway epithelia from them, but not from the mice completely lacking Cftr. The mice told us that we could make the defective Cftr work to allow chloride to move, but they don't tell us if the same thing will happen in humans, or more importantly, whether increasing Cftr's activity will have an impact on a CF patient.

The same year we were carrying out the experiments with the mice, Laura Milgram, M.D., came into the lab to carry out research related to her fellowship in pediatric pulmonology. Laura tried some projects in molecular biology and electrophysiology, but ultimately chose to work with patients. Guided by Tom Kelley, she applied the electrophysiology she had learned while working on mice to humans. She was interested in seeing if the drugs that increased chloride transport in mice would, in fact, do the same in patients. Dr. Milgram is now a Pulmonary Division member, a faculty member at CWRU, and is continuing this project.

Another offshoot of the mouse experiments was the unexpected observation that numerous other biochemical pathways were altered in CF cells. Dr. Kelley found that when he took a closer look at the pathways on which our drugs were working, there were some interesting differences between the CF and non-CF mice. The drugs we found to work in the frog eggs and mouse airway inhibit a type of enzyme called cyclic nucleotide phosphodiesterase. As Tom examined the pathways through which some of these enzymes are naturally regulated, he found that another enzyme, nitric oxide synthase, is drastically reduced in CF epithelial cells. This observation led Tom to keep following the pathways back even further. He continues to find differences between the CF and non-CF cells. Tom follows these pursuits at CWRU, as he too has joined the Pediatric faculty in the Pulmonary Division.

One of the important lessons about finding other alterations in the CF cells, besides altered chloride transport, is that we had taken for granted what causes the disease symptoms. We had assumed that since the primary defect causing the disease involves defective chloride transport, all we would have to do is restore chloride transport to a more normal level. The splash of cold water on this assumption is that with all these other pathways altered, any or all of them could be the culprit(s) in causing many of the CF symptoms, and we can't just assume that fixing the chloride will cause these other pathway to be restored. As an analogy, if you get a flat tire while you're driving, and that causes you to wrap your car around a telephone pole, fixing the flat tire may not do much toward putting the car in driving condition again.

As a result, we continue to try to identify ways to restore normal chloride transport, but we are working in other areas as well. We are using mice that have naturally occurring differences in sodium and chloride transport across their airway surfaces and breeding these mice with each other as the first steps toward identifying genes regulating these processes. We have also found that different mice regulate their Cftr genes differently, and these differences are inherited. Therefore, we are also trying to find the "control switches" for Cftr itself.

We are not only concentrating on mice; we are also looking at human genes that naturally differ among individuals to determine if any of these genes might make the disease a little better or a little worse. The products of certain genes are important in preventing infection, and others are needed to fight off the infection once it is established. Many of the genes encoding these proteins have variants that cause slight changes in the protein's function, or the amount of protein. Many of these changes have no effect on the majority of people and their ability to cope with infectious agents, but we are investigating whether in the context of CF, where even subtle changes may be critical, these genes may play an important role.

All of the experiments to identify more genes have a common goal: if we can find genes that are important in the CF disease process, those genes provide us with new targets for drugs. In this way, we can increase our potential armory against CF by finding multiple ways to intervene, whether it be toward CFTR itself, or some other process that contributes to the lung or gastrointestinal disease. Whether the experiments are designed to find a new gene or to inhibit a pathway, our hope is that by understanding as much as we can about CFTR and its effect on the epithelium, we will figure out better ways to restore the CF epithelium to a state closer to non-disease and substantially reduce the severity of CF.

References

1. Kerem B, Rommens JM, Buchanan JM, Markiewicz D, Cox TK, Chakravarti A., Buchwald M., and Tsui L-C. "Identification of the cystic fibrosis gene: genetic analysis." *Science* 1989;245:1073-1080.
2. Riordan JR, Rommens JM, Kerem B, Alon N, Rozmahel R, Grzelczak Z, Zielenski J, Lok S, Plavsic N, Chou JL, et al." Identification of the cystic fibrosis gene: cloning and characterization of complementary DNA." *Science* 1989;245:1066-1073.
3. Rommens JM, Iannuzzi MC, Kerem B, Drumm ML, Melmer G, Dean M, Rozmahel R., Cole JL, Kennedy D, Hidaka N. et al. "Identification of the cystic fibrosis gene: chromosome walking and jumping." *Science* 1989;245:1059-1065.

7

Intravenous Treatment: Where We Are and How We Got There

Robert C. Stern, M.D.

By 1938, the year that the modern description of CF was published by Dorothy Andersen,[1] the theory and practice of giving fluids and drugs by intravenous (IV) infusion or injection already had a long and rich history. Techniques to achieve IV access continued to evolve, but were not of great importance to CF patients in the 1940s and 1950s, because their treatment rarely required IV drugs. The treatment of CF, at the time, was limited to oral pancreatic enzymes, oral vitamins, and oral (and later intramuscular) antibiotics, and airway clearance. There were infrequent cases of acute dehydration which required administration of IV fluids and electrolytes and the rare patients with acute staphylococcal pneumonia treated with intravenous penicillin. However, for almost 30 years after Andersen's landmark paper, the continuing improvement in IV access and the progress of mainstream CF treatment were evolving separately. These two time lines were about to collide when I graduated from medical school in 1963, and came to Babies and Children's Hospital (B & C Hosp) Cleveland to begin my pediatric internship and residency. What happened after that is the main subject of this chapter.

History of IV Therapy Before 1965

The idea that a disease of a major organ could be treated by injecting a drug into a blood vessel in the periphery of the body (i.e., far away from the diseased organ itself) was not at all obvious, and, in fact, no serious attempt to try it was made before 1628 when William Harvey published the results of his experiments[2] (Figure 7.1). These brilliant experiments showed that the blood must circulate, i.e., it must leave the heart (through the arteries), travel throughout the body, and return to the heart (through the veins). Harvey died in 1657 four years before Marcello Malphighi discovered the anatomic structures (capillaries) which actually connect the arteries to the veins.[3] By then, Christopher Wren had already given the first intravenous injection of a drug.[4,5] In 1656, Wren, in an experiment carried out at the home of the French Ambassador to England, Le Duc de Bordeaux, used a "syringe," made by attaching an animal (urinary) bladder to a quill, to inject a solution of opium into the vein of a dog. Not surprisingly, the dog became stuporous, establishing that the drug had traveled far beyond the site of injection. Less than 10 years later, Richard Lower demonstrated successful blood transfusion in an animal, and within a year Jean Denys performed a successful transfusion in a human.[6] There is some controversy here as some historians feel that Hannibal Potter may have tried blood transfusion by 1652. In any case, "various accidents, ... soon occurred ... and the Parliament of France and the Sovereign Pontiff almost simultaneously issued edicts prohibiting its repetition."

Nothing much happened for about 150 years. Then, in the early 1800s, François Magendie demonstrated the safety of blood transfusion between animals of the same species, and, shortly thereafter, Blundell treated uterine hemorrhage successfully with transfusion.[7] Other substances, including opium, were soon injected intravenously into humans, and were said to be helpful for the treatment of tetanus, a potentially fatal disease in which a bacterial toxin causes muscle spasms. Intravenous injection was adopted quickly by veterinarians, especially in Denmark, where no other mode of medicine administration was used for animals as the IV route had more success and allowed economy of consumption of drugs.

Finally, during the 1831-1832 cholera (an infectious disease which causes severe and often fatal diarrhea) epidemic in England, there were a few physicians who were ready to abandon the worthless blood-letting and induction of vomiting which dominated the recommendations for treatment (and doubtless contributed to the deaths of many patients).[8] William Brook O'Shaughnessy, a 22 year old Edinburgh physician, suggested, "to restore the blood to its natural specific gravity ... can only be effected by ... imbibition (i.e., drinking) or by injection of aqueous fluid into the veins ... in desperate cases ... the injection into the veins of tepid water holding a solution of the normal salts of the blood," i.e., infusion of an approximation of what is now called normal saline.[9] Five months later, Dr. Robert Lewins reported that Dr. Thomas Latta had administered 6 pints of a solution of electrolytes (sodium, potassium, and chloride) with excellent immediate results to a woman who was dying of cholera.[10] Other cases followed, and 8 of the first 25 moribund (i.e., close to death) patients who were treated with IV fluid recovered.

Lewins commented, "Verily, Sir, this is an astonishing method of medication, and I predict will lead to wonderful changes and improvements in the practice of medicine."[10] The Lancet, itself, in an editorial, gushed with, " ... the patient underwent a change more like the workings of a miraculous and supernatural agent, than the effect of the interposition of medical science ... the case thus alluded to is we think one of the most interesting recorded in the annals of our profession."[7] The treatment of "hypovolemic shock" with large amounts of intravenous fluid was launched.

In addition to a sounder physiologic basis (e. g., from O'Shaughnessy), Latta and his contemporaries had better equipment for intravenous injection. Wren's "Quill and Bladder" had given way to Latta's use of "Read's Patent Syringe" (a small silver tube attached to a flexible injecting tube). This syringe, said Latta, "must be quite perfect so as to avoid the risk of injecting air ... and ... the vein

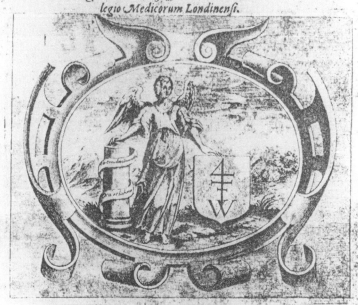

Figure 7.1. *It all started here! Title page of Harvey's classic book in which the movement of the heart and the circulation of the blood were first described. Although the title is often abbreviated to De Motu Cordis ("on the movement of the heart"), that "... sanguinis ..." in somewhat smaller print refers, of course, to the blood. Blood which is in the peripheral veins is on its way back to the heart, where it (and whatever the physician has added to it) will eventually reach all the vital organs.*

treated with much delicacy to avoid phlebitis"[11] (inflammation of a vein, due either to infection or to mechanical or chemical irritation).

By the mid 1920s, Florence Seibert had solved the long standing[12] (since 1865) mystery of occasional fevers caused by IV fluids with the demonstration that it was caused by bacterial contamination of distilled water.[13] This led to markedly increased use of IV fluids and medications, especially for very sick patients. IV fluids with added electrolytes were often used, but a rigorous scientific basis for calculating the concentration of these additives for IV fluid treatment awaited the elegant investigation of serum electrolytes and the physiology of dehydration, begun by James Gamble in the 1920s.[14] Finally, the advent of mass-produced steel, later, stainless steel, needles including specially crafted slightly blunted "scalp vein" needles with constant hub sizes allowed the use of interchangeable glass syringes, and these components and some of the plastic IV tubing could be autoclaved and reused. Nonetheless, parenteral (i.e., not by mouth) administration of fluid to very sick patients (especially premature infants) was still occasionally done by intraperitoneal injection, intraosseous (i.e., directly into the bone marrow), subcutaneous injection ("clysis", i.e., injections of fluid into the soft tissue of the inner thigh or back), a technique that was still in use when I was a medical student and then a pediatric resident in the early 1960s.

The idea of using plastic intravenous catheters instead of steel needles in peripheral veins was introduced in 1945.[15] The femoral vein was most often used, and, perhaps for that reason, catheters were not used extensively for many years. When peripheral IV access was impossible, a "cutdown" (surgically finding and cutting into a vein, usually at the ankle) was done to insert a catheter which was then secured with sutures. This solved the immediate problem but, because the distal vein was ligated (i.e., tied), resulted in the permanent loss of that vein.

This was the general situation, with regard to IV therapy, just prior to the development of the aminoglycoside antibiotics and the new penicillins in the mid-60s. These antibiotics, which were effective against *Pseudomonas aeruginosa*, were best administered by intravenous infusion. For CF patients, most of whom would eventually need frequent and often prolonged courses of treatment, venous access would suddenly become an important issue.

Treatment of Cystic Fibrosis in 1963

The early 1960s were exciting times for CF in Cleveland. Dr. LeRoy W. Matthews had instituted a "comprehensive treatment" approach in 1957. This meant addressing all manifestations of the disease, and applying every reasonable treatment modality then available. All patients, whether they had manifested any pulmonary symptoms or not, received anticipatory treatment, including airway clearance, respiratory decongestants, aggressive use of antibiotics, and mist tents. Mist tent therapy was later abandoned, partly because it was impossible to show that the mist tent was a critical part of the comprehensive care program, and partly because of theoretical arguments, based on mathematical constructs of pulmonary physiology, which predicted that mist could not possibly reach the distal airways. This issue has never been scientifically settled (i.e., by controlled trials) and the mathematical constructs proved to be flawed. However the mist tent went out of vogue and (whether it was really helpful or not) will probably never return. Pancreatic insufficiency, electrolyte deficiencies, etc. were also aggressively treated. Matthews, together with Dr. Carl Doershuk (who had joined him 4 years later), had achieved substantially better survival and quality of life than had been possible before. They were still about one year away from publishing their results.[16,17]

A beneficial role for antibiotics had been known for many years,[18] and the fact that *Staphylococcus aureus* and *Pseudomonas aeruginosa* were the main pathogens (microorganisms which can cause [human] disease) isolated from the lungs of patients with advanced CF lung disease had also been established. Although oral antibiotics, especially tetracycline[19] and chloramphenicol, were clearly effective, many patients had progression of disease despite their use, and eventually only parenteral treatment was effective. At that time, the only anti-pseudomonal drug which could be given only parenterally was colistin, and it was given only by intramuscular (not IV) injection.

Getting Hooked

I began my internship at B&C Hosp in 1963 with four 6-week rotations: pediatric outpatients; laboratory training (reading x-rays and electrocardiograms, hands-on experience with microbiological techniques, etc.); pediatric surgery; and newborns. Interns and residents were not involved with CF outpatients at that time, and so I had not even seen a Cleveland CF patient until I began my in-patient rotations in January 1964, about a month after my 25th birthday. (CF was described and I was born in the same year [1938].)

During that first half-year, I had heard some of my fellow interns and their supervisory residents groaning about "all those CF patients" on the wards. Some, but by no means all! One of my fellow interns, Christopher Heller, said about LeRoy Matthews, "what he's done for those patients ... makes me want to ... give him a great big hug." I was already more than ready to see some CF patients, but hearing that made me all the more excited. Chris had gone to medical school at Johns Hopkins, and it was good to hear that my previous experience with CF had apparently been little different from his. What interested me most about this groaning, though, was that there actually were living CF patients on both the "pre-school ward" (up to age 6) and the "older kids ward" (ages 7 and up), in addition to those who were still infants.

I was actually looking forward to seeing these "old" patients. My entire medical school education about CF had literally been two sentences in a 90-minute talk about gastrointestinal diseases in childhood (I went back and confirmed this with my lecture notes later): "Cystic fibrosis [is an] autosomal genetic disease with an incidence of about 1 in 2500 births. [It causes] pancreatic insufficiency with malabsorption [and the] patients die of lung disease before age 3." As a medical student I had seen, but not taken care of, two CF siblings who were about ages 1 and 3, and both were ghastly sick.

The first CF patient I saw in Cleveland was Barbara Oswalt, a delightful 10 year old girl who had CF-related liver disease (cirrhosis) complicated by enlargement of the spleen. She was recovering from splenectomy (surgical removal of the spleen). I was to begin my ward rotations a week later, and was "scouting out" how the in-patient service worked. Barb was doing well and was about to go home. I was impressed with her energy and healthy appearance, and, although she was atypical in that she had had a relatively unusual course and a relatively rare complication of CF, to me, she was the first in-the-flesh proof that a revolution was in progress. It's now almost 38 years later; Barb's 48 years old and now has been my patient for almost 30 years!

The first CF patient I actually was responsible for was an 11 year old girl (on the pre-school ward because the ward for older children was too full) who was admitted for increasing lung symptoms. She looked pretty good to me. She had actually walked in, although with a limp from having had polio in early childhood. She gave much of her own history, and was not desperately breathless at rest. I also liked her.

Then, as now, *Pseudomonas aeruginosa* infection was the main clinical problem. As noted earlier, there was only one reliably effective injectable antibiotic, colistin. Colistin (polymyxin E) had been discovered in 1950[19] and was thought to be more effective against *Pseudomonas aeruginosa* than its close relative polymyxin.[20] The colistin vial (and the package insert) stated explicitly, "for intramuscular injection only." My patient's hospitalization went well, as did those of the other CF patients that month (all the others were pre-schoolers). But they hated those shots. IM colistin hurt "like the very devil himself."

I liked all my CF patients. They stayed long enough for me to get to know them, and they all had amazingly good humor. Furthermore, here was a disease where something exciting was happening. The prognosis for survival (perhaps 7 years) was still not terrific, but these were not ghastly-sick 2 year olds either. They were vibrant and appealing youngsters for whom optimal medical care could make a difference. I was hooked!

Intravenous Colistin: The Time Lines for IVs, CF, and My Career Meet

My next ward assignment was older kids, which extended, at that time, to about 21 years of age. Most patients had leukemia or another malignancy, CF, hemophilia, congenital heart disease, or rheumatic fever. A few had kidney disease or diabetes. The older CF patients were sicker than the pre-schoolers had been, but most got better after several days of colistin, and the rest of their treatment program, including airway clearance, aerosols etc. It was clear, though, that the thought of all those colistin injections had caused a substantial number of them to delay their admission longer than they should have.

Toward the end of my rotation on that ward, a desperately sick, probably terminal, 7 year old girl with CF was admitted. She was started on the usual in-patient treatment program (including IM colistin). But she had one additional obstacle to treatment, she was cachectic (emaciated) and had virtually no muscle mass. The nurses had more and more difficulty even finding a site for the colistin injections.

In those days, interns were on call for at least 36 straight hours, then off for at most 12 and then back on for another 36. Our main work area was only 50 feet from her room. Every 8 hours for 36 hours (i.e. for 5 of every 6 of her colistin doses), I heard her penetrating blood-curdling scream when the nurse injected the colistin. I didn't know what I could do to help, but I did go in with the nurse on a couple of occasions to watch. The second time, I remember thinking, "there's got to be a better way," a thought I've had many times in medicine, but, in most cases, only to find that there usually isn't a better way, or at least not one that I could devise. I looked around the room, and suddenly realized that, unlike most CF patients, she was receiving continuous IV fluids to prevent dehydration, as she was too sick to drink, and was having consistent episodes of vomiting after coughing. Of course, I was the one who had ordered the IV fluids and inserted the IV, but the fact that she was getting colistin by intramuscular injection while she was receiving fluids by IV infusion somehow didn't click until I was actually in the room survey-ing the scene.

I went back to our work area and announced to the senior resident (my supervisor) that I was going to give the next dose of colistin intravenously. I had already had a long-standing fascination with the wonderful potential of the IV infusion. Almost anything (I decided in medical school) could be given through it, unless the medication had to "work" in the muscle (e. g., vaccines, where the intent is for the drug to stay at the injection site, and the body to send immune cells into the muscle). I almost always avoided intramuscular injections for children if there was any way around it.

This is my recollection of the ensuing conversation (the italicized portions are verbatim or close to it—the rest reflects actual ideas but may not have been the exact words):

RCS: There's just no place to give those shots any more. She's misera-ble. *This is ridiculous. I'm going to give the next dose IV.*

Sr. Res: That drug can only be given IM.

RCS: How do you know? Look, the drug acts in the lung ... *it must get to the lung somehow from that muscle. I suspect it gets there in the blood.* Every 8 hours we give a dose of colistin; *presumably, every 8 hours one dose gradually enters the blood from the muscle and some of it goes to the lung. I'm going to infuse the dose over 8 hours ... how will her body be able to tell if it's entering the blood from the muscle or from* [an infu-sion into] *her vein?*

Sr. Res: I suppose that's OK if it's over 8 hours.

A few hours later, the first regular (non-research) dose of intravenous colistin ever given in Cleveland (and perhaps in the world) was added to the patient's next 8-hour supply of IV fluid. By 8 hours later, a new age had dawned, at least in Cleveland. After the initial success, we gradually sped up the infusion rate. The only comment that anyone (family or nurses) ever said to me was, "... why didn't you/anyone do that before?!" IM colistin continued to be used, at least for patients who did not need IV fluids, for a while, but, when carbenicillin entered medical practice, it became obvious that the IV route was here to stay. As far as colistin was concerned, even the package insert and the drug label eventually was changed to say that colistin could be given by IM injection or IV infusion.

New Problems-New Solutions: The One-Man "IV Team"

Intravenous antibiotics were not used much for CF between 1965 when I left Cleveland to complete my pediatric residency and have my last fling at New York City and 1968 when I returned after two years in the United States Air Force. Much had happened in medicine during the two years I had been at Bunker Hill Air Force Base in Indiana (e.g., furosemide [Lasix^R] had entered medical practice and techniques for measurement of blood gases had become practical for wide-spread use).

The main change in CF treatment, one which affected virtually every hospitalized patient, was the widespread use of gentamicin, which preceded tobramycin, and the early use of carbenicillin, as an experimental drug, but also as an illegal import from Britain and other countries. Ticarcillin and then piperacillin followed soon thereafter. Whereas colistin doses (at most 1 ml or 75 mg could be, and usually still were, given by IM injection at 8-hour intervals, gentamicin and tobramycin doses (often as much as 150 mg or slightly under 2 ml every 8 hours) were theoretically possible, but not feasible because of the pain of the injection and the inadequate muscle mass. And the advent of the new and very potent carbenicillin, with doses frequently as high as 5000 mg every four hours, made IM treatment completely impossible.

So, instead of blood-curdling screams at the 8-hour colistin intervals, I returned to two new problems: 1) CF physicians had long worried about giving IV antibiotics, because the patient had to be "hooked up" to "keep open" fluids 24 hours a day in order to get their antibiotic doses every 8 hours, and the doctors worried that restriction of activity would have a detrimental effect on the lungs. The medical establishment thought the patients would stay in bed all day if they were receiving continuous IV fluid; and 2) many patients were in constant panic, worrying about how long their IV lines were likely to last and, equally important, who was going to replace them.

The second problem was fairly easy to solve. After seeing one 17-year old in tears ("The most devastating flood known to man is a woman's tears." - Bert

Murray) after having had 6 unsuccessful IV attempts, I started inserting all the difficult IVs for all the CF patients. It wasn't long before every IV was deemed "difficult" by the patients (and the nurses) and, for all practical purposes, I became the CF IV team. I have been doing IVs ever since, and have actually not found it to be much of an added burden. It also resulted in my maintaining my interest in the general area of IV access.

New Problems-New Solutions: The Heparin Lock

I continued to think about the first problem, the nuisance of "keep open fluids," and began experimenting with ways to disconnect patients between doses. The first idea that actually worked well enough to call it a "solution" was to connect, to the IV access needle, a 3-way stopcock into which a syringe of heparinized saline (100 units/ml) was inserted. At dose times, the IV was connected to the remaining stopcock terminal, and the dose was infused; at the conclusion of the dose, the IV was disconnected and a plug placed over the terminal; heparinized saline was then injected from the other terminal and the stopcock controller then rotated to the plugged terminal. The equipment was a little heavy and cumbersome, but was a definite improvement over staying in bed all day and watching non-therapeutic fluids drip into the vein. Patients were up, out of bed, and active again.

Shortly thereafter, I realized that the now familiar "heparin lock," which was already being used to give repeated doses of heparin to adults, could be used instead of my makeshift 3-way stopcock contraption. Continuous "keep open" IV fluids disappeared from Babies and Childrens Hospital. Ironically, it took well over a decade before the idea of using the heparin lock for medications other than heparin had made it back to the adult area of the hospital where I had first seen it, even though all the component hospitals of University Hospitals of Cleveland were physically connected by tunnels and bridges. Although we published our initial experience with the heparin lock for the antibiotic therapy of CF patients fairly soon after we started to use it,[21] again it took quite some time before it achieved widespread use at other CF Centers.

There have been trivial changes in our use of the heparin lock since that time. The main one was the reduction in the concentration of heparin to the totally innocuous 10 units/ml from the probably equally innocuous, but more expensive, 100 units/ml. Not all these innovations have been good. Some nursing protocols recommend using only normal saline for between-dose maintenance. Although this usually is sufficient, it occasionally allows clot formation in the IV line, which often necessitates changing the IV line, but also can be a health threat if it results, as I think it does, in an increased risk of clot formation in the vein itself. However, saline is cheaper than heparinized saline.

The heparin lock is now used, in both CF and non-CF patients, for many other purposes, including repeated blood sampling (e. g., "tolerance tests"), maintenance of IV access in a patient who is doing well, but is at risk for an unexpected, but potentially catastrophic, complication; intermittent blood sampling; or to allow

IV insertion by one physician/technician (e. g., pediatrician/internist) for use later by another physician/ technician (e. g., anesthesiologist, radiologist), etc.

Like most tertiary pediatric services, Rainbow Babies and Childrens Hospital often had many hospitalized CF patients on the same ward. The need for prolonged IV antibiotic courses, together with the development of the heparin lock, which allowed the patients to be much more mobile, resulted in a groups of patients who were comparing notes on IV treatment, and gradually becoming more bold in taking over some of the nursing procedures themselves. They "hooked themselves up," disconnected IVs after medications, observed IV insertions, offered ideas as to improvements in medications times, wrapped their own, or a friend's, IV site to take showers, etc. Some even attempted to insert their own IV needles. These activities would have been much less likely to occur on adult services where patients generally stayed in their own rooms, and relied on medical professionals to manipulate the IV equipment. In retrospect, these CF patients were laying the groundwork for home IV treatment.

If It Ain't Broke, Don't Fix It

Intramuscular antibiotic injections for the treatment of CF pulmonary exacerbations were pretty much gone for good by 1969. Difficult venous access, and the anxiety and uncertainty of IV insertion, replaced inadequate muscle mass and the pain of IM injections as minute-to-minute and admission-to-admission concerns of patients/families and physicians. A steady stream of journal articles had warned about infection and other problems associated with long-duration IV needles[22] and catheters.[23] However, like almost all pediatricians, I would never remove an IV line unless: 1) the insertion site was clearly infected (local inflammation and pus), but infection of IV sites was virtually unknown in CF patients, although it was a theoretical possibility; 2) the infusion was too painful (a decision made exclusively by the patient); 3) there was extravasation (leakage) of fluid into the subcutaneous tissue outside the vein (infiltration); 4) fluid was leaking at the insertion site; or, occasionally: 5) the patient requested its removal because the present IV would prevent his/her participation in a ward activity, or a leave-of-absence (LOA). Although there were a few articles[24]/letters[25] which showed no correlation with infection and duration of IV use, the pediatricians were relying mainly on their own experience and "common knowledge" that IV duration did not substantially increase risk. Duration of IV needle/catheter was probably one risk factor; duration of continuous use of the same IV infusion tubing and other equipment was another equally or more important risk factor.

In any case, however, by the early 1970s, a large series of papers (added to and summarized by Maki et al[26]) about the risk of potentially dangerous infections, resulting from long-duration IV catheters in adults, led some Departments and even entire hospitals to establish rigid criteria for routine replacement of "old" IVs. These "guidelines" generally forced removal of even non-problematic IV lines that were older than 48–72 hours. I was not convinced that the results of these studies should be applied to CF patients. Needless to say, the patients were not enthusiastic about removing perfectly functioning IVs just because they were "old" either!

Many of these studies, which included all adults regardless of diagnosis, did indeed suggest a rising incidence of infection with time. In fact, some patients such as those with hematologic malignancies (e. g., leukemia) were even more likely to develop infectious complications of IV needles and catheters. Ironically, the observation that this group did worse actually should have suggested that the guidelines were not universally necessary, and that there might be a way to exclude CF patients from their requirements. What was missed in the analysis of previous studies, in my view, was the obvious, but unstated and perhaps unnoticed conclusion: if some patient groups did unusually poorly with regard to long-duration IVs, there must be other groups who did unusually well with long-duration IVs to account for the "average results" from previously published studies of unselected patients. CF patients, I felt, constituted one such group.

By that time, I had already inserted and nursed along hundreds and perhaps thousands of IV lines. There had not been a single case of serious infection either at the IV insertion site itself or elsewhere in the body that was related to IV treatment. In the late 1970s, a medical student, Sally L. Hodder, and I did a prospective study of long-duration IV lines in CF patients.[27] These involved exclusively stainless steel "butterfly" needles (plastic catheters were not yet in wide use). The study included patients from 5 to 35 years of age. The results were unequivocal. Clinically important infections of IV catheters did not occur during the study, and were obviously (based on years of previous experience) very rare, in CF patients. Bacteriologic results were not related to duration or to local inflammation. Another medical student, Linda K. Rossi, and I did a similar study with plastic catheters several years later; it yielded identical results but was never published.

Although case reports of uncomplicated use of very long duration plastic IV lines had appeared, most previous studies of the safety/risk of IV lines involved durations measured in hours and days; our IV durations were measured in days and weeks. The longest duration IV (remember these were stainless steel needles, not plastic) was in place for 46 days. 39 of a total of 246 IVs in the study were in place for 11 days or longer. I developed names for these long duration IVs: 8 days = "masterpiece"; 16 days = "antique"; 24 days = "ancient relic"; 32 days = "fossil"; greater than 40 days = "big-bang remnant." The patients demanded that these labels be placed on their IVs as they reached the appropriate milestones. Some patients actually wanted to extend their hospital stays to keep their IVs in longer and get more prestigious labels, and, perhaps, set a new record.

The results supplied the "ammunition" we needed to spare our CF patients from routine time-determined IV removals, and would later make home IV treatment for CF considerably easier. And not a minute too soon, because failure to change IV sites every 48 hours was already being condemned as a "violation of good nursing procedure" in pediatric journal editorials.[28] For CF patients, youth and general immunologic competence were probably important reasons for their excellent tolerance of IV lines. In addition, however, their IV infusion equipment was changed at frequent intervals, thus further reducing the risk of infection.

The CF Patient Who Has Very Difficult or No Venous Access

If the patient had any hint of a "do-able" vein, I was almost always able to get an IV into it, but, by the end of the 1970s, there were an increasing number of patients for whom peripheral IV access was simply impossible. Foot veins were rarely acceptable (too much pain to insert them; risk of thrombosis; short duration of use until venitis occurred). "Cutdowns," with permanent loss of a major vein, seemed a bit drastic, and had not been done for years. Intraosseous infusions, a standard emergency measure for critically ill infants since 1934,[29] and widely advocated in the United States after 1940,[30] was too drastic, impractical for repeated use, and not applicable much beyond infancy.

We turned to the surgeons for help. For patients who would need prolonged IV treatment, a Broviac line was usually placed. For other patients, they recommended a percutaneously (i.e., inserted through the skin) central catheter (PICC). A central catheter is one in which a long plastic tube is inserted so that its tip, where the medicine emerged and entered the blood stream, was in one of the large veins in the chest close to or at the entrance to the heart. The bigger the vein, the more volume of blood was going through it. A large volume of blood dilutes the medicine so quickly that it cannot injure the walls of the vein and cause venitis and/or penetration of the vein wall with infiltration and/or bleeding. These lines usually entered the skin just under the clavicle (i.e., collarbone) and the catheter itself was threaded through the subclavian vein so that it reached near to or barely inside the heart. This procedure was not new to medical practice, and in most non-CF patients usually could be done without complication. Unfortunately, CF patients who had reached this stage of their disease had very overinflated lungs which "wrapped around" the clavicle, so that attempted insertion of the IV "introducer" needle often resulted in pneumothorax. With a pneumothorax, air leaks out of the lung (due to disease or injury) and into the chest where it can restrict the expansion of the lung or even result in its total collapse.

After two of our first three percutaneous subclavian line placements had been complicated by pneumothorax, I set out to find a safer solution. Armed with a sample of every piece of IV equipment used in the hospital, and my medical school anatomy book, I retreated to my office and began assessing "what fits into what" and where a line could be safely placed. The goal was to avoid the risk of pneumothorax, by not attempting to enter the vein in the chest, and still maintain maximum freedom of movement (i.e., avoid entering the vein in the neck) or interfering with movement of a joint (i.e., the elbow, shoulder, or wrist). The basilic vein, which runs along the inner part of the upper arm between the biceps and triceps muscles, looked like the straightest route to the heart from the arm, although the cephalic vein, which runs on top of the biceps and is particularly large in weight lifters, was theoretically usable but it was somewhat smaller and its route was more circuitous.

The basilic vein in most normal people is buried deep in the crease between the muscles of the upper arm, and is overlain with fat so it is difficult to see or feel. Fortunately, in CF patients, at this stage of the illness, there is usually not much fat and this vein is often easily felt, and occasionally it can be seen through the skin as a cylindrical bulge in the inner upper arm if a tourniquet is applied. I developed a method of percutaneous line insertion which allows the introducer (the initial short, but large, plastic catheter) to remain in place even after the longer "central catheter" is threaded through it. This permits greater flexibility in "repairing" lines which have become non-functional for one reason or another. Furthermore, this method did not require sutures (stitches), which I felt made the skin unstable and subject to yeast and other infections. Within a year or so of starting to use this technique, it was clear that patients much preferred these new lines (over those inserted by the surgeons), and they were cheaper to insert and were virtually completely safe. I inserted my first central catheter in about 1980. It was an instant success, and these lines essentially solved the IV access problem almost completely for about 10 years. I have now inserted about 2000 of these lines without a single major complication, i.e., no pneumothoraces, no line infections, no disseminated infections, no line breakage, and no clot formation in the large veins of the chest. The technique is described in detail elsewhere[31] or can be requested from the author.

Of course, I was not the only physician who thought of using percutaneously inserted central catheters (including those which are not inserted directly into a chest vein). In most other methods, however, including one reported in 1985 for CF patients,[32] the "introducer" was inserted into an antecubital vein (i.e., "the elbow vein" which is often used for blood sampling). Antecubital central catheters are now widely used in CF, but are rarely inserted by CF physicians. In general, other methods are much more expensive than mine. These entail a trip to either the radiology department or the operating room, and at least 3 people (operator, assistant, nurse, and if it is done in the operating room, an anesthetist). Unfortunately, I have not been very effective in my attempt to export my method, which under ideal circumstances takes me (with no assistant) about 10 minutes in the patient's room, although some other Centers are beginning to use it.

Even under relatively ideal circumstances, PICC placement eventually becomes impossible due to scarring of peripheral vein at the entry point or narrowing of vein between the insertion site and the central veins, which blocks the threading of the central catheter. At that point, with continuing and frequent need for courses of IV antibiotics, a more definitive method is needed.

Several semi-permanent implantable devices have been used, including those where the entry point for treatment is in the arm (e. g., Pasport[R]), or the chest (Mediport[R], Infusaport[R]). They can also be placed below the skin of the abdomen with the catheter itself threaded up the femoral (leg) vein through the inferior vena cava to the right atrium of the heart. These devices were originally developed for the delivery of cancer chemotherapy, but have been applied to many other diseases. There has been substantial variability in the success of these methods for CF and there are occasional serious complications (such as thrombosis of the central veins).[33] However, they work well for most CF patients,[34] although they are often not happy with them for cosmetic reasons. Central catheters were another major advance in IV treatment.

On The Way to Home IV Treatment

"Listen to the patient," said one of my medical school teachers; "Listen to the patient - he's trying to tell you what's wrong." This is valuable advice for any young physician who is worried about making the correct diagnosis. But my CF patients have helped me expand on it.

Patricia (Patty) Gelin lived on Yorkshire Road in Cleveland Heights, just 5–10 minutes from Babies and Childrens Hospital. I already knew what was wrong with her, CF, but, for many years, she "told me" what was right. Like many young CF patients, she never unnecessarily surrendered any aspect of life to disease. She was a successful athlete and a social star throughout her school years. All her friends and her whole school knew about CF. I called her, "Patricia the First of Yorkshire," otherwise known as "Patty the Great."

Most patients try to tell the doctor what's wrong with them. The Great Patricia and many other patients showed me what was right. Basically, it was this: Don't give an inch to disease that you don't know for sure that you have to give! Patty was one of many trailblazers. There are, of course, thousands of Pattys now. But in the late 1960s and 70s, many Centers and physicians were still officially recommending too many unnecessary restrictions on CF patients.

In the early 1970s, Patty was in the hospital for IV antibiotics. One day, she casually asked me if it would be OK for her to wrap her heparin lock in an ace bandage, so she could "leave the hospital for a few hours to work at the Pronto Room as a waitress that afternoon. It took me less than a second to realize that a new age had dawned. Off she went to the Pronto Room, and off I went an hour later with my camera (see Figure 7.2). The reason I include this picture (which is technically not very good and has not stood the test of time very well) is not to show that it is possible to work while under treatment with IV antibiotics for CF lung disease. It is to show that, in 1973, I thought that the idea, although it was new, was so obviously important, that it was worth my leaving the hospital to record it on film. Patty's original idea was to use the ace bandage to avoid "grossing out" her customers, but, of course, by the time I arrived with my camera, she had the ace bandage off and was discussing her IV with one of her afternoon diners. She put the bandage back on only at my request so I could take the picture.

Patty was the first Cleveland CF patient to work or pursue any normal out-of-hospital activity, with the physician's approval, while receiving IV antibiotics (and, I suspect) one of the first anywhere. She had simply extended, to the "real

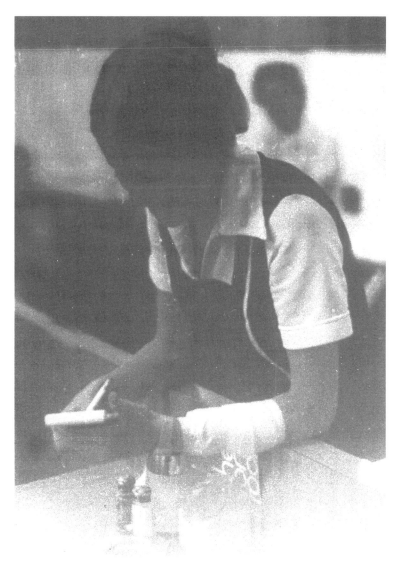

Figure 7.2. *A 15 year old waitress, Patricia Gelin, at work while on leave of absence (LOA) from Babies and Children's Hospital in Cleveland, Ohio. The patient's heparin lock is under the ace bandage. She was (in this picture from about 1973) an early, if not the first, "pioneer" who self-administered IV medications while continuing to work and pursue other normal out-of-hospital activities, thus helping to pave the way for the home therapy movement of the 1980s and 1990s. Courtesy of Dr. Robert Stern.*

world," the experience that she and many CF patients had acquired in the hospital over the preceding few years (See Demystification of Medical Procedures above). In retrospect, Patty Gelin and her heparin lock, and her fellow patient pioneers in Cleveland and at other Centers,[35] were sowing the seeds of CF home-care. And, probably, accelerating the use of home IV antibiotics throughout all of pediatrics and medicine.

Controversies

Long Range Vein Plans: Since venous access is clearly critically important to CF patients, it would seem logical to make every attempt to preserve them. However, in recent years, physicians have increasingly chosen, or have been forced by economic considerations, to rely on ancillary medical personnel (nurses, technicians, etc) for IV placement and "vein planning." I have failed miserably in my attempt to convince young doctors that planning how each patient's veins are used (and even, for some patients, taking personal responsibility for the insertion and removal of IV lines) is sufficiently important in serious chronic illness to become the job of the physician. "IV nurses" and many house officers/residents are interested mainly, and often only, in inserting an IV that will function for the remainder of their work day or for residents, their tour of duty. Issues such as how much the IV restricts the patient's movements, whether it is likely to last more than a few hours, and whether it is desirable to "use up" that particular vein are rarely considered.

Similarly, I have failed in my attempt to prevent the use of antecubital (elbow) veins for routine (non-emergency) IV drug administration. These veins will be needed by the patient for a lifetime of blood sampling, and may be needed for emergency access during a true emergency. Similarly, in my view, veins in the upper arm should be "saved" for potential central line insertion, a strategy rarely followed, and, often, intentionally violated (e. g., with "mid-line" catheters which extend into and often sclerose (scar) the veins in the mid-upper arm.

Rational Use of Local Anesthesia: Subcutaneously injected local anesthetic is minimally painful when carefully done, is extremely effective (prevents pain and generally increases success rate), and, mainly, almost guarantees the patient that all IV attempts, whether successful or not, will cause about the same amount of discomfort. This eliminates the dread of the treatment room, and "IV phobia" which is not unusual in CF patients.

I also have failed, thus far, in my attempt to ban EMLA cream (a mixture of local anesthetics) and similar products from use before routine IV insertion in CF patients. I believe it sends the wrong message, that insertion of an IV, even with injected local anesthesia, is so painful that no one can stand it. Since EMLA takes at least an hour to numb the skin area, this leads to hysteria when the patient has to have an IV inserted quickly. In addition, EMLA causes reduction in local blood flow, making the veins harder to find.

I believe, as discussed previously, that it is helpful to demystify the treatment room. I invite the patient to bring other patients or their friends or family members with them for IV insertion. Cheerleaders and friendly support always help.

What's Next In IV Treatment?

There is always room for improvement. IV treatment is not perfect. IV access continues to be a challenge for many patients and lack of IV access can be a significant obstacle to care. All of us hope that future surveys of IV treatment in CF will include some or all of the following "wish-list" items:

1. A "perfect" IV catheter. Such a catheter: 1) would not stimulate local inflammation and scarring which eventually causes local pain, and, more important, narrowing or even loss of the access vein; and 2) would not stimulate thrombosis (clot formation) or other hematologic toxicity/injury. Catheters are better in this regard than they used to be, but even the best catheters are still far from perfect.

2. Truly painless insertion. The "perfect" local anesthetic has not been developed. It would provide instant anesthesia of the skin and underlying soft tissue, including the vein itself, it would not cause local vasoconstriction (spasm in a blood vessel) which would make IV insertion technically difficult, and it would be non-toxic. Progress is being made, but we're not there yet.

3. Permanent "invisible" micro-access device. An implantable device which would provide easy access when it is needed, would not "wear out," and would not be visible at all when not in use.

4. Tissue-specific or organ-specific drug delivery. A system which would allow specific targeting of drugs to the organ which needs them. In CF, for example, this would mean developing drugs which can be injected intravenously and thus circulate in the blood, but then only leave the blood to enter the lungs and no other organ. There is some research in this area, but no clinically useful results yet.

Summary

Parenteral treatment of CF related lung infection has come a long way since the terrible intramuscular colistin injections of the 1950s and 1960s. The introduction of more potent anti-pseudomonal antibiotics, which could be given in very large dose by intravenous infusions, resulted in more effective, less painful, and more convenient treatment of pulmonary exacerbations. CF patients of the last 30 years were fortunate in that 150 years of IV treatment preceded their need for prolonged venous access. On the other hand, however, CF patients and their physicians have helped improve the technique of IV treatment, which has improved IV treatment throughout medicine. Furthermore, the experience of CF patients in the early 1970s helped make home treatment possible for them and for patients with other conditions which previously had required very prolonged and expensive hospitalizations.

References:

1. Andersen DH. "Cystic fibrosis of the pancreas and its relation to celiac disease: A clinical and pathologic study." *Am J Dis Child* 1938;56:344-399.
2. Harvei G. *Exercitatio anatomica de motv cordis et sangvinis in animalibvs.* Francofvrti: Sumptibus Gvilielmi Fitzeri, 1628.
3. Malpighi M. "De pvlmonibvs observationes anatomicæ." *Bononiæ: Typis Io.* Baptistæ Ferronij, 1661 (Original manuscript submitted as a letter from Marcello Malpighi to Giovanni Alfonso Borelli).
4. Wren C. [letter to Petty 1656], in *Parentalia,* ed. C. Wren, London, 1750 p 228.
5. Keys TE." Historical Vignettes. Sir Christopher Wren." *Anesthesia & Analgesia* 1974; 53:853.
6. Webster C. "The origins of blood transfusion: a reassessment." *Medical History* 1971;15:387-392.
7. Editorial 2 June 1832, *Lancet* 1832;I:284-286.
8. Cosnett JE. "The origins of intravenous fluid therapy." *Lancet* 1989;1:768-771.
9. O'Shaughnessy WB. Letter to *Lancet.* 1831;II:30 Dec.
10. Lewins R. "Injection of saline solutions in extraordinary quantities into the veins in cases of malignant cholera." Letter to *Lancet* 1832;2:243-244.
11. Latta T. "Aqueous injections into the veins for the treatment of malignant cholera." (Letter 23 May 1832) *Lancet* 1832;I:274-276.
12. Holt EC, Penfold WJ. "The dangers of saline injections." *Lancet* 1911;II:1589-1591.
13. Seibert FB." Fever producing substances found in some distilled waters." *Am J Physiol* 1923;67:90-104.
14. Gamble JL. "Dehydration." *New Engl J Med* 1929;201:909-917.
15. Meyers L. "Intravenous catheterization." *Am J Nurs* 45:930-931, 1945.
16. Matthews LW, Doershuk CF, Wise M, Eddy G, Nudelman H, Spector S. "A therapeutic regimen for patients with cystic fibrosis." *J Pediatrics* 1964;65:558-575.
17. Doershuk CF, Matthews LW, Tucker AS, Nudelman H, Eddy G, Wise M. "A 5-year clinical evaluation of a therapeutic program for patients with cystic fibrosis." *J Pediatrics* 1964;65:677-693.
18. Shwachman H, Crocker AC, Foley GE, Patterson PR. "Aureomycin therapy in the pulmonary involvement of pancreatic fibrosis (mucoviscidosis)." *New Engl J Med* 1949;241:185-192.
19. Koyama Y, Kurosawa A, Tsuchiya A, Takakuta K. "A new antibiotic, colistin, produced by spore-forming soil bacteria." *J Antibiot* Tokyo 1950;3:457.
20. Nord NM, Hoeprich PD." Polymyxin B and colistin. A critical comparison." *New Engl J Med* 1964;270:1030-1035.

21. Stern RC, Doershuk CF, Matthews LW. "Use of a heparin lock to administer intermittent intravenous drugs." *Clin Ped* 1972;11:521-523.
22. Lowenbraun S, Young V, Kenton D, Serpick AA. "Infection from intravenous "scalp-vein" needles in a susceptible population." *JAMA* 1970;212:451-453.
23. Druskin MS, Siegel PD. "Bacterial contamination of indwelling intravenous polyethylene catheters." *JAMA* 1963;185:966-968.
24. Crossley K, Matsen JM. "The scalp-vein needle: a prospective study of complications." *JAMA* 1972;220:985-987.
25. Lloyd-Still JD, Peter G, Lovejoy FH. "Infected "scalp vein" needles (Letter)." *JAMA* 1970;213:1496-1497.
26. Maki DG, Goldman DA, Rhame FS. "Infection control in intravenous therapy." *Annals Internal Medicine* 1973;79:867-887.
27. Hodder SL, Stern RC. "Safety of long duration heparin-lock needles for administration of antibiotics to cystic fibrosis patients." *J Pediatrics* 1981;99:312-314.
28. Nelson JD. "Oral antibiotic therapy for serious infections in hospitalized patients." *J Pediatrics* 1978;92:175-176.
29. Josefson A. "A new method of treatment: intraosseous injections." *Acta Med Scand* 1934;81:550-564.
30. Tocantins LM, O'Neil JF. "Infusion of blood and other fluids into circulation via the bone marrow." *Proc Soc Exp Biol Med* 1940;45:782-783.
31. Stern RC. "Treatment of Pulmonary Disease in Orenstein DM and RC Stern (Editors): The Hospitalized Cystic Fibrosis Patient" *Lung Biology in Health and Disease Series.* Marcel Dekker 1997.
32. Canni RL, Shutack JG, Schuler PM, Christie D, Holsclaw DS. "Peripherally inserted central venous catheters for treatment of cystic fibrosis." *Pediatric Pulmonology* 1985;1:328-332.
33. Sola JE, Stone MM, Wise B, Colombani PM. "Atypical thrombotic and septic complications of totally implantable venous access devices in patients with cystic fibrosis." *Pediatric Pulmonology* 1992;4:239-242.
34. Morris JB, Occhionero ME, Gauderer MWL, Stern RC, Doershuk CF. "Totally implantable vascular access devices in cystic fibrosis: A four year experience with fifty eight patients. "*J Pediatrics* 1990;117:82-85.
35. Rucker RW, Harrison GM. "Outpatient intravenous medications in the management of cystic fibrosis." *Pediatrics* 1974;54:358-360.

8

Pediatric Flexible Bronchoscopy: The Inside Story

Robert E. Wood, M.D., Ph.D.

Early in my career, had anyone suggested that cystic fibrosis (CF) would become an important part of my life, I would have thought them crazy. When I decided to become a physician during my last year in high school, I had absolutely no interest in clinical medicine and actually felt frightened of the idea of having to deal with patients. Rather, I wanted to do research – specifically research with clinical implications. I knew that I should go to medical school in order to have a proper perspective from which to do clinically relevant research, but I *really* wanted to stay in the laboratory. I decided to enroll in both a Ph.D. *and* an M.D. training program. I knew that it would also be important to have several years of post-graduate clinical training (to get my "union card", so to speak), and also that it would be important to plan to spend further time at the National Institutes of Health (NIH). One Saturday afternoon in January 1959, I outlined the next 15 years of my life. With that roadmap in hand, it was clear what was required to reach my goals.

After graduating from Stetson University in Florida with a major in chemistry, I went to Vanderbilt University in Tennessee and pursued a dual degree program, receiving my Ph.D. in physiology before completing my M.D. degree in 1970. Since I continued to be uncomfortable with patient contacts and still could not picture myself as anything other than a laboratory person, imagine my surprise when I awoke one morning to realize that I wanted to become a pediatrician. Even then, however, my thinking was that I would do only enough clinical training to define my research goals.

My graduate work related to the regulation of membrane transport in bird red blood cells. I was fascinated by the idea of metabolic diseases, and avidly studied arcane metabolic pathways and enzyme kinetics. Upon completion of my Ph.D., I returned for the last three years of medical school. As graduation neared, I needed to make definitive plans for the next several years and went to the library in search of a researchable metabolic disease. I found CF in Stanbury's *Textbook of Metabolic Diseases*, and was immediately intrigued but I had seen only two CF patients up to that time.

Now that I had an interest in CF, I was pleased to learn, upon application to the NIH, that one of the potential openings was in the CF laboratory of Dr. Paul A. di Sant'Agnese. Paul had been responsible for the discovery of the sweat electrolyte defect in CF, and was an amazing man. I applied to his program and crossed my fingers. Shortly after beginning my internship, I was accepted in Paul's program, to begin two years later. I was delighted.

I went to Duke University Medical Center for my pediatric internship and residency. Duke had a very large CF clinic, led by Dr. Alexander Spock (a cousin of the more famous Dr. Benjamin Spock). Al was a very dynamic man, who paid great attention to detail in caring for his patients. During my two years at Duke, I took a particular interest in CF patients, sometimes having as many as 10 CF patients under my direct care. In those days, relatively few CF patients survived adolescence, and I had many sad experiences with death of adolescent and pre-adolescent CF patients. I was very impressed, however, with their attitude towards life and their knowledge of their own disease and its care.

In the early 1970s, the care of CF patients was relatively unsophisticated. Patients were seen in the clinic at intervals of several months, were admitted to the hospital only when they developed serious pulmonary disease, and were generally expected to die early. Dr. Spock took a particularly aggressive stance with his patients near the end of their life, and I was impressed to see him place trans-tracheal catheters for direct instillation of antibiotics, saline, and mucolytic agents (Mucomyst^R). I spent many hours performing transnasal deep tracheal suctioning with these patients. Unfortunately, however, even though we were able to remove seemingly large quantities of secretions, we saw little beneficial effect. Dr. Spock had also been involved with very large volume lung lavage in CF patients (washing one lung at a time with many liters of saline). This procedure was very difficult, usually performed in a hyperbaric oxygen chamber, and was also of somewhat uncertain clinical benefit. I began to wonder if there might be a better way to clear the lungs of CF patients, and whether we should begin this procedure earlier in the disease.

In 1972, I completed my two years at Duke and went to the NIH Clinical Center in Bethesda, Maryland as a trainee in Paul di Sant'Agnese's clinical associate Program. What a difference from Duke! While I had seen only three or four adult CF patients during my residency training, at the NIH there were more than 100 adult or teen-aged CF patients. The very first week I was there, a 24 year old young woman with CF died. I was about to learn a new face of CF. I was also about to learn a lot more about myself. With Paul's guidance, I discovered that I was comfortable with being a clinician after all and that my primary career focus would combine clinical medicine and research.

Shortly after arriving at the NIH, I admitted a 45 year old man with CF for treatment of atelectasis of the left upper lobe. After working for two weeks with vigorous chest physical therapy, antibiotics, etc., I had been unable to achieve any improvement. I consulted my colleagues in adult pulmonology. "Simple," they said, "we'll bronchoscope him." "Oh, no, you don't," I cried, thinking of rigid bronchoscopy and the anesthesia required. "No, no. You don't understand. Now we have this new *flexible* bronchoscope. Come and watch." I was amazed to see my patient walk into the procedure room, have his nose and throat sprayed with lidocaine to numb the very sensitive airways, and a flexible bronchoscope passed through his nose and into his lung. After the procedure, the patient got up, said, "Thank you," and walked back to his room. "Wow," I thought. "What a research tool!"

Several weeks later, I overheard a conversation between two radiologists in the elevator. They had purchased a flexible bronchoscope (these instruments had first become available in 1971, and were still relatively unknown) to use for bronchogram studies (instilling contrast material into selected bronchi for radiologic diagnosis). They had found it too complicated, and were not going to use the instrument any more. I immediately got off the elevator and went to the office of Dr. Doppman, Chairman of the Department of Radiology. After a brief conversation, I found myself the proud owner of a flexible bronchoscope. Little did I suspect what would happen to me as a result of this acquisition.

I began to learn to use the flexible bronchoscope under the guidance of my adult pulmonary colleague. After several weeks, it was a surprise to learn that he was leaving the NIH, and that there would be no one, other than myself, with any experience with a flexible bronchoscope. For the next year and a half, I did most of the bronchoscopies at the NIH Clinical Center and on patients from the Cancer Institute and other clinical programs. While I was able to perform bronchoscopy on a 10 year old patient, my experience was essentially limited to adults. Flexible bronchoscopes in those days were too large (about 6 mm in diameter) for use in most pediatric patients.

My initial interest in the flexible bronchoscope had begun as a research tool. I was impressed with the ease and apparent safety with which one could access the bronchi, and a number of research applications were evident. But at the same time, several papers had been published reporting the use of rigid bronchoscopy with instillation of fluids and vigorous suctioning for treatment of lung disease in patients with CF. As a result, I began to experiment with bronchial lavage and suctioning to see whether this might help CF patients. While this made good sense on theoretical grounds, it did not prove to be useful clinically. Some patients requested repeated procedures, but neither I nor anyone else could document objective evidence of any lasting benefit.

Shortly after I began to use the bronchoscope, I was fascinated by a research conference presented at the NIH by Dr. Marvin Sackner. He and his colleagues, including Dr. Adam Wanner, had developed a technique to measure the rate of mucociliary transport in the trachea and central bronchi by observing the movement of uniformly sized teflon disks which were deposited onto the tracheal wall through a flexible bronchoscope. With Adam's help, I arranged for a study in CF patients at the NIH. We were able to show that the rate of mucociliary transport in CF patients was only about 10–15% of the rate seen in control subjects. The transport rate could be doubled when the drug, terbutaline, was administered. This was exciting and I had found the focus for my research after I left the NIH.

This was the focus I had been searching for. Pediatric pulmonology was not a recognized subspecialty at that time (1973–4), and there were few training programs available. I knew of the Cleveland CF program through Dr. Thomas

Boat, a previous di Sant'Agnese clinical associate trainee at the NIH and now a young faculty member at Rainbow Babies & Children's Hospital (RB&C Hospital). When I arranged for an interview for a fellowship position, Tom asked me to bring the bronchoscope to demonstrate its use on a patient at the time of my interview. He had a 14 year old CF patient with a mucoid impaction of the bronchi and thought bronchoscopy might provide useful information and perhaps a treatment intervention for the patient. We set up to do the procedure and the room was filled with observers. I was nervous (not nearly so much as the patient, however), and for the first (and last) time in my career found myself unable to pass the bronchoscope through the nose. I was inexperienced enough at that time that I failed to have the confidence to do what was needed. After about an hour, only Tom Boat was left in the room. Twenty five years later, I met that patient Bruce Baskin at Carl Doershuk's retirement celebration, and we laughed heartily about "the Nose from Hell." Despite my fiasco, I was offered the fellowship. (Editor's note: Alive over thirty years later, Bruce contributed Chapter 19 to this book.

I applied for my first NIH research grant, which was funded to begin with the start of my fellowship. The aim was to study the effect of adrenergic agents, such as terbutaline, on mucociliary transport in CF patients. When I left the NIH, there was no one who would be using the flexible bronchoscope, so Paul di Sant'Agnese generously allowed me to borrow it to begin my work in Cleveland. The first week I was there, I took the bronchoscope (and a new one purchased by the hospital) to Respiratory Therapy and asked to have them sterilized in the "gas autoclave." "No problem, Doc." The next morning I found a note on my office door. "Please see Dr. Doershuk immediately." Carl asked me if I had seen my bronchoscopes that morning. "I think you'd better go have a look," he said quietly. Unfortunately, these very expensive bronchoscopes had been processed through the *steam* autoclave, rather than the ethylene oxide gas sterilizer. Both had *melted* and were now useless. Carl never said another word about it, realizing that I would punish myself much more than he could for such a stupid mistake. I have tried to ensure that no one else would repeat my mistake, either.

When I applied for permission to begin my studies of mucociliary transport in CF patients at Rainbow Babies & Children's Hospital, the idea of investigational bronchoscopy was virtually unheard of, especially in pediatric patients. In preparation for presenting my protocol to the Institutional Review Board and before leaving the NIH, I had myself bronchoscoped by a physician I had trained to take over from me as I left the NIH and had a movie made of the procedure. When the IRB required that I present my proposal to the entire committee, I did so and showed them the flexible bronchoscope. Then I showed the movie to show what the flexible bronchoscopy procedure was like. When the movie ended, there was a stunned silence. Finally, the Chairman turned to me and said, "Dr. Wood, I think you may proceed with your proposal." I don't think they even took a formal vote!

With a new bronchoscope, I continued my studies on the possible therapeutic effect of localized lung lavage as well as the mucociliary transport studies. Despite trying numerous techniques, even completely filling one lung with saline and washing it repeatedly with a total of up to 40 liters, it was not possible to demonstrate useful clinical benefit from lavage. It seemed that once the patient had developed significant bronchiectasis, there was no way we could reverse the process, even by the direct instillation of antibiotics into the bronchi. On the other hand, as a result of this effort, I was able to develop a method for unilateral lung lavage in patients with alveolar proteinosis who are too small for the large double-lumen endotracheal tube. My original patient for this bronchoscopy lavage procedure is still alive more than 25 years (and many lavages) later. The procedures performed on CF patients provided a rich source of material for the research labs and a number of research projects were built around this new capability. It also proved practical to obtain large numbers of alveolar macrophages from normal subjects for use in other research projects. Quite a number of nurses and students thought being a research bronchoscopy subject was a neat way to earn an extra $50.

In the mid 1970s, flexible bronchoscopy in pediatric patients remained mostly a research procedure in teenagers and older subjects. I began to appreciate the vast potential of the technique for clinical applications in younger children, but the physical limitations of instrument size prohibited this. A smaller 3.5 mm flexible bronchoscope became available in 1975, but it had no suction port, thus making it of only very limited utility. It was intended to be used as a flexible telescope, passed through a rigid bronchoscope. I purchased one, and decided to see if I could add a suction channel to the outside by attaching a length of plastic tubing to the bronchoscope with Teflon pipefitting tape. To my delight, I could now perform quite useful procedures in children as young as 18 months of age and presented this experience at the first World Congress of Bronchoscopy in 1976. Later that year when I visited the headquarters of the Olympus Corporation of America and told them of my work, I gave them some design specifications and asked them to make a pediatric flexible bronchoscope. They probably thought that this was a crazy request and seriously doubted there would ever be a commercial market for such an instrument. Nevertheless, in November 1978, they provided me with the first pediatric flexible bronchoscope.

Suddenly, I found that there were an enormous number of children who could benefit from flexible bronchoscopy. As a result, my research program suffered because I became very busy with clinical procedures. From some 30 to 40 research procedures a year, I was now performing 350 to 400 clinical procedures a year. I presented my initial experience with young children at the American Bronchoesophagological Association meeting in Palm Beach. In the discussion that followed my presentation, I was accused of "medical voyeurism" and "gross medical malpractice" for performing flexible bronchoscopy in infants and children. The next day I found myself sitting with Dr. Henry Heimlich (he of the "Maneuver" and no stranger to controversy), and told him about my presentation and its reception. After he stopped laughing, he clapped me on the back and gave me this sage advice. "Bob," he said, "if at any time in your career you find that your peers are all comfortable with what you are doing, you may as well hang it up. You're no longer being creative." I have found this to be good advice.

The next several years passed quickly, as I gained experience with bronchoscopy and its applications to infants and children. I was amazed at how often I found surprises in the airways of children. For example, one percent of the first 1,000 children that I bronchoscoped had a clinically unsuspected foreign body. There was no pediatric otolaryngologist at the hospital, and Dr. Michael Gauderer, a pediatric surgeon, and I developed a serious interest in children with subglottic stenosis and tracheostomies. I clearly perceived that pediatric pulmonologists with interests in the airways and bronchoscopy now had access to the airways and could play a very important role in the management of patients with airway problems.

Patients with CF continued to fascinate me. I soon discovered that bronchoscopy was a very good way to determine whether the lungs of younger patients were infected or not. Younger patients could not be expected to expectorate sputum and cultures taken from the upper airway did not always correlate with the results of washings taken from deep within the lungs. There were many patients who had obvious lung disease but from whom no pathogenic bacteria could be isolated by conventional techniques. Yet on bronchoscopy, the lungs were discovered to be heavily infected and the results from the bronchoscopy cultures could be used to direct specific antibiotic therapy. In other patients, who clinically appeared to have minimal (or even no) lung disease, bronchoscopy revealed serious infection and inflammation. In a few patients, bronchoscopy revealed that the lungs were sterile, even though there were copious, thick secretions obstructing the airways (some of these patients were found to have significant gastroesophageal reflux). In infants, bronchoscopy indicated that there was early evidence of airways disease, as manifest by the presence of airway casts in the fluid returned from bronchoalveolar lavage, even in the absence of infection. Another interesting and illuminating discovery was that many CF patients had little or no abnormality on physical examination of their chest, but bronchoscopy would reveal amazing quantities of extremely thick, purulent tracheobronchial secretions. These secretions were so thick that perhaps they generated little extra noise during the respiratory cycle. The bronchoscope taught me that most CF patients have much more lung disease than anyone might suspect on purely clinical grounds.

One of the things I learned from LeRoy Matthews was the importance of an aggressive, comprehensive approach to the treatment of CF *starting very early in life*. The ability to more accurately define the nature and extent of the lung disease in CF patients, even infants, by bronchoscopy opened new doors to slowing the onset of irreversible lung disease. I advocate performing bronchoscopy on any non-sputum producing CF patient who undergoes anesthesia for a surgical procedure as a way of monitoring the lower airway bacterial flora and disease state. Whether routinely scheduled bronchoscopy in younger CF patients can significantly alter the course of the disease remains to be established. But clearly, when there is clinical indication for antibiotic therapy, bronchoscopy can provide vitally important information to guide the selection of the most appropriate antibiotics and, in some cases, to monitor the results of therapy.

Flexible bronchoscopy is a technique that must be learned, and requires a certain level of mechanical aptitude, as well as a sense of three-dimensionality. When the Olympus Corporation brought the 3.5 mm pediatric flexible bronchoscope to the market in 1981, virtually no one in pediatrics knew how to use one. I began to receive many calls from physicians asking to come to Cleveland for training. After the first such experience in 1982, when Dr. Bettina Hilman and Dr. Michelle Cloutier spent several weeks with me, I realized that I would be unable to keep up with the requests. This experience led to the organization of a formal postgraduate course to teach physicians the techniques of flexible bronchoscopy in children and the fundamentals of bronchology. The course has been held every year since then, and has been the primary introduction to bronchoscopy for more than a thousand pediatric physicians from more than 40 countries. Many of these physicians have gone on to utilize what they learned in the care of CF patients and in CF related research. Since 1989, the course has also been held in Davos, Switzerland (every other year) with Dr. Martin Schöni as the local host.

The flexible bronchoscope proved to be, as I had suspected, a boon to research. Safe and easy access to the lower airways enabled a variety of research applications never before possible. A number of research projects involving bronchoscopy, most of them related to CF, were initiated. The introduction of the smaller, pediatric flexible bronchoscope dramatically expanded the potential. Gratifyingly, investigators in a number of other institutions also began to apply the techniques to CF related research. Although there are serious limitations on the use of children for medical research, much was learned from the study of material obtained in the course of clinical procedures.

In 1982, Dr. Boat was recruited to the University of North Carolina at Chapel Hill as Chairman of the Department of Pediatrics. The Department had no pulmonary division and Tom asked me to come with him to establish a pulmonary program. It was difficult to leave RB&C Hospital and my mentor, Carl Doershuk, but I was soon immersed in the new program and its challenges. Pediatric bronchoscopy was essentially unheard of in Chapel Hill, except for anesthesia and rigid bronchoscopy to remove an aspirated foreign body. Soon, however, the skeptics were converted and the value of bronchoscopy came to be recognized. It was the source of considerable amusement to me to see Dr. Floyd Denny, Tom's predecessor as Chairman and a renowned infectious disease expert with a particular interest in pulmonary disease, begin to inquire as to whether the patient on whom he was being asked to consult had undergone bronchoscopy. "Why not?" he would often ask. "That's where the answer will come from."

The CF program at UNC was very small when I arrived in 1983 (fewer than 50 patients). It was a very exciting place to be, however, because of what was going on in the adult pulmonary program. Dr. Rick Boucher and Dr. Mike Knowles had developed a strong interest in CF, and their research program was expanding. As the research program grew, so did the size of their adult CF patient population and the pediatric population also grew rapidly. By the time I eventually left Chapel Hill in 1999, the UNC-CH CF Center was one of the two largest CF Centers in the US. I have once again followed Tom Boat, this time to Cincinnati where I will be involved in developing a multidisciplinary program for the diagnosis and treatment of children with complex airways and swallowing disorders, continue to support CF related research, and teach young physicians to perform flexible bronchoscopy.

And what of bronchoscopy and CF? I believe that the future of CF and pulmonary research lies in the application of molecular biology techniques to patients. The natural history of CF with conventional therapy is now so slow that many years are required to document a change in the survival of patient groups as a result of a new therapy. Likewise, conventional measures of lung function, which reflect airway obstruction and destruction, are insensitive and relatively indirect. The future of CF research will necessarily involve observations and sampling from deep within the lungs and this can only be done with bronchoscopy. Major advances in CF will begin in the laboratory, but proving their efficacy will be done in the bronchoscopy laboratory. It has been a source of great pride for me to have played a seminal role in the development of the instrumentation and techniques of bronchoscopy in children and to disseminate them to the pediatric community.

9

Neonatal Screening: Toward Earlier Diagnosis and Improved Outcome

Philip M. Farrell, M.D., Ph.D.

> Every physician's first duty is to diagnose — accurately and promptly.

> Diagnosis is the first step of treatment!

The principles stated above represent core values in the medical profession. Medical students learn them during their clinical practice introductory experience. Ironically, however, improving the diagnostic aspect of care has received relatively limited attention in the field of cystic fibrosis (CF). This is both surprising and troubling, especially since new treatments are likely to be most beneficial to patients identified early, before irreversible lung pathology supervenes. The rationale for routine early diagnosis of CF through neonatal screening and my personal perspectives follow. Detailed information and many references on neonatal screening can be found in review articles.[1-4] As described in the "Future Directions" section, I believe that a transformation of CF diagnosis and treatment will soon occur and that future management will emphasize disease prevention, which can only be fully effective on a population basis when coupled to neonatal screening programs.

Several studies have documented that beneficial effects of screening on nutrition and lung function persist to at least 13 years of age.[3-5] This information, when analyzed in the context of delayed diagnosis beyond one year of age and the attending risk of multisystem involvement, emphasize the potential for newborn screening for CF.

My commitment to investigate early diagnosis through neonatal screening for CF began during 1981 when I visited Cleveland to participate in a site visit of the prototype CF Center at Case Western Reserve University. At the time, I was serving as CF Center Director at the University of Wisconsin. After an inspiring series of research presentations at Rainbow Babies and Children's Hospital, I was walking along Adelbert Road with Dr. Tom Boat enjoying a conversation about the challenges of diagnosing CF in early childhood and thinking about the potential advantages of neonatal screening. By the end of the day after more reflection, I decided to begin shifting my research focus from pulmonary surfactant metabolism to CF neonatal screening, and this eventually became a two-decade commitment.

Before describing CF neonatal screening per se, I would like to summarize relevant background information about my career development and explain how I was blessed with a series of outstanding opportunities and mentors. Just as science advances in an incremental fashion, individual scientists must develop stage by stage.

My career development experiences relevant to CF neonatal screening actually began while I was a student in the MD/PhD program at St. Louis University. During graduate training in biochemistry, I was studying vitamin E deficiency and became keenly interested in laboratory medicine. Undoubtedly, my wife's concurrent training program in medical technology stimulated this interest, along with a fondness for clinical chemistry. In my last year of combined medical and graduate school, I was in the process of interviewing for a pathology residency when, what I've called a "pediatrics thunderbolt," struck me one day while working in an ambulatory care clinic for children. This transforming experience immediately inspired me to change plans and apply for a pediatrics residency. The great biochemistry programs at the University of Wisconsin, its strengthened pediatric residency program, and the personal attractions of the Madison community led me to Dr. Charles Lobeck's Department of Pediatrics. While serving as a resident, my experiences in CF care with Drs. Lobeck and John Mangos were outstanding. Shortly before my residency began, I had an opportunity to visit the National Institutes of Health (NIH) and interview for a fellowship as suggested by my major professor in graduate school, the Chair of Biochemistry at St. Louis University, Dr. Robert Olson. My academic career course was set firmly in place when Dr. Paul di Sant' Agnese called me while I was busy making resident rounds in July 1970 at Madison General Hospital. To my great advantage, Paul selected me for a once in a lifetime opportunity to become a clinical associate and research trainee at the NIH.

Also of note, while interviewing for the position at the NIH Clinical Center in 1969, I first met Tom Boat and learned from him how uniquely valuable the training would be, how much I would enjoy Paul's tutelage, and how well I would be prepared for a research career. Tom and I, therefore, knew each other from similar training experience under Dr. di Sant'Agnese at the Pediatric Metabolism Branch of the National Institute for Arthritis, Metabolism and Digestive Diseases of NIH where I stayed from 1972 to 1977. As we walked on Adelbert Road, we both recognized the difficulties of caring for CF patients whose diagnosis had been delayed and who already had either severe malnutrition or progressive lung disease. Tom's research by 1981 had focused on the newly emerging field of pediatric pulmonology, while I was engaged in a combination of neonatology and pulmonology--applying nutritional and biochemical techniques to study pediatric respiratory disorders, particularly in newborn infants.

My faculty role with the University of Wisconsin Department of Pediatrics beginning in 1977 included not only serving as Director of the Madison CF Center but also as a neonatologist. This was a somewhat unusual combination of responsibilities, and one which offered me what I considered "the best of both worlds" (the excitement of two rapidly advancing fields, namely neonatology and pediatric pulmonology--both intensive and "high-tech" while also being "high-touch"). My clinical experiences in neonatal intensive care units gave me a deep appreciation of the power of newborn screening tests[1] and the importance of treating meconium ileus (intestinal blockage seen at birth in some CF newborns) aggressively. At the same time, my work as a CF physician brought me many referrals of infants and young children who had suffered from a delay in diagnosis and showed either severe malnutrition (even kwashiorkor) or progressive lung disease. These CF center experiences were troubling to me because the referrals typically came from highly skilled, general pediatricians I knew well from my training as a resident in Madison earlier in the decade (1970–72). It became increasingly apparent to me that delays in diagnosing CF by the standard method (a sweat test because of signs and/or symptoms) offered limited hope for the average patient.

My experiences in neonatal intensive care also led me by 1980 to recognize that there were many infants with delayed passage of meconium (babies at risk for meconium ileus). These infants usually could not be diagnosed with a sweat test until they reached at least one month of age-a delay that caused parental anxiety and physician uncertainty. I began to use the meconium albumin test myself at crib side and found that in individual cases, it could be valuable. However, a literature review showed that it was not satisfactory as a population-based screening test.[2] Nevertheless, the attractiveness of early diagnosis through neonatal screening had become obvious to me, and I stayed informed about other developments such as Crossley's report of a retrospective study on immunoreactive trypsinogen (IRT) levels in stored newborn blood specimens.[6] This report was, in retrospect, "the shot heard around the world" in the field of CF neonatal screening.

To complete the summary of my background information, I had two other compelling experiences. First, when I began my residency in 1970, Dr. Harry Shwachman published a paper that was very encouraging with regard to the prognosis of CF patients who experienced early diagnosis.[7] Most significantly, children diagnosed before three months of age had a mortality rate that was much less than those diagnosed later. While I was at the NIH from 1972–977, I met Harry many times and often heard him comment about how important it would be to diagnose all patients at a young age. He was such a strong advocate for early diagnosis and was so firm in directing those comments to me personally that Harry actually "planted seeds" that later "sprouted." It struck me at the time that it would only be fair to individual CF patients if each one had a "healthy start." [3] My conviction about this is even stronger today.

Secondly, I've always remembered vividly the critical comments about the sweat test by Dr. di Sant'Agnese, discoverer of the sweat electrolyte defect in CF. Paul often said that sweat electrolyte analysis was inherently not such a good test but it worked because of the wide separation of chloride values between CF and non-CF populations, as long as physicians had the insight to order a sweat test. So my mind was well prepared on the day of that fateful walk with Tom Boat. I was also blessed with the skill set that enabled me to organize and lead what was des-

Table 9.1. Special/Unique Features or Outcomes of the Wisconsin CF Neonatal Screening Project

1. First controlled investigation of newborn screening for any congenital disease

2. First use of population-based DNA testing to screen for a congenital disorder

3. Unique design to avoid selection bias with "unblinding" and surveillance

4. Largest prospective pediatric research project since the 1954 polio vaccine trials

5. Most comprehensive and expensive clinical trial in children with cystic fibrosis

6. Longest controlled epidemiologic study of children with cystic fibrosis

7. Most accurate delineation of CF incidence in a regional population

8. Largest CF Center database involving a cohort of enrolled subjects with CF

9. Most extensive sweat test experience with infants at risk for cystic fibrosis

10. Most successful nutrition support program applied to children with CF*

---

*   Demonstrating that malnutrition can be prevented by a combination of early diagnosis and effective nutritional management.

---

tined to become a unique investigation (Table 9.1) and the largest prospective pediatric research project since the polio vaccine field trials of 1954.

The Trypsinogen Test and the Plan to Study its Potential Value

The IRT test was developed using radioimmunoassay micro-technology[6] for application to dried newborn blood specimens obtained within a few days of birth, as with other newborn screening methods.[1] The test relies on measurement of immunoreactive trypsinogen, the level of which is increased in newborns with CF (presumably because of obstructed pancreatic ductules causing a leakage of digestive enzyme precursors into the bloodstream). When the seminal publications emerged from New Zealand [6] and others followed,[5,8] some advocates argued that it would have been reasonable to implement trypsinogen based newborn screening for CF immediately on a routine basis. Indeed, the State of Colorado did so.[8] Colorado and New South Wales, Australia have been leaders in the field of IRT screening services for almost two decades.

My temptation to implement rather than study CF neonatal screening would have been stronger except for one of the other lessons I learned under Dr. di

Sant'Agnese. In essence, Paul taught me that once you begin to use a diagnostic or therapeutic intervention, you could never study it properly. In fact, Paul helped me complete a series of key investigations on human vitamin E deficiency by waiting until my arrival at the NIH to begin clinical studies of this nutrient in CF patients. At the time, i.e., in the early 1970s, alpha-tocopherol had only recently been established as a vitamin. The recommendation by Dr. LeRoy Matthews, et al, that vitamin E supplementation could be helpful for CF patients was based on deficiency reports in the literature, but convincing evidence that it was needed was lacking. Consequently, Paul had decided that clinical studies should be performed before routine treatment was implemented at his CF Center. It was an unforgettable experience for me to arrive at the NIH and recognize what a unique opportunity he saved for me to pursue the definitive clinical study [9] on a vitamin that drew me into basic research originally. Returning to the IRT test, it should be noted that in the early 1980s, there was clearly a national dilemma with regard to CF neonatal screening. Ironically, the same situation still applies today, although the issues are somewhat different. In 1983, the Cystic Fibrosis Foundation (CFF) convened a task force and published a position paper urging caution and recommending research.[10] The stage was then set for Wisconsin's two CF Centers to begin investigation of neonatal screening using the trypsinogen test to generate a group of children with CF who would have an early diagnosis.

Planning for the study occurred in 1983/84. Recognizing that diagnostic, therapeutic, and health policy decisions should depend upon a comparison of benefits and risks, we decided to perform a comprehensive investigation ultimately entitled "Assessment of the Benefits, Risks and Costs of Neonatal Screening for Cystic Fibrosis," as the project expanded to include a wide range of epidemiologic, financial and health policy issues. Designing the study was a challenge because only a randomized clinical trial would generate the comparison or control group to test the hypothesis of interest, namely "early diagnosis of CF through neonatal screening will be medically beneficial without major risks."

We determined that the Wisconsin Centers, Madison and Milwaukee (the latter directed by my good friend, Dr. W. Theodore Bruns), would collaborate on all aspects of the project. We considered the possibility of a two or three state study and I reviewed this option in Minneapolis with Dr. Warren Warwick, who directed the University of Minnesota CF Center and was an advocate for early diagnosis. In the final analysis, we concluded that the complexity of adding another state would in the long run outweigh any advantages (and time proved that this was a wise decision). This decision was facilitated by the realization that only a long-term investigation that could maintain uniform treatment would produce the consistently high quality data to allow us to address the key hypothesis. In addition, my conviction about the need to resolve neonatal screening controversies unequivocally had become deep enough that our research team prepared for the "long haul" with a commitment to maintain cohesiveness and ultimately achieve closure.

Table 9.2 Problems Potentially Associated with Delayed Diagnosis of Patients with Cystic Fibrosis*

1. Malnutrition severe enough to cause wasting/stunting and altered brain growth

2. Pulmonary disease and complications

3. Possibly preventable deaths (e.g., hyponatremia and kwashiorkor)

4. Biased diagnoses that include under recognition in minority groups

5. Parental anxiety (obviously sick infant/child left undiagnosed)

6. Parental frustration with the health care delivery system

7. Parental loss of trust and confidence in the medical profession

8. Parental uninformed reproductive decision making

9. Avoidable health care costs for diagnosis and treatment

10. Underutilization of the CF Center network (limiting access to optimal care)

* Suffering of patients, parents, and siblings and adverse effects on health care delivery systems.

The Diagnostic Imperative

The morbidity and mortality of CF are so great, and the treatment so specialized and necessary, that diagnosis is imperative to assure that patients have full opportunity to benefit from clinical management in CF Centers. Some experts have speculated that a sizeable proportion, perhaps 10%, of CF patients die without being recognized/diagnosed.[4] Data supporting this concern are limited, but unquestionably some patients do succumb without being recognized. Causes of such deaths include: undiagnosed meconium ileus, acute kwashiorkor, hyponatremic dehydration, spontaneous pneumothorax, rapidly progressive pneumonia, and on rare occasions severe deficiencies in vitamin K (causing hemorrhagic disease) or vitamin E (causing severe hemolytic anemia). Although one would think that the severity of the foregoing manifestations would regularly and promptly lead to a diagnostic sweat test, often this is not the case. Indeed, Lai et al. determined that close to half of the CF patients diagnosed in the United States are severely malnourished at the time of the positive sweat test.[11] Table 9.2 lists some of the other problems associated with delayed diagnosis. Parental suffering certainly accompanies that of the affected child. Every CF specialist has had experiences with families who changed from physician to physician trying to obtain a diagnosis for their sick child.

It has been obvious for decades that delays in diagnoses are common in North America. The data for the United States and Canada are similar when one examines patients identified by standard diagnostic methods, i.e., a positive sweat test recommended for either symptoms or recognition that CF has occurred previously in a family member. The most recent data available from the United States based on 906 patients reported to the CFF Registry in 1998 reveal that the average age of diagnosis was 3.0 years and the median 6 months. These values are very similar to those of the past two decades (e.g., 1988 CFF data for 840 newly diagnosed patients revealed a mean of 2.8 years and a median of 7 months age at diagnosis). Of significance, recent years have not been associated with improvement in the age of diagnosis despite great research advances, an excellent CF Center network, an impressive amount of publicity about the disease, and existence of sophisticated parents and health care professionals. Of even greater significance, about one-half of those patients diagnosed in their first year of life are recognized because they have either meconium ileus or a positive family history for CF, thus they are not inherently difficult to detect. Thus, the average age of patients identified after signs and symptoms of CF have developed is even later in life than the overall reports indicate.[3,4]

The Problem with the Traditional, Standard Method of Diagnosis

In my judgment, there is no reason to expect lowering of the age of diagnosis through standard diagnostic methods; indeed, the opposite is more likely in the managed care era. Frankly, we've all been naïve, and perhaps irresponsible, to think that recognition by primary care physicians of signs and symptoms suggesting CF would lead to a promptly obtained sweat test. Even the most astute pediatricians have followed infants and children in their practice for many months before obtaining the sweat test, during which time deterioration and even irreversible changes occurred. As mentioned previously, the sweat test is only good for diagnosis when someone remembers to order it. In addition, the sweat test remains imperfect because there are patients with inadequate sweat or borderline results that require another appointment for retesting. One of every twenty CF patients can have a sweat chloride value below 60 mEq/liter. There are additional CF patients with false negative results, borderline values that are overlooked, or sweat chloride levels in the presumed normal range, i.e., less than 40 meq/liter. And some 100 negative sweat tests are likely to be performed for every true positive.[2]

Also, the cost and skill levels needed to perform a sweat test are high. Our informal surveys suggest that the price range varies from $50 to $200 in the United States. The direct cost alone to perform a single sweat test during 1999 in our laboratory was $177, taking into account the hourly wage and fringe benefits of our technician, the supplies, and the ancillary expenses. These data allow one to estimate a national cost in the US for sweat tests; assuming 100 such tests for each patient diagnosed and a conservative average cost of $200 per sweat test leads to an estimate of $20 million for diagnosing 1000 CF patients. The laboratory cost of routine CF neonatal screening could be lower.[2]

Therefore, the central diagnostic problem is that CF will never be accurately and promptly diagnosed in pediatric populations as long as we continue to rely on the standard method, i.e., ordering the sweat test *after* signs and/or symptoms are already present, or there is a positive family history. Consequently, it is impossible to ensure each child a "healthy start" given the limitations of our current standard diagnostic method (which has significant deficiencies, as noted earlier). On the other hand, the IRT method—coupled to DNA analysis—provides a method to identify at least 90% of CF patients in the first few weeks of life.

Design of a Unique Randomized Clinical Trial

The greatest challenge in planning for the Wisconsin CF Neonatal Screening Project was designing a study that could accrue sufficient patients while avoiding selection bias. The number of CF patients needed in each group was determined using internal observations of the Madison CF Center and data reported by the Cleveland Center,[12] their retrospective assessment of 16 sibling pairs that showed the younger children diagnosed before one year of age had better pulmonary outcomes. We recognized from the beginning that an early diagnosis (screened) group could be inherently better off than a group of ill patients diagnosed largely on the basis of signs and symptoms. We also recognized that each CF patient, once diagnosed, would need to receive the same high quality treatment. Ethical considerations demanded no less therapy for the control group, and it was imperative to isolate the early diagnosis variable to the extent possible. Consequently, the only acceptable design was one in which we could completely identify the standard diagnosis (control) group and offer them the same treatment immediately following a positive sweat test.

Two possible approaches occurred to us: 1) save the dried blood specimens from newborns randomized to the control group and analyze them later for trypsinogen (and after 1991 for CFTR mutations); or 2) perform the IRT and DNA analyses on the control group during the neonatal period but remain blinded as to the results by computer storing of the raw data for four years and then using an "unblinding" process[3] to identify CF patients in the standard diagnosis group. We selected the latter strategy because of storage limitations and the instability of trypsinogen during storage. Four years of age was chosen for "unblinding" because: 1) four years was the approximate average age at which children with CF were diagnosed, both in the US as a whole and in Wisconsin,[2] and 2) locating IRT or IRT/DNA positive children and obtaining sweat tests would become increasingly difficult at older ages when children were in elementary school, despite our surveillance methods.[3] The term "unblinding" refers to a sequence of procedures applied to control children at 4 years of age in which the IRT data are computed and reported, DNA testing for the ΔF508 mutation is performed (in another laboratory), primary care physicians are contacted, parents/children located and informed, and sweat tests obtained at a Wisconsin CF Center. In practice, newborn dried blood specimens whose laboratory accession numbers ended in an odd digit were tested for trypsinogen (the IRT test) and the results reported immediately (screened group), whereas those ending in an even number constituted the control group that would be completely identified ("unblinded") by four years of age.

Nevertheless, there was a major concern from the beginning about the ethical aspects of using this strategy for randomized screening. There were two critical, inter-related questions that were addressed in a prize winning paper by Fost and Farrell.[13] [and are summarized below]

> "Did the withholding of neonatal screening from the control group violate any ethical obligation?"

> "Did the withholding of information from the parents of control infants violate any ethical duty?"

Our analysis led to the conclusion that negative answers could be given to each question because: 1) control group infants would not be denied anything of proven value; 2) standard treatment also involves potential risks, both medical and psychosocial; 3) without the control group, there would be no study, and without the study, there would be no screening; and 4) "volenti, non fit injuriae" (with consent, there is no moral injury). Obtaining parental consent required a brochure that explained the research project along with providing background information on CF and disclosing options available to parents (including the opportunity to refuse the CF "research test" and another option to obtain the screening test results if they wished to know). The second ethical question about withholding information was critical because of the need to use an experimental design that would avoid selection bias even though it meant not informing parents about screening test results in babies randomized to the control group. Obviously, withholding information from experimental subjects is not new or unusual. Many randomized clinical trials involve a double blind design in which patients and physicians are denied access to information unless some urgent reason to break the code arises. The justifications for these withholdings are always the same, patients are not being denied anything of known value; disclosure may cause harm; or the subjects consented to the conditions of nondisclosure. Although we had reached our conclusion independently about not violating ethical obligations, a decision by the two funding agencies (CFF and NIH) to require a comparable, unbiased control group as a condition of awarding grants provided another justification.

Starting the CF Neonatal Screening Project

Once the experimental design was determined, the ethical issues addressed, and the preparations completed by Wisconsin's two CF Centers, there were four remaining challenges as listed below.

1. Obtain institutional review board (IRB) approvals for randomized screening.

2. Generate sufficient research grant support from the CFF and/or NIH.

3. Establish the State Laboratory of Hygiene's CF screening procedures within the Wisconsin Newborn Screening Laboratory.

4. Implement the method for consent in all Wisconsin hospitals with obstetrical services.

Obtaining IRB approvals was more difficult than anticipated because so many institutions (the UW-Madison Human Subjects Committee, and the review board that approves research projects for the Children's Hospital in Milwaukee and the Medical College of Wisconsin, and several community hospitals) wanted to review and approve the investigation before allowing their nurseries to participate. This was acceptable as we expected, in fact insisted, that the newborn screening brochure be given to parents as the consent instrument. It would have been difficult to accomplish this project if any Wisconsin hospital IRB disapproved the protocol; however, all the approvals were secured within about a six-month period. This broad spectrum of reviews turned out to be quite helpful since one IRB suggested that we include an "escape clause" that would allow parents to contact us and obtain the IRT test results no matter to which group their baby was randomized.[13] I remember attending that committee meeting and having a clergyman suggest we might want to allow such inquiries; he then asked me if we would have any objections. I answered "No," and left the room thinking that this was another example of a constructive revision in a research project achieved through peer review.

The Wisconsin CF Neonatal Screening Project obviously could not be initiated without research grant support. Our initial grant application was submitted to both the NIH and the CFF, and the latter organization awarded us a grant of $869,660 following a site visit in the fall of 1983. Soon after, the NIH approved and funded the project ($1,056,082 initially for 5 years). The only serious concerns expressed by the NIH study section were related to ensuring avoidance of selection bias and achieving success in locating the control group subjects when they reached age four years. We were able to return most of the CFF grant, but it got us started and we have always credited that organization with the start up phase of our project. Indeed, later on in 1988 when difficulty emerged in a NIH competitive renewal, the CFF stepped in again with leadership by Dr. Robert Beall and provided funds for supporting continuation of the randomized screening, a component of the project eventually extended from the anticipated 3–4 years to almost 9 years.

The Newborn Screening Laboratory start up phase included establishing the trypsinogen testing method, implementing quality control mechanisms, and reaching a conclusion about an initial cut-off level (ultimately determined to be 180 ng/ml). We decided to rely on the experience of the Colorado screening program, and are deeply grateful to Keith Hammond for serving as a faithful and effective consultant. On his advice, we used the Sorin kit as in Colorado. To establish the

180 ng/ml cut off, we analyzed 10,000 consecutive newborn blood specimens (blindly), determining the distribution of values and calculating the 99.8 percentile. Although there was some concern about analyzing 10,000 specimens blindly, this was approved by our IRB before randomized screening began. Again, the critical point in the ethical analysis was that newborn screening had not been established convincingly as beneficial and therefore early diagnosis through screening could not be considered compelling on clinical grounds.

During this start up, our Policy and Data Monitoring Board began to meet. This group has served us well in an oversight and advisory capacity as they monitored the results presented by biostatisticians and dealt with a variety of issues. It has been chaired throughout the years by Dr. Charles Lobeck and has continued to benefit from diverse membership, including Robert Beall, Jeffery Davis, David DeMets, Norman Fost, and Keith Hammond, all voting members.

Wisconsin's newborn screening brochure, a publication of the State Division of Health, has been critical to success of this project. The Division of Health leaders have been enthusiastic about collaborative efforts to improve the language and the distribution of the brochure, and we used it during randomized screening to obtain implied consent from parents on maternity wards of all Wisconsin hospitals that have obstetrical services. This collaboration became a mutually beneficial relationship between a research team and a state organization with a public health service mission as we rewrote the brochure and included information on the CF "research test." The Division of Health made sure that community hospitals discarded the old version and used the new brochure, which was made distinctive with a picture of an infant on the cover. An important part of this effort involved the nurse of the Division of Health with responsibility for Maternal-Child Health programs. She visited the larger hospitals with obstetrical services to explain the new brochure, assure that the old version was discarded, inform perinatal nurses about the State's expectations for brochure distribution, and answer questions that might arise. Even during the start up phase, this research project was already enhancing communication around the state and contributing to better health care through a public/private partnership. We augmented our communications by sending letters to every primary care physician in Wisconsin and publishing articles in the *Wisconsin Medical Journal*.

We were ready to initiate randomized screening by April 1, 1985, but we decided to avoid "April Fool's Day" and chose a date everyone would remember, namely April 15th. Screening proceeded with our expectation that an incidence of one CF patient for every 2,000 live births would allow us to generate the 45 patients needed in each group within 3 to 4 years. This target was determined by an analysis of statistical power needed to demonstrate significant differences in two categories of potential benefit, namely nutritional status (especially length/height and weight) and pulmonary outcomes based on PFT data and quantitative chest radiology.

Problems Encountered

Since there had never been a randomized clinical trial of any newborn screening test, and in view of the limited knowledge in 1985 about the epidemiology of CF, we were in a pioneering role and encountered many unexpected problems. One of the first was evident during 1986 when it became apparent that the incidence of CF we were encountering was much less than the 1:2,000 textbook figure and closer to the 1:4,000 incidence of CF we eventually demonstrated for North American newborn populations.[3] In addition, we observed almost twice the frequency of CF patients with meconium ileus compared to the proportion predicted from the literature. Previous studies generally reported that about 10% of CF patients were born with meconium ileus, but our screening program showed the actual proportion to be about twice as high in the US, yet another example of initial erroneous epidemiologic data.

Another early problem was the relatively high randomized assignment of patients with meconium ileus to the control group leading to almost twice as many CF patients who had neonatal intestinal obstruction in the standard diagnosis (control) group. Since such patients were invariably diagnosed early, these subjects were not helpful for assessing benefits and risks of early diagnosis through neonatal screening. The only solution to the problem of imbalance of patients in screened and control groups was to continue randomized screening until we had at least 45 subjects without meconium ileus in the screened group. Fortunately, when we reached that point, the proportions with meconium ileus were statistically the same between the two groups.

One potential issue did not turn out to be a problem. The "escape clause" for parents did not lead to any difficulties. We screened 650,341 newborns over nine years and only 195 families (0.03%) contacted us to ask for the IRT or IRT/DNA results. This is especially remarkable since a much greater number of UW-Madison Pediatrics clinical staff had babies during 1985–94, and most of them knew about this project and its "escape clause." Thus, the fear of grant reviewers that this provision would invalidate the study did not materialize. Also, the vast majority of parents did not express concern in general about neonatal screening tests.

The Combined Trypsinogen-Gene Test Method

The trypsinogen test was used for randomized screening until 1991 when we expanded to the combination of trypsinogen and DNA (ΔF508 mutation) method as follows. We were awaiting publication of an accepted manuscript on trypsinogen levels[14] when the breakthrough identification of the ΔF508 CF gene mutation was reported[15] in 1989. We had already noted the need for a two tier testing strategy (as used for congenital hyperthryoidism[1]) and subsequently revised that statement to a prophetic commentary: "With advances in technology and the recent identification of one of the cystic fibrosis mutations and the identification of other mutations to soon follow, we believe that the strategy for cystic fibrosis newborn screening will need to evolve into a true two-tier screening test. The first tier would be the IRT assay; if the IRT assay is positive, the second tier would be performed on the same original blood spot, and it would be a probe for the cystic fibrosis mutations. The implementation of cystic fibrosis screening, however, should be delayed until a clear benefit of newborn screening has been identified."[14]

In fact, this two-tier approach has proved to be even more attractive than we anticipated and now is accepted widely as the best method.[3, 4] Typical North American populations have more than 90% of CF patients with at least one ΔF508 mutation and about 50% have two such alleles, so the sensitivity can approach 100% using the procedures implemented in Wisconsin.[16] In addition, the IRT/DNA method has the highest positive predictive value of all current newborn screening tests[16] and thus minimizes the challenge of false positive infant tests. The DNA analysis can be performed with minimal additional cost[2] on the same dried newborn blood specimen, whenever trypsinogen levels exceed a conservative cut-off point. One of the greatest advantages is the ability to positively establish the genetic diagnosis of CF in at least 50% of patients with this screening test before babies are one week old by demonstrating the presence of two ΔF508 alleles through DNA analysis.

Results of the Randomized Clinical Trial

Ultimately, our randomization period extended to 9 years, resulting in two groups that were well balanced with regard to gender, meconium ileus, and Center. The size of the two groups was similar (74 screened and 75 control patients). Experience with the patients of the control group who did not have meconium ileus revealed an average age of diagnosis (107 weeks) similar to national data for 1985–94,[11] and much older than the screened group average of 13 weeks (p<.001). Sixty (80%) of the control patients were detected through signs, symptoms, or a positive family history, while 15 patients (20%) were detected by unblinding as they were some-what mildly affected with CF symptoms at age four years. However, the control group was, by chance, relatively better off than the screened patients, having less pancreatic insufficiency (67% versus 91%) and fewer ΔF508 genotypes (82% versus 100%).

Our strategy for addressing objectives related to testing methodologies, benefits, risks, and costs has depended on setting research priorities in a time framed fashion. The chronological sequence for benefits assessment has been as follows: 1. Establish and study the IRT and IRT/DNA screening tests while proceeding with patient accrual from 1984 to 1989 (IRT test) and from 1990–1994 (IRT/DNA test); 2. Concurrently emphasize nutritional assessment with the rationale being that the signs and symptoms of malnutrition appear early and that the endpoints are clear, allowing us to utilize well defined outcomes; 3. Collect data on pulmonary outcome measures but defer analysis since (a) lung disease occurs later and has a more variable onset than malabsorption/malnutrition and (b) reliable pulmonary function tests (PFT's) can not be obtained until children reached at least 5 years of age. In addition, it became obvious in 1990 that demonstrating pulmonary outcome differences would be more challenging because the measures available such as chest radiographic scoring systems needed improvement.

Therefore, in the analysis of outcomes, our attention focused first on nutritional status in relation to screening. The biochemical indicators of nutritional status such as levels of retinol, tocopherol, and linoleic acid are profoundly influenced by treatment, so they were only useful for comparisons at the time of diagnosis. Both the screened and control groups showed a high proportion of patients with similarly low blood levels of these nutrients. But the one noteworthy difference was the length of time that severe biochemical deficiencies persisted, with the screened patients' duration of deficiency almost 2 years shorter on the average. For longitudinal comparisons, anthropometric indexes are of greater interest and are more valuable in assessment of the long term nutritional status of CF patients. We concentrated on length/height and weight and expressed the data as percentiles during sequential analysis of results. After diagnosis, caregivers were uninformed about group identity, and all investigators except the statisticians were blinded as to the outcome measure comparisons between the two groups. The biostatisticians used state of the art "repeated measures" analytical methods and stratified the data by group and by gender during the sequential analyses. The latter stratification was done because of previous observations suggesting that female patients were worse off than males. Stratification in this fashion, however, had the effect of reducing statistical power until the combined results were analyzed after 45 subjects were accumulated in the screened group. This analysis demonstrated a statistically significant difference in the anthropometric indexes at the age of diagnosis and in follow up; the screened group was better in both height and weight as reported in 1997.[17]

Throughout the longitudinal assessment period the differences in length/height have been most impressive, especially in the subgroups of patients with either one or two ΔF508 alleles and/or pancreatic insufficiency.[17] In addition, to our surprise, the head circumference values were significantly less in the control group. This abnormality had been reported before as accompanying malnutrition in infants with CF, but not as in association with age of diagnosis.[3] The implications of reduced head (and presumably brain) growth are currently being studied in our project.

The demonstrated group differences in height and weight led our Policy and Data Monitoring Board to recommend accelerated unblinding of the control group on the basis that we had demonstrated a significant nutritional benefit of screening and had generated no evidence of any significant adverse impact.[3] Unblinding for all patients was completed in April 1998, and a definitive statistical analysis performed in April 1999 revealed even greater differences in growth with the screened group showing significantly better weight and height throughout 13 years of follow up.[3] Our conclusion is that permanent stunting and inadequate weight for height can occur as a consequence of early malnutrition in children with CF secondary to delayed diagnosis.

The magnitude and duration of differences in the screened group compared to controls provides a singular demonstration of a long term benefit to CF patients. Dr. Frank Acurso of the Colorado CF Center, during the 1997 Centers for Disease Control Workshop,[18] emphatically pointed out that this intervention, early diagnosis, has resulted in the most significant beneficial effect with the longest duration in the history of CF research. His observation should not seem surprising since diagnosis is the first step toward treatment and clearly the majority of CF patients continue to have symptoms and findings of the disease before they are identified.

The other outcome measures being examined in our project include surrogates that extend to the time of diagnosis, such as respiratory symptoms, chest radiograph scores, Shwachman-Kulczycki scores, and hospitalization for pulmonary treatment. Other measurements include repeated spirometry and lung volume determinations and epidemiology of respiratory infections with *Pseudomonas aeruginosa*. Of special interest, serial chest radiographs may be the most valuable indicators of lung disease since abnormalities accumulate over time and may not be reversible. This observation is based on analysis of quantitative chest radiology data which revealed that the first chest film taken on 54 screened patients (at 5.9 months and without history of meconium ileus) was significantly better than the corresponding scores of 47 controls who had their first chest radiograph at 27 months on average. Thus, we tentatively conclude that a delay in diagnosis leads not only to malnutrition but also more severe lung disease.

Results by Others

Observational studies begun 5 to10 years before ours, report that CF neonatal screening leads to long term better pulmonary outcomes. These include observations in the Netherlands where a screened cohort born from 1973–1979 showed better pulmonary function and life expectancy [19] and Australia where neonatal screening in New South Wales with trypsinogen and more recently with DNA methods has found improved nutritional and pulmonary outcomes, as well as less hospitalization over 10 years of follow-up evaluation.[5] The growth of the early diagnosis group (median age 1.8 months) in Australia was significantly greater than a non-screened birth cohort from the previous 3 years (1978–1981) who were diagnosed at a median age of 6.2 months. The screened subjects also had better pulmonary function than the historical controls with significantly higher forced expiratory volume at 1 second and forced vital capacity data at both 5 and 10 years of age.

Developing Policy For CF Neonatal Screening

It would be ideal if health policy decision making could be driven exclusively and rapidly by incontrovertible scientific evidence. This rarely occurs and has never been the case for any newborn screening test. History shows that the phenylketonuria (PKU) test was widely implemented in the 1960s because of parental and legislative pressure following development of the combination of dried newborn blood specimen technology and the Guthrie test for phenylalanine levels.[1] Other newborn screening tests were implemented soon thereafter without first being established convincingly through research. Currently, however, the value of some tests is being challenged and all such tests have technical limitations.[1]

In the case of CF, with the trypsinogen/DNA method now being well established,[4] the challenge is to determine if there are sufficient benefits and cost justification to implement routine screening based on published criteria for routine implementation as reviewed elsewhere. [2-4] Wisconsin dealt with this question when congenital adrenal hyperplasia (CAH) screening was first being contemplated and specific criteria were developed for adding newborn screening tests.[1] When nutritional benefits of CF neonatal screening were demonstrated, the same criteria were used by applying the "evidentiary model" to develop policy.[2] We believe the time has come that "the burden of proof is on those who argue against newborn screening for cystic fibrosis."[3] We are proud that Wisconsin was the first state in the US to implement routine IRT/DNA screening for CF.[15] Other states have contacted us and are now considering this strategy as suggested by the CDC statement that "sufficient evidence exists to recommend pilot, state-based demonstration programs."[18]

Conclusions

The Wisconsin CF Neonatal Screening Project was initiated as a randomized clinical trial of early diagnosis, but it eventually evolved into a definitive investigation of the epidemiology of childhood CF. The advantages of longitudinal evaluation coupled to systematic therapy became obvious early in the project. One of the most significant features has been the study of defined patient populations. This has allowed us to uncover the truth about CF epidemiology in an unbiased fashion and avoid interpretative errors and misperceptions that develop with anecdotal based inferences and cross-sectional, observational studies. Many new clinical insights have emerged from our database, ranging from defining the true CF incidence, to identification of some of the risk factors for malnutrition and pseudomonas acquisition.

This project could not have been successful, and indeed would not have been feasible, without modern computing and biostatistical methods. The database we've generated now contains over 988,000 observations accumulated over a period of about 15 years. Fortunately, we've been blessed with outstanding, dedicated biostatisticians who gain insights while remaining unbiased and maintaining the integrity of the study (assured only because healthcare providers and those who generate laboratory data have been kept blinded about statistical analyses throughout the project). I am especially indebted to Dr. Michael Kosorok who has been our leader in data management and analysis while serving on the faculty of UW-Madison's Department of Biostatistics and Medical Informatics.

This study has also benefited greatly from having so many other excellent collaborating investigators on the UW-Madison campus and at the Medical College of Wisconsin. At each juncture in the investigation, whenever a pivotal issue emerged, we have always been able to identify an enthusiastic, experienced faculty member with the expertise needed to address a particular research question. In addition, the CF Center Directors in Madison (Drs. Elaine Mischler, Chris Green, and Michael Rock) and Milwaukee (Drs. Ted Bruns, and Mark Splaingard) have been the *sine qua non* of this investigation. It is incredible in retrospect, that so much talent and interest would be available and that so many loyal coworkers would sustain their interest and commitment in this project.

In closing, to return to a more personal perspective, I've felt fortunate and privileged to be able to lead this investigation while serving in administrative roles as Chair of Pediatrics and Dean of the University of Wisconsin Medical School. I've always said that "a steady diet of administration is nauseating," and this led me to sustain my academic/clinical role as both a priority and a pleasure. Much of the pleasure has been derived from the thrill of discovery, the gratification of research productivity, and ultimately being able to make a difference in our care of patient populations and in our understanding of CF, creating knowledge along the way by generating and interpreting population derived data.

In addition, the Wisconsin CF Neonatal Screening Project has provided the perfect academic/clinical opportunity for convergence of my various interests; cystic fibrosis, neonatology, laboratory medicine, nutrition, pulmonology, epidemiology, biostatistics, ethics, and patient/parent communication. As the evolution of this project developed toward epidemiologic research, I benefited greatly by having the opportunity to train at two exceptional public health schools, namely University of Michigan (summer epidemiology courses) and the London School of Hygiene and Tropical Medicine, University of London (advanced epidemiology and biostatistics). It is ironic in retrospect that my earlier dilemma about a residency training program in clinical pathology (before being struck by a "pediatrics thunderbolt") was resolved by the ability to work in the field of laboratory medicine as applied to children at risk for CF.

References:

1. Allen DB, Farrell PM. "Newborn screening." *Adv Pediatr* 1996;43:231-70.
2. Farrell PM, Mischler EH. "Newborn screening for cystic fibrosis." *Adv Pediatr* 1992;39:31-64.
3. Farrell PM, et al. "Improving the health of patients with cystic fibrosis through neonatal screening." *Adv Pediatr* 2000;47:79-115.
4. Wilcken B and Travert G. "Neonatal screening for cystic fibrosis: Present and future." *Acta Pediatr* 1999; 88 suppl 432:33-5.
5. Water DL, Wilcken B, Irwig L, Van Asperen P, Mellis C, Simpson JM, et al. "Clinical outcomes of newborn screening for cystic fibrosis." *Arch Dis Child Fetal Neonatal Ed* 1999;80:F1-F7.

6. Crossley JR, Elliott RB, Smith PA. "Dried-blood spot screening for cystic fibrosis in the newborn." *Lancet* 1979;1:742-4.

7. Shwachman H, Redmond A, Khaw KT. "Studies in cystic fibrosis: report of 130 patients diagnosed under 3 months of age over a 20-year period." *Pediatrics* 1970;46:335-43.

8. Hammond KB, Abman SH, Sokol RJ, Accurso FJ. "Efficacy of statewide screening for cystic fibrosis by assay for trypsinogen concentrations." *N Engl J Med* 1991;325:769-774.

9. Farrell PM, Bieri JG, Fratantoni JC, Wood RE, Fischer VW and di Sant'Agnese PA. "The occurrence and effects of human vitamin E deficiency: A study in patients with cystic fibrosis." *J Clin Invest* 1977; 60:233-241.

10. Ad Hoc Committee Task Force on Neonatal Screening, Cystic Fibrosis Foundation. "Neonatal screening for cystic fibrosis: position paper." *Pediatrics* 1983; 72:741-5.

11. Lai HC, Kosorok MR, Sondel SA, et al. "Growth status in children with cystic fibrosis based on the National Cystic Fibrosis Patient Registry data: evaluation of various criteria used to identify malnutrition." *J Pediatr* 1998;132:478-85.

12. Orenstein DM, Boat TF, Stem RC, Tucker AS, Charnock EL, Matthews LW, Doershuk CF. "The effect of early diagnosis and treatment in cystic fibrosis." *Am J Dis Child* 1977; 131:973.

13. Fost NC, Farrell PM. "A prospective randomized trial of early diagnosis and treatment of cystic fibrosis: a unique ethical dilemma." *Clin Res* 1989;37:495-500.

14. Rock MJ, Mischler EH, Farrell PM et al. "Newborn screening for cystic fibrosis is complicated by age-related decline in immunoreactive trypsinogen levels." *Pediatrics* 1990;85:1001-07.

15. Kerem B, Rommens JM, Buchanan JA, et al. "Identification of the cystic fibrosis gene:: Genetic analysis." *Science* 1989;245:1073-80.

16. Farrell PM, Aronson RA, Hoffman GL, et al. "Newborn screening for cystic fibrosis in Wisconsin: First application of population-based molecular genetics testing." *Wisc Med J* 1994;93:415-21.

17. Farrell PM, Kosorok MR, Laxova A, et al. "Nutritional benefits of newborn screening for cystic fibrosis." *N Engl J Med.* 1997;337:963-69.

18. Centers for Disease Control and Prevention, "Newborn Screening for Cystic Fibrosis: A Paradigm for Public Health Genetics Policy Development." *Morbidity and Mortality Weekly Report.* U.S. Department of Health and Human Services, Vol. 46, No. RR-16, Dec. 1997.

19. Dankert-Roelse JE, te Meerman GJ. "Long term prognosis of patients with cystic fibrosis in relation to early detection by neonatal screening in a cystic fibrosis center." *Thorax* 1995;50:712-18.

10

Applying the Center Concept: Progressive Benefits from the Network

Pamela B. Davis, M.D., Ph.D.

The development of a national network of Cystic Fibrosis Care Teaching and Research Centers has had a major impact on survival of patients with cystic fibrosis (CF). Details of the origin and organization of the Center Program are in Chapters 11, 16, and 17. When the disease was first described in 1938, survival was thought to be about 6 months, and death came from severe malnutrition or overwhelming pneumonia. This dismal state of affairs continued with only minor improvements following the introduction of antibiotics to the civilian population following World War II, and the advent of pancreatic enzyme supplements in the form of powdered animal pancreases. In 1949, a major heat wave in New York City led to an epidemic of heat prostration in infants, who have a high surface area to volume ratio. Dr. Paul di Sant'Agnese at Babies Hospital made the astute observation that the proportion of infants with CF among those with heat prostration was very high, and inferred that there must be some abnormality of the sweat in these infants. He was the first to demonstrate that the salt content of CF sweat was elevated fivefold over normal. This abnormality has proven to be quite consistent among patients and to be a valuable clinical discriminant for the disease. This abnormality turned into a new diagnostic test for the disease, the "sweat test," which allowed the identification of patients with milder disease. By the 1960s, as the sweat test came into wider use, the median survival age for patients with CF was estimated at about 5 years. This was before Dr. Warren Warwick started the Patient Registry.

At four separate locations, pioneering physicians gathered patients together for care and research. Harry Shwachman at Boston Children's Hospital, Paul Patterson in Albany, Paul di Sant'Agnese at Babies Hospital in New York (and later at the National Institutes of Health), and LeRoy Matthews at Babies and Children's Hospital in Cleveland began to collect patients, learn from them both in clinical observational studies and in the laboratory, provide encouragement and advice to the families, and most of all, manage a program of intensive symptomatic treatment of these patients. Families, desperate for hope, followed complicated daily treatment plans for their children that involved attempts to moisten the desiccated secretions in the airways, assist in removal of the secretions, treat infectious exacerbations with antibiotics, and administer pancreatic enzyme supplements and vitamins. The best documented program was by Matthews in Cleveland. By the late 1950s, he had such remarkable results (no one died in the first two years following initiation of the comprehensive treatment program) that it attracted still more patients from distant locales.

The directors of these four early Programs, Patterson, di Sant'Agnese, Shwachman, and Matthews, also became the "founding fathers" of a parents' organization designed to facilitate communication with families, provide emotional support, give hope, and provide an outlet for the families' desire to do more for their children. The founding fathers knew that even the most intensive symptomatic treatments would ultimately fail, and research was the hope for better understanding leading to definitive therapies. Thus, they encouraged the parents to raise money for research, to allow their children to participate in studies, and to participate themselves. The desire and dedication of the families and their friends had led to a voluntary health organization, originally called the National Cystic Fibrosis Research Foundation and later simply the Cystic Fibrosis Foundation (CFF). This Foundation came to represent the ultimate in professionalism and success in fund raising, public policy, and forward looking to the cure or control of a disease.

These prominent programs had the opportunity to observe the disease under treatment and make inferences about its pathobiology, which contributed critical information to our understanding of CF. They were a nidus for the formation of the Care Teaching and Research Center Program started by the Foundation in 1961. For many years, the clinical observations were all we knew for sure about the disease. Reports of the clinical manifestations of the disease, especially when they surveyed dozens or hundreds of patients, gave valuable information about the extent of the disease and its fundamental nature. Moreover, the observational studies formed the basis for therapeutic investigations as well.

Over the next twenty years, there were great variations in survival around the country. At institutions like Rainbow Babies and Children's Hospital/University Hospitals of Cleveland, and the Hospital for Sick Children in Toronto, where aggressive treatment was the order of the day (though treatment was not necessarily identical at every site), median survival age skyrocketed to the mid-twenties and beyond, especially for males. At the same time, some of the Centers established by the CFF after 1961 still felt that treatment was ultimately futile and concentrated their efforts on patient comfort and easing dying. Thus, the median survival age for CF patients nationwide was only in the early to mid teens in the late 1960s and early 1970s. From its beginnings with the first few Centers associated with the CF Foundation, the Center network grew to 53 Centers reporting nearly 5,300 patients by 1966, and by 1973, over 10,000 patients were reported by 106 Centers.

As the network developed and information could be shared, it became clear that aggressive care was not necessarily incompatible with compassionate care. More and more Centers adopted the aggressive, comprehensive approach to CF patient care. The principles of CF care enunciated by the early Centers have endured. They were: 1) attention to nutrition, 2) removal of the tenacious secretions from the airway (with mechanical and pharmacologic assistance), and 3) vigorous antibiotic therapy of the lung infection. Over time, the specifics of the care changed. Enzymes improved, mist tents went out of favor, various devices to assist clearance of secretions became available which obviated the need of another person to clap the chest by hand, new mucolytics were released, and newer, more potent antibiotics became available. Newer formulations of pancreatic enzymes came to replace the powder and pressed tablets. Complications of the older formulations, such as allergic sensitization to the powder and the hyperuricemia associated with the tablets, simply vanished. The Foundation supported regular Center Director's meetings where information and new treatment approaches could be shared, and the patients benefited.

At first, when the CF Foundation began to sponsor the Center network, financial support was minimal. After all, the Foundation had as its primary goal the conquest of the disease, and emphasized research for the future rather than care for the here and now. However, as the CF Foundation grew and prospered financially under the strong leadership of Robert J. Beall, Ph.D., first as Medical Director 1980–83, then as Executive Vice President, and finally, since 1994, as President and Chief Executive Officer, there was enough money to go around, so the financial support for the Centers improved. This improved support, rendered in the form of grants to the Centers, gave the CF Center Directors new stature in their Pediatric Departments. Money talks. In turn, they were able to command resources from their hospitals and Departments, and this improved the care for patients with CF still further. In addition, groups of patients with a similar disease, enthusiastic about research and backed by a Foundation that offers grants for research, became more visible in the research community, and attracted new investigators to the field.

CF Centers were a boon to patients and families, as well. The association with other patients, the sense of not being alone, the sharing of strategies for coping, and the sense of hope were all of great help to the patients. The variety of personnel to whom they could turn, besides the physician, was also a great help. The nurse, social worker, respiratory therapist, dietician, and genetic counselor, all became resources for the family, who might be reluctant to "bother the doctor" with a "stupid question." Hospitalization at a CF Center associated hospital assured access to knowledgeable caregivers. Care was planned, and could be observed to be effective as patients aged into their teens and twenties. This gave hope and inspiration to the parents of younger children, who rededicated themselves to vigorous daily prophylactic care. Participation in the CF Foundation, fund raising and consciousness raising, as well as participation in clinical research, gave the sorrow and anger over the diagnosis of a fatal disease some acceptable focus and outlet. The advantages to being associated with experts in the disease were considerable.

However, as time went on, it became clear that there were risks associated with Centers as well. Although early data suggested that there was little, if any, person to person transmission of bacterial infection by CF patients, in the late 1970s and early 1980s it became clear that at least one organism, *Burkholderia cepacia*, which was quite dangerous for CF patients, was transmitted in precisely a person to person manner. Commerce among patients in waiting rooms, hospital rooms and playrooms, CF Foundation functions, social occasions, support groups, and fundraisers was sharply curtailed in order to prevent spread of this organism. This necessity changed the complexion of the support structure that had grown up in the Centers. The support structure began to be focused on the relation between patients and their families and the caregivers, and much less on the exchange among the patients and families. Patients with CF rarely were hospitalized in the same room any more, and even casual contact in the playrooms was discouraged. Patients who were infected with *B. cepacia* became hospitalized separately from those who were not, but since infection could have occurred since the previous culture was reported, even contact between ostensibly uninfected patients was not encouraged. The intellectual and clinical advantages of the CF Center remained for families, but the social advantages diminished. Further concerns over transmission of *Pseudomonas aeruginosa* from person to person, particularly from infected to uninfected patients, have further heightened concerns about the clinic setting and may compel further changes in Center structure and function. This may impact especially on newly diagnosed patients, who are less likely to harbor *Pseudomonas aeruginosa*, but more likely to need the support and encouragement of other "CF families."

A big step forward came when the CF Foundation began to site visit and accredit Centers on a regular basis. This required the setting of standards for staffing, laboratory testing, and clinical care. These standards provided Center Directors with leverage in their institutions to demand appropriate support services and coverage. For example, by specifying acceptable and unacceptable means of performing the sweat test, a key diagnostic test for the disease, and by withholding accreditation (and therefore money) if the methods used at the hospital were not acceptable, the CF Foundation was able to assure diagnostic standards for detection of the disease, at least at their accredited Centers. Examples abound of misdiagnoses of CF from sweat tests performed in nonstandard fashion at hospitals not accustomed to rigorous quality control of the process. Another important standard has been the periodic outside testing of microbiology laboratories with a panel of test samples, in order to assure that they can detect rarer organisms such as the *Burkholderia cepacia*. The accreditation site visits proved important in assuring that the Centers have available the appropriate spectrum of ancillary health care providers, including social workers, dedicated nurses, respiratory therapists, and nutritionists, since documentation of their participation in patient care was required for accreditation. The knowledge that the Center would be reviewed periodically encouraged the hospitals to continue Center support. The Center accreditation grew to include reviews of randomly selected charts, which ensured that the frequency of patient contact, documentation of cultures and pulmonary function tests, and participation of nonphysicians such as social workers or nutritionists in patient care actually occurs. Standards everywhere were raised. A similar process has occurred more recently with the establishment of adult CF Centers, focused on the care of adults with CF.

In 2001, over 110 CF Care Centers, which have 30 Affiliate Programs in 46 states, the District of Columbia, and Puerto Rico, are accredited by the Foundation, along with some 90 Adult Pulmonary Centers.

Impact on Care

There is considerable evidence that collecting patients for care into Centers improves survival, though since this is the norm in the United States, much of the supporting data comes from Western Europe. Moreover, there is good evidence that the intensity of care, apart from the specifics of care, improves survival and slows the rate of decline of pulmonary function. The initial evidence for this came from a still unpublished study performed by Robert Wood, M.D., Ph.D., who was able to select three Centers of comparable size, tenure of Center Director, and demographic characteristics. Yet each of these Centers had vastly different median survival ages, one twice and one three times the median survival age of the worst Center. The Center with the best survival had the greatest intensity of care, as defined by the number of outpatient visits per patient and number of cultures, pulmonary function tests, and hospitalizations, despite the fact that one would predict that the Center with poorer survival might have sicker patients, who would require more intense care. Subsequent studies, with a much larger database of over 19,000 patients, show that the slowest rates of decline of FEV_1, a measure of rapidity of decline of pulmonary function, are found in the Centers with the most intense care, as defined by the most pulmonary function tests, the most cultures, the most hospital days, and the most time on antibiotics. The collection of patients into Centers allows such data to be collected efficiently and the impact of practice patterns on outcomes to be determined.

The impact of Center care on survival is now clearly evident. The median survival age for patients with CF in the United States has been hovering between 29 and 32 for the last five years, a definite improvement compared to 20 years ago, when only select Centers had survival that good. As more and more Centers nationwide have adopted an aggressive clinical approach, it is clear that the patients have benefited. As calculated by the CF Foundation patient registry, median survival age best represents the median survival age a child born with CF in the United States today can expect. Of course, some individual patients will not achieve this median age, and some individual patients will live much longer, but the increase in the median survival age is strong evidence that, on the whole, patients with CF do better now than they did before the Center network took hold. This patient registry documented great increase, compared to forty years ago when the Centers program began in just a few sites, is a therapeutic triumph.

Research and the Center Program

The latest phase entered by the Centers is that of research. This has occurred at several levels and the need had been anticipated and plans made (see Chernoff Chapter). The most obvious connection to the clinical Centers has been their participation in multicenter studies of drugs for patients with CF, which require large numbers of patients to be recruited nearly simultaneously. In order to determine efficacy within a reasonable time (in an industry for which time is money), hundreds of patients meeting entry particular criteria had to be accessed, enrolled in a short time frame, followed appropriately, and the data retrieved by the data monitors in timely fashion. The Centers now came full circle. Whereas when the Centers began, the observational studies conducted in them provided the basic information for development of hypotheses to be tested in the laboratory, now the availability of well characterized and willing patients in the Centers allowed new therapies developed in the laboratories to be tested in patients. The CF Foundation had mandated their access to many diagnostic tests useful for clinical monitoring that now became important as outcome measures - for example, pulmonary function testing, other laboratory testing, microbiology, or sweat testing. These tests now became outcome measures for clinical trials, and were already available and met certain quality standards. Patient records had already been centralized in order to be reported to the vital CF Foundation Patient Registry, so it was possible to access patients meeting particular criteria without undue records searching. The patient registry continues to serve as an invaluable resource.

It was the Center network that allowed enrollment of over 950 patients in a three-arm trial of recombinant human DNase aerosols and completion of a six month drug trial within a year's time. These results were the critical data which led to approval of this drug by the Food and Drug Administration (FDA) for use in patients with CF. Rapid access and deployment in the Centers reduces the costs of clinical testing for a pharmaceutical developer, and this, combined with the provisions of the Orphan Drug Act, makes CF an attractive target disease among "orphan" diseases (that is, diseases which affect too few patients to guarantee profit from specific drug development). The network of clinical centers has also conducted a multicenter trial of amiloride, a study of aerosol tobramycin, a study of alternate day steroid therapy, and a study of high dose ibuprofen for CF. The amiloride trial failed to show benefit, in contrast to a widely publicized pilot study published in the *New England Journal of Medicine*, and has not yet been published. The alternate day steroid trial uncovered adverse effects which were not predicted by the pilot trial, and forced this strategy to be abandoned. On the other hand, the alternative anti-inflammatory treatment, high dose ibuprofen, emerged as both effective and safe in a four year study published in the *New England Journal of Medicine*. The trial of high dose aerosol tobramycin led to the release of this formulation of the drug by the FDA for use in CF. Thus, one entirely new drug and one reformulated antibiotic have come to patients as a result of extensive and intensive Phase III testing in the Centers, an "old" drug (ibuprofen) has found a new application to CF, and two potential new therapies, both of which seemed quite promising in the pilot studies, have been put aside as either ineffective or too dangerous. As this research function of the Centers becomes increasingly important, the CF Foundation has added participation in clinical trials as a criterion for accreditation.

Another example of effective use of the clinical Center network was in the discovery of the CF gene. Several active research groups, some supported by the CF Foundation, in competition to find the CF locus by positional cloning, needed access to DNA from families with multiple affected siblings. In order to accumulate a sufficient number of these families, many Centers had to be accessed, and cooperate in obtaining blood samples for analysis. The work done in the laboratories of

Dr. Ray White in Utah, Dr. Robert Williamson in London, and the actual discoverers, Drs. Lap-Chee Tsui, Francis Collins, and Jack Riordan, could not have been accomplished without this valuable resource. Moreover, convincing themselves and the community at large that they had found the real CF gene required demonstration of the expression of the gene in affected cell types. A sweat duct cell cDNA library, derived from cells from patients, figured prominently in the discovery of the gene. These clinical samples required the cooperation and collaboration of physicians to establish.

At another level of research, the Center network has become the basis of an even more sophisticated network of research centers and clinical research centers initiated by the CF Foundation. Some of the early clinical Centers had directors gifted with vision, who recognized that however assiduous they were with symptomatic care, real progress would depend on better understanding of the disease process. They encouraged a generation of bench scientists to turn their attention to CF and fostered the training of the next generation of educated and committed clinicians. di Sant'Agnese and Matthews were in the forefront of this effort. di Sant'Agnese moved to the National Institutes of Health to set up a research program in coordination with a clinical program, where I had the privilege to train when it was in its heyday. This clinical associate program not only provided a model of bench to bedside science, but also trained many of the leaders in CF and CF research. These included Thomas Boat, M.D., Lynn Taussig, M.D., Robert Wood, M.D., Ph.D., Philip Farrell, M.D., Ph.D., Richard Grand, M.D., Richard Talamo, M.D., Lewis Gibson, M.D., Robert Schwartz, M.D., Lucy Lester, M.D., Allen Lapey, M.D., and Van Hubbard, M.D., Ph.D., among others, as well as other prominent academic pediatricians such as Stuart Handwerger, M.D. Matthews set out to study the properties of mucus, assembling a group of Ph.D. scientists to help, and obtained first a program project grant in CF in 1964, and later Dr. Carl Doershuk obtained a Core Center Grant in 1983, which supported individual R01 grants. I had the opportunity to assume leadership of the Cleveland program in 1985, as it developed from a program focused on mucus to a broader based program exploring the cell and molecular biology of the basic defect as well as its downstream consequences in the lung. Both Drs. di Sant'Agnese and Matthews began to train physician-scientists and physicians in CF and pediatric pulmonology long before the subspecialty was constituted and recognized by the American Board of Pediatrics.

These Centers pioneered the cross fertilization of the bench scientist and the clinician, and served as the model for the CF Foundation's Research Development Program (RDP), which competitively established research centers around the country, beginning in 1981 at the University of Alabama. This RDP program, established under the leadership of Dr. Robert Beall by the Cystic Fibrosis Foundation, was a product of the Strategic Plan (see Chernoff Chapter). It required extensive new funding and was backed by an aggressive fund raising campaign headed by Doris Tulcin. Doris was a parent of a child with CF and herself a past President and a major contributor to the CF Foundation, who evolved into its most effective fundraiser. The program expanded rapidly with a peak number of 13 such Centers.

However, once the gene was discovered the Centers engaged in gene finding moved on to other areas, and the principal investigators and their groups moved and shifted interests, so that at the present time the RDP program consists of 10 Centers. These Centers are now located at the University of California at San Francisco, Case Western Reserve University in Cleveland, Children's Hospital Medical Center in Cincinnati, the University of Iowa at Iowa City, the Johns Hopkins University School of Medicine in Baltimore, the University of North Carolina at Chapel Hill, the Institute for Human Gene Therapy at the University of Pennsylvania in Philadelphia, the University of Pittsburgh, and the University of Washington in Seattle, accompanying the University of Alabama at Birmingham. These Centers have a variety of scientific foci, ranging from the cell and molecular biology of cystic fibrosis transmembrane conductance regulator (CFTR), to the developmental biology of the lung and to the pulmonary infections and inflammation that are the proximate cause of death in CF.

These Centers consisted of a senior scientist as Director, with several other scientists working in concert on problems related to CF, and included a training component. Although some of these Centers were predominantly laboratory based, over time the CF Foundation began to insist on connections with a clinical CF Center in order to provide motivation and stimulation for the bench scientist and clinician alike. As the RDP Centers flourished, the CF Foundation prevailed upon the National Institutes of Health to offer grants for research centers in CF. Many of the established RDP Centers then competed successfully for this federal funding. Eventually this network of Centers supported by both the National Institute for Diabetes, Digestive, and Kidney Diseases (NIDDK) (currently at Case Western Reserve University, the Hospital for Sick Children in Toronto, the University of Alabama, and the University of Pittsburgh) and the National Heart, Lung, and Blood Institute (NHLBI) (currently at Case Western Reserve University, the University of California at San Francisco, the University of Iowa, and the University of North Carolina at Chapel Hill), grew up, and have been quite productive for the field. The program for the large annual North American Cystic Fibrosis Conference and for the smaller, by invitation, the annual Williamsburg meeting sponsored by the CF Foundation are heavily populated with investigators from the RDP and NIH supported Centers. These Centers, and the participants in the RDP, have been the driving forces for progress in CF, with their synergy between different disciplines and their bench to bedside approaches. They have provided information on structure and function of the CFTR molecule, interaction of CFTR with other proteins, the electrophysiologic properties of the CFTR channel, the propensity toward airway infections, the inflammatory response in CF, and the first gene therapy experiments in CF patients. Most recently, the NIH has supported Centers for Gene Therapy with a focus on CF, in a program which has proven highly competitive and highly productive, and currently supports Centers at Cornell University Medical College, the Institute for Human Gene Therapy at the University of Pennsylvania, the University of Florida, the University of North Carolina at Chapel Hill, and the University of Washington in Seattle. Clearly, for these Centers especially, access to a patient population and excellent clinical collaboration is essential.

The overall success of the CF research enterprise, the cloning of the gene in 1989, the identification of the nature of the basic defect by Dr. Paul Quinton in the early 1980s, the increased knowledge of the downstream consequences of the CF defect in epithelia and organs from then on, combined with the growth of biotechnology have all served to spawn new opportunities for drug development for CF. Some of these drugs were aimed at either correcting the basic defect by activating various mutant alleles, or at controlling the excessive inflammatory response in the CF airways. Direct biochemical or physiological assessments of drug effects in these areas required exacting, highly standardized in vivo measurements. For drugs presumed to affect ion transport, in vivo physiologic efficacy could be assessed by nasal potential difference measurements, a technique previously used only for research purposes. For drugs directed at the inflammatory response, bronchoalveolar lavage (BAL) can sample the lower airways and allow direct measurement of inflammatory mediators and cells. This procedure had also been used predominantly for research purposes. These, and other highly technical procedures, are quite useful for Phase I and Phase II testing of new therapeutics, if they can be standardized among sites. In order to provide a group of Centers with technical skills to perform these studies as well as access to large numbers of well-characterized patients for Phase I and Phase II testing, the CF Foundation in 1998 established the Therapeutics Development Network, which now consists of eight cooperating Centers who agree to standardize methods of data collection and acquire the necessary skills for such testing. These Centers, located in Baltimore, Boston, Chapel Hill, Cincinnati, Cleveland, Denver, Palo Alto, and Seattle are geographically disperse and may draw patients from the neighboring clinical centers for study. This highly specialized center network represents the next level of clinical CF centers, pioneering the new therapies of the future. This network represents the final stage in the "bench to bedside" approach to this disease.

All in all, the development of CF Centers, at many levels and with a breadth of different focuses, has catalyzed many of the important improvements in CF care and research of the last few decades. It has been a privilege to observe this process from a ringside seat at the Center in Cleveland, which participates in the RDP, the NIDDK and NHLBI Centers, as well as the Therapeutics Development Network and the Clinical Center network. By the beginning of 1999, there were 19,513 patients reported under care at the Clinical Centers, with over 9,000 adults. The collection of patients in these locations that can provide the necessary expertise, support personnel, and experience with the disease has undoubtedly improved survival and quality of life for patients with CF. These Centers have also nucleated research programs in CF, which have produced dazzling advances in the last decade especially. Finally, they have also served as the basis for tour de force clinical studies which have raised the level of clinical research conducted in patients with CF and facilitated new drug development and approval for patients with CF.

How Has the Community Helped
With Care and Research?
Volunteers Organized to Work Together

11

Origin and Development of the Cystic Fibrosis Foundation

Evelyn and Milton Graub, M.D.

> The Cystic Fibrosis story is built on the struggles and anguish of all Cystic Fibrosis families. The success of the Cystic Fibrosis Foundation is directly attributed to their efforts

Early Years

It was 1950 and we had just visited the Babies Hospital of Columbia University in New York City. Our son Lee was 2 years old and had been coughing since birth, in addition to having abnormal stools. We had visited local pediatricians and the consultants at the Philadelphia Children's Hospital but I was not satisfied with the diagnosis. I was told that our son had a syndrome, which the Germans called "Exudative Diathesis." It was recommended that irradiation of the nasopharynx would help; but of course it did not. Our daughter Kathy was born the following year and also had the disease.

Being a neophyte pediatrician, I searched the literature and realized that Lee might have a fatal and rare disease, Cystic Fibrosis of the Pancreas. The pediatric text hardly mentioned the disease. The one who had described the disease in the US in 1938, was Dr. Dorothy Andersen, a pediatric pathologist at Columbia University Medical School. She documented the microscopic changes in the pancreas, associated with severe pulmonary changes. Dr. Andersen was a bright compassionate and sensitive scientist who was also a chain smoker. Not many years later she died of pulmonary carcinoma.

I was so distraught I called Dr. Andersen, on a Sunday morning and found her in her laboratory office. She listened to the medical history of my son and saw him the next day. These were the pre-sweat test days. The diagnosis was much more difficult and was made, primarily on clinical findings plus analysis of duodenal secretions. These were done and the diagnosis of cystic fibrosis of the pancreas was established. Since Dr. Andersen was a pathologist, she referred Lee for further clinical care to Dr. Paul di Sant'Agnese. He was a pediatric specialist, and a delight. Soft spoken, reassuring, and supportive. In the next few years, he and associates would identify the sweat electrolyte defect that led in turn to development of the iontophoresis sweat test to simplify the diagnosis of cystic fibrosis (CF).

In late 1951, I received a call from Dr. Lesnick, a local pharmacist who told me he had a relative in Los Angeles, California who had lost a grandchild with cystic fibrosis (CF). I was able to contact her and she confirmed that indeed not only had she lost a grandchild but had formed a small group of families and friends to advance the CF cause. It was named the "Jenny Lesnick Fund" in memory of her grandchild. **I believed that this was the first group to organize in the fight against cystic fibrosis.**

In 1952, a few families met for the first time in Philadelphia to join together to share our common problems and possibly do something more for CF. We were a small and very diverse group. A mother, Mrs. Betty Mosser; a truck driver and his wife, Mr. & Mrs. Bill Bamford; a builder, Mr. Barney Moss; a lawyer and his wife, Mr. & Mrs. Robert C. Allen; and my wife, Evelyn, and myself. We met in the Girard Trust Bank Boardroom. Robert Allen was a vice president and was interested in helping but was not a parent. We met monthly thereafter and tried to devise ways of identifying new families. We were unsophisticated and rank amateurs in fund raising and public relations; however, we had great enthusiasm. Our major problem was identifying more CF families and encouraging their support. To accomplish this, Evelyn and I visited every newly diagnosed family personally, to inform them that a support system was available and that we needed their help. Some families were as far as 100 miles distant. We continued this effort until we were well established.

The disease was almost unknown to the public or even to the medical community. No one had heard of cystic fibrosis of the pancreas or CF. Locally we were successful at public relations due to the efforts of Sy Shaltz, who was a PR Professional. He was a special human being. He had just lost a twelve-year-old son due to leukemia. When I approached him to publicize this unknown CF disease, he readily accepted the challenge. He did not bill us for his agency services but also he had a fund of $1,200, contributions in memory of his son, which he generously contributed to our Foundation. Within a few years we had 13 local volunteer branches all raising funds, an office, and an Executive Director.

In 1954, Evelyn ran our first major fund raising event. We called it the "Friends of Cystic Fibrosis." It was exciting to see how supportive friends and families could be. There were 250 persons present. Most of them had never heard of this disease. I would never forget how proud I was to announce that we had raised $14,000, a huge sum in 1954, for a budding organization. This fundraiser continued for 42 years. Our guest speaker was Dr. Wynne Sharples, a local socialite and non-practicing pediatrician who was also the mother of two CF children. She was married to Dr. Robert Denton, a pediatrician who was involved with mucus chemistry. Dr. Sharples had the time, motivation, and resources to devote to this cause; she was to become our first National Cystic Fibrosis President. During the many years that Evelyn ran our major CF function, many notable entertainers performed. Among those were Joey Bishop, Roberta Peters, Rodney Dangerfield, Dick Van Dyke, David Brenner, Connie Stevens, Wayne Rogers, Theodore Bikel, and Dick Shawn.

Nationally, the visibility was much more difficult. However, our enterprise was not diminished. A dear friend, Nate Horrow was very close to Bert Parks, the Master of Ceremonies for the Miss America Pageant in Atlantic City. Berk Parks agreed to do anything he could. It was our plan that Mr. Parks go to the White House in Washington D.C. and in the presence of President Eisenhower kick off our national campaign. We were able to arrange all these details. Our CF President, Dr. Sharples, would be present. As you can imagine we were ecstatic. We would get national coverage. Lo and behold Dr. Sharples was pregnant and therefore changed her mind about the event and it was cancelled. We were devastated. Bert Parks, Mr. Horrow, and our contact in Washington were all disappointed. We needed that exposure so badly.

The following was another valiant attempt to obtain more recognition. My brother Dan married Nessa Weinstein in 1954. Her father, Charles Weinstein, was president of the Amalgamated Clothing Workers Union. He was a dedicated, sensitive human being. His foremost objective was to be supportive to his union members. He was truly an idealistic person. The Union was powerful and had great contacts. The William Morris Agency, a national talent agency, represented them. Nessa and Dan prevailed on her father to get the agency to obtain a Celebrity to represent our Foundation. Eddie Cantor, the popular Broadway and Hollywood celebrity, was a client of the agency. He was ill at the time and therefore suggested that Eddie Fisher be our Celebrity. Mr. Cantor had discovered Eddie Fisher and said Eddie would cooperate if he asked him. A meeting was set up on the West Coast. Bob Natal, my dear friend, and Mr. Weinstein were delighted. So, my brother Dan and I went.

We first had to meet with Eddie Cantor at noon in Los Angeles. We planned to take the entire trip in 36 hours if possible. Remember these were pre-jet days. The trip took 14 hours to the West Coast. We went directly to see Eddie Cantor in Beverly Hills and I could see he was not well. He immediately phoned Eddie Fisher who was performing in Las Vegas at the Sands. This was great as Eddie Fisher who was at the peak of his popularity and was married to Debbie Reynolds. He had just received a $1,000,000 TV contract from the Coca-Cola Company- the highest ever.

We arrived at the Sands Hotel in Las Vegas at 10 PM and went directly to Eddie Fisher's dressing room. While he was preparing for his next show, I asked him to be our national celebrity and to cooperate with our public relations efforts wherever possible. He accepted graciously. What a great coup. He insisted we see his show although we had to catch a midnight flight. When we were leaving he asked me if I ever gambled and I replied no, but my brother had a $10 chip. So Eddie Fisher said, "lets go partner at the dice table for a few minutes." It became especially exciting when we realized he was using $500 chips, but within 5 minutes he had lost $5,000 plus Dan's $10 chip. We made our plane on time, but often nothing goes as planned. One week later Debbie and Eddie agreed to split and we were advised not to use him in any of our PR efforts.

In my attempt to identify CF families to increase our numbers, in 1960 I sent a personal letter to each pediatrician in the area asking them to please identify any CF patients in their practice, so that we could tell them of our new organization and activities. I received no replies and did not realize until many years later that this type of activity was frowned upon by many of my pediatric colleagues. This came to my attention approximately ten years later. A good friend of mine, Dr. Pat Lucchesi, who was a prominent pediatrician and politician, informed me that he had been a member of the grievance committee of the County Medical Society. The committee indeed had received two letters of criticism that I was trying to steal some of their patients. I was devastated when he told me this, but he had known of my family's involvement with CF and therefore nothing came of these complaints. This incident indicates the uncooperative outlook that my medical colleagues had in those primitive CF days.

I had developed a thriving pediatric practice which was all consuming; and it was during this period that Evelyn and I came to a serious crossroad in our lives. It occurred to us one evening while traveling to the shore to see my parents, that we were confronted with: should we sit back and direct all our efforts to the support and care of our children or we should take that extra giant step and go beyond the ordinary and seriously devote all our efforts for research to possibly save our and other children's lives. We chose to get completely involved and never dreamed how overwhelming and consuming this decision would be.

In 1953 during our many hospital stays in New York City, we met other CF families. Margie & Vic Blitzer and Martha & Milton Satler from Bayside, New York who became our good friends, as was Bob Natal, a neighbor of theirs. He was a non-parent who became a devoted worker. We exchanged many ideas and Evelyn especially was very helpful in suggesting to them new helpful ideas. Bob Natal was an executive in a trucking firm and assumed early leadership not only in their new local organization but was also to become the second President of the National Foundation. He was exceptionally devoted, tactful and made many contributions to Foundation.

Birth of the Foundation

In 1955, during a routine visit to Dr. di Sant'Agnese, I found that an effort to form a National Foundation was in process. Dr. Sharples informed us that a Charter had been obtained and invited us to join in a national effort to fight this disease. As Philadelphia Chapter President, I was designated to represent our local organizations at a Founder's meeting to be held in New York City. I can recall how excited I was, as only in greater numbers and organizations would we be stronger and succeed. This Charter provided the legal structure for a Cystic Fibrosis Foundation but there was no Board as yet. This was the purpose of our New York City meeting. It was held in the offices of Dr. Rustin McIntosh, physician and Chief at Columbia Presbyterian Babies Hospital. Dr. McIntosh chaired the initial Founder's meeting.

Dr. Sharples was present, as were five representatives, one from each of the known organized chapters in the country. These were:

Mr. Robert Natal, New York business executive and non-parent

Mr. Charles Hardison, Los Angeles public relations executive and parent

Mr. Jim Dailey, Hartford businessman and parent

Milton Graub M.D., Philadelphia practicing pediatrician and parent

And a Boston businessman and parent

Also, there was a corporate lawyer from Philadelphia who accompanied Dr. Sharples and Dr. McIntosh.

Dr. Sharples immediately proposed that the Board of Trustees be made up of outstanding citizens whom she would designate. She was in an excellent position to do this as her father; Philip T. Sharples, was an industrialist and had the associations to obtain such a Board. Dr. Sharples envisioned an elitist Board with the chapters raising the funds, but without representation. Bob Natal, Charles Hardison, and myself immediately objected to this structure. There was much argument until it became clear a major compromise was necessary. **Chapter representation was mandatory.** After 2 years of struggle in Philadelphia, I very well knew that unless there was deep and continuing commitment from involved individuals on the Board, it would not survive. There had to be more personal involvement on the Board for so young an organization to succeed.

After much discussion I insisted that the chapters must have 50% representation on the Board of Trustees. Dr. Sharples was very displeased, as she had not anticipated any resistance to her proposed plan. There appeared to be a stalemate. Dr. McIntosh and the legal counsel finally advised that equal representation seemed fair. With the support of Dr. McIntosh, the compromise was accepted and the Foundation came into being. **Thus, through the enterprise and determination of Dr. Sharples and many CF families the National Cystic Fibrosis Research Foundation (NCFRF) was born in 1955.** Dr. Sharples was designated the new President. Each of the five chapters was to have 2 representatives and Dr. Sharples would appoint 10 members making a total of 20 members. At-large representatives who came to the Board were:

Joseph Heston, lawyer and parent from Sacramento, CA

Abe Birenbaum, shoe manufacturer from Philadelphia and grandparent

George Frankel, oil entrepreneur from Greenwich, Conn. and grandparent

Philip T. Sharples, industrialist from Philadelphia and
grandparent

Lawrence Saunders, medical book publisher from Philadelphia
and non-parent

The first CF scientific meeting I can recall was held around 1955 in Iowa
City, Iowa. It was called by the NCFRF and Dr. Charles May, Chairman of the
Department of Pediatrics at the University of Iowa. Many of the dedicated CF
physicians were trained initially either at Columbia University with Dr. Dorothy
Andersen or with Dr. Harry Shwachman at Boston Children's Hospital. The invi-
tees were all active physicians in the field. Some of those present were:

Harry Shwachman, M.D., Boston Children's Hospital

Paul di Sant'Agnese, M.D., Babies Hospital, New York

LeRoy Matthews, M.D., Babies and Children's Hospital,
Cleveland

Paul Patterson, M.D., Albany, New York

Gordon Gibbs, M.D., Lincoln, Nebraska

Giulio Barbero, M.D., Children's Hospital of Philadelphia

Warren Warwick, M.D., University of Minnesota

Wynne Sharples, M.D., President of the Foundation

Milton Graub, M.D., Hahnemann Medical College and
Hospital, Philadelphia

Dr. Barbero informed me that the meeting was to take place. I had not
been invited, but I decided to go as an uninvited guest. Keep in mind, I had two
sick CF children. I was gung-ho to get any research going and so little was known
of this disease. I was a member of the Board of Trustees and I felt a responsibility to
know medically all that was going on. I was determined and I went. The meeting
accomplished little except to identify all the medical leadership in this new and
challenging disease.

Early on I became acquainted with Dr. Matthews from Cleveland. His
enthusiasm, commitment, warmth, and intensity were so great that we entrusted
the ongoing care of our children to him. Evelyn and the children flew to Cleveland
every six weeks for their ongoing care. I believe that this is the type of confidence
and trust that every CF physician has exhibited through the years.

Early Decisions

The Board of Trustees initially met in Philadelphia, but soon realized that the corporate world was in New York City and it would be advantageous to move our
office there. Mr. George Frankel became a wonderful resource. Not only did he

have excellent contacts but he also offered space in his offices gratuitously on Fifth Avenue for the National offices. We utilized these offices for many years. One of Mr. Frankel's close friends was Basil O'Connor, the dynamic President of the National Infantile Paralysis Foundation (the Polio Foundation). The Polio Foundation had been in existence for many years and was eminently successful. Mr. O'Connor was a dear friend of President Franklin Delano Roosevelt, who had supported the Polio Foundation for many years. Mr. Frankel consulted with Basil O'Connor and was able to guide us in many of our early activities. Out of this close relationship with the Polio Foundation an offer was made to the NCFRF to merge. This was a momentous point in our history as the CF Board chose to maintain its identity and autonomy and go it alone. We certainly would have been swallowed up. Time has proven our wisdom in making this decision.

In Philadelphia, we had a similar offer from our United Way, to become part of them, participate in no fundraising, and receive $20,000 annually. Our function thus would be education and care. This offer was wisely rejected. The following year we raised $75,000 and had a bright independent future. Of course, this can be contrasted to the experience in Cleveland, where they not only remained an independent productive Chapter but also in addition were able to attract large sums from their United Way for support of their excellent research and care program headed by LeRoy Matthews.

The first years of the Foundation were a struggle but were very successful in that many new Chapters were added. Most significantly, a network of CF Centers was established in 1961 under the direction of Dr. Kenneth Landauer. Dr. Landauer had set up a similar national network of treatment centers at major medical institutions for the Polio Foundation. This concept proved to be very successful. Our CF Centers were to be located only at medical teaching facilities and were to encompass three most important attributes namely:

Care, Teaching, and Research, and came to be known as CTR Centers

Whereas previously we had devoted all of our resources to research, we now broadened our mandate to include care and education. The Centers have served as the corner stone for our patients and physicians until this day. Later we dropped the research title in our Foundation name and became the National Cystic Fibrosis Foundation. Much of our present day therapeutic and clinical research programs utilize extensively the patient registry information collected annually from our clinical Centers.

The early problems were raising enough funds to support our CF centers and finding sufficient funds for the meager research that was being done. There were many years when our program extended beyond our means and we had to ask our Centers to cut back their budgets after they had been approved. Our philosophy in those days was that even if we didn't have the research funds to budget, we would approve exemplary research and worry about the funding later. Our CF physicians through those tough years were magnificent; they were not only supportive and deeply committed to their patients but remained loyal and steadfast to the Foundation.

My Years as President of the Foundation

Mr. Robert Natal followed Dr. Sharples as President. He was a bright, efficient, and dedicated executive. His tact and common sense were refreshing, as was his genuine dedication. Unfortunately, Bob developed colon carcinoma and resigned after a few years. I was vice-president and became President in 1964. I realized that our research was too clinical. Our medical committees were composed primarily of pediatric clinicians, an observation not a criticism. The instrumentation and techniques were still too primitive to produce the basic answers we were seeking. *At this time our Foundation was not supporting one basic research fellowship.* These basic science fellowships are the heart of most research programs.

Although we were short of funds, I felt that we must go ahead and develop this program. I therefore called George Frankel, our trustee, and went to New York and had lunch with him at the Roosevelt Hotel. Bob Natal was ill but asked to come along. George Frankel was curious, as I had not told him what I wanted. What I wanted was $87,500 for our first research fellow. He was astounded. Bob Natal was startled, as this was a huge amount in those days. George was curious as to how I had ever arrived at such a figure. I explained that a basic research fellow at the National Institutes of Health (NIH) was getting $17,500 per year and that it takes a least 3–5 years for most research projects to be completed. George understood. He did not blink an eye and agreed. He even went a giant step further and exclaimed that he would not commit this for 5 years but would commit it in PERPETUITY. It was my turn to be astounded. This had been my first experience requesting a large grant and I felt I was in the presence of greatness. Later his legal counsel advised that the commitment be for 5 years and be renewed every 5 years. This grant was renewed for many years.

In order to expand our basic science expertise, I sought the guidance of Louis Sarett, PhD. and President of Merck and Companies Research Division. He was a dear friend of George Barrie, our National Executive Director. Dr. Sarett, through his offices, was in a position to call on almost any biological scientist consultant. He suggested that we meet to identify the basic scientific needs to solve the CF problem. We met at the Harvard Club in New York City and he brought James Watson, a Nobel Prize winner. George Barrie was also present. After I presented an overview of the disease, Dr. Sarett suggested and Dr. Watson agreed that what was needed was a cadre of outstanding basic scientists to be available to our Foundation for consultation. At Dr. Sarett's direction such a group was identified. It included:

Joshua Lederberg, Arthur Kornberg, and James Watson.

Each of these scientists was a Nobel Prize awardee. And there were six other consultants of varying expertise.

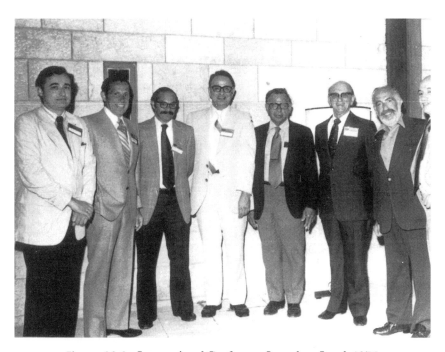

Figure 11.1. *International Conference, Jerusalem, Israel, 1976. Left to right, Richard C. Talamo, M.D., Johns Hopkins University, Baltimore; Milton Graub, M.D., Hahnemann University, Philadelphia; Kurt Hirschhorn, M.D., Mt. Sinai Hospital, New York; John Mangos, M.D., University of Florida, Gainesville; Harry Shwachman, M.D.; Jack Karpas, M.D., Hadassah Hospital, Jerusalem; Sam Ajl, Ph.D., National Polio Foundation. Courtesy of Dr. Milton Graub.*

Over the next few years, Joshua Lederberg and Arthur Kornberg organized and attended a CF genetics conference at the Weizman Institute in Israel. This was followed by another International Conference there in 1976. (Figure 11.1) The contribution that these scientists made was not scientific but rather that particular problems had to be solved in step by step fashion by selected groups of qualified investigators who the CF Foundation would support. I remember presenting this idea to Dr. Giulio Barbero and Dr. Warren Chernick. They agreed whole heartedly, but they cautioned that our clinically oriented medical council might not be sympathetic to competing projects. This was proven to be true when, the American Academy of Pediatrics met in Philadelphia and most of our Center Directors came to Philadelphia for these meetings. I invited approximately 20 of them for dinner to my home. After dinner, Dr. Barbero, in a very positive way, presented the New Program called **The GAP Conference** plan. The letters stood for Guidance, Action, and Projection. GAP was to fill in the gaps in our knowledge. Each GAP conference would be on a narrow particular problem with primarily young basic scientists in attendance. As predicted, many directors were outspoken and averse to the idea. Dr. Shwachman and others were not happy. Where would the funds come from for the new projects? Would the Center directors be involved in deciding who the grant recipients would be? The benefits were so obvious that the GAP Conference concept became a Foundation activity and, in form, remain until today. The funding for these meetings initially came from the Frankel family. Doris Tulcin subsequently provided a restricted fund from the Frankel Foundation to support these conferences for many years.

George Barrie was the Executive Director during the major part of my Presidency. He was a bright and knowledgeable person, had graduated from Harvard, and had gotten interested in the health field after his daughter had contracted polio. His background was with the Polio Foundation where his fund raising and administrative skills were honed. George was very astute but his major failing was that he was somewhat impatient at times with the average volunteer. This resulted in him not being the most popular. In spite of this deficiency, he was a very enterprising, creative, and effective organizer.

George was the first lay person to initiate contacts with the European Community to organize the International Cystic Fibrosis Association. At this time the only other countries that had any volunteer structure were Great Britain and Canada. France, Germany, Italy, and the Scandinavian Countries had small and scattered parent groups. The first meeting was held in Paris. George had visited Europe previously to arrange for this initial meeting. General Vacon of France was elected the first President; he was a genuine General and had no family ties with CF. The organization had a strong medical component headed by American, Dr. di Sant'Agnese; however, many physicians from Great Britain and other European Countries attended. Because the Lay representation was so unsophisticated, George Barrie was able to make a significant contribution in organization and fund raising to many of the countries just getting started. Most of the countries in Europe, Canada and eventually South America benefited from the direction that the International Association offered. Today, the North American CF Conference, initiated by Bob Beall and our own CF Foundation, is the focus of world CF interest—medical and lay.

In 1965, through the efforts of our Executive Director, Anne Capalino Brewer, and Pennsylvania Senator Hugh Scott, I was invited to the White House with our poster girl to take photos with President Lyndon Johnson. We had been disappointed in the past with President Eisenhower but now felt we could get some excellent PR; it was exciting. I was permitted to bring Evelyn and our daughters, Kathy who had CF, and Pearl. We met in the East Room of the White House where President Franklin D. Roosevelt had given his fireside chats. Lady Bird greeted us and told us the President was unfortunately detained. U Thant, the Secretary General of the United Nations, had just come in by helicopter for an emergency meeting, with our President. We watched as the Secretary General alit on the lawn and disappeared with President Johnson. Lady Bird was delightful, patient, charming, and gracious (Figure 11.2). Also present, was Kathryn Granahan, the Treasurer of the United States. We knew her previously as she came from Philadel-

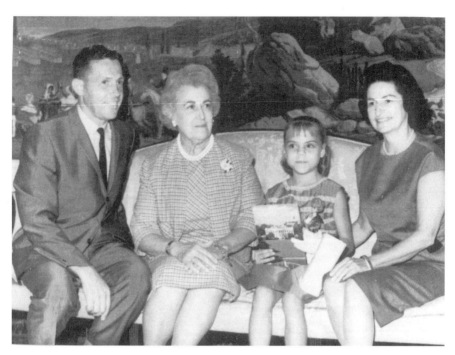

Figure 11.2. *Left to right, Milton Graub, M.D., President of the Foundation, Kathryn Granahan, Treasurer of the United States, CF Poster Child, Lady Bird Johnson, First Lady of the United States, in the Blue Room, 1966. Courtesy of Dr. Milton Graub.*

phia. We loved the intimate meeting but best of all the publicity was great for our CF cause.

When my first term as President of the Foundation ended in 1967, I was appointed to President Johnson's Committee on Employment of the Handicapped. This was a timely assignment since the committee was just starting to be presented with the problem of health insurance for those such as our CF young adults. In 1968, I was named to The National Health Council, a Presidential Committee on which I represented our Foundation with all of the other national Health Agencies.

Funding Research

The 1960s were days when the NIH supported most of the research funds in the US. At this juncture, we had few funds and as President I felt that we must tap into these NIH funds. We therefore sought out Colonel Luke Quinn, a lobbyist who was active on the Hill. He had been General Eisenhower's Aide during the Second World War. He was very influential and knew the important congressional health legislators. Few grants had been awarded for CF prior to this time.

His first act was to get our Foundation an audience with Mr. Daniel Flood. He was head of the subcommittee on Health in the House of Representatives. This committee was responsible for the allocation of 2 billion dollars for health each year. Serendipity was working in our favor. Mr. Flood came from Wilkes-Barre, PA and was a dear friend of my brother in law's aunt—Mollie Abramson. Also on his committee was Mr. Bob Michel from Peoria, IL. His secretary had three children with CF. Mr. Flood was a real character. He had been an actor and loved to dramatize. Dr. Matthews, Dr. Barbero, and Colonel Quinn were also present. Mr. Flood, who tried to be intimidating, asked me, "What is so important to be taking up his time." He knew nothing about CF. After telling him of the great prevalence and seriousness, I told him we were asking for 2 million dollars as a **line item** in the budget for basic research in CF from the National Institute for Arthritis and Metabolic Diseases (NIAMD). This Institute was responsible for CF at the NIH (as CF was listed within the metabolic diseases at that time). He exploded. In a loud voice he exclaimed, "How can you waste my time asking for 2 million dollars, when I have 2 *billion* dollars to allocate? Not only that, but no categorical disease has ever had a line item in the national budget." We were startled, but soon realized it was all part of his thespian act. He really was a gentle and cooperative person. Mr. Flood immediately arranged for our Foundation to testify before the entire appropriation subcommittee. The head of the NIAMD was in attendance. I told of our needs and Dr. Matthews described the research areas. Our testimony was written into the Congressional Record. Colonel Quinn shepherded our request through many obstacles and we prevailed. **We became the first categorical disease entity to have a line item written into the budget.**

Thus the National Institute for Arthritis and Metabolic Diseases (NIAMD) was directed to spend the 2 million dollars on CF related basic science. This grant was renewable yearly. We were anxious the next year to see how the 2 million dollars had been spent. We therefore requested this information from the NIAMD, but they were reluctant to release it. After much cajoling a list was produced. We were aghast that the grants were indeed basic science oriented, but they had little or no relationship to CF. Colonel Quinn, Mr. Flood, and the entire Committee were furious. Thus, when our Foundation testified in the following year, the NIAMD was admonished for not carrying out the mandate of the Congress and the grant was renewed with the understanding that the funds go for CF related basic research.

The science remained primitive for many years with no real insight until the genetic abnormality was revealed. There were many red herrings, i.e., abnormalities in the mucus which were really break down products, a "Spock" factor which we thought directly affected ciliary activity, and for so many years sodium was thought to be the culprit until the abnormal chloride transport was identified by Paul Quinton. The institution of the Basic Science Program was a major step forward. However, it remained for the tenure of President Doris Tulcin, who developed a close working relationship with the NIH, for the tenure of President Robert Dresing, who brought corporate participation which enabled us to fund the scien-

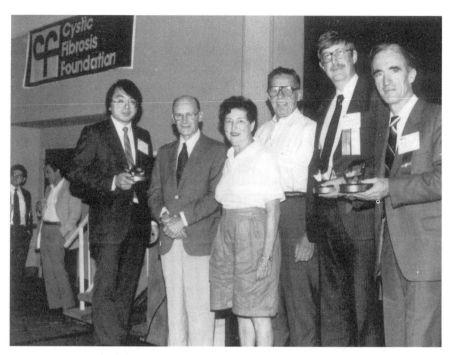

Figure 11.3. *CF Gene Elucidators. Left to right. Lap-Chee Tsui, Francis Collins, and John Riordan, along with Paul di Sant'Agnese, Evelyn Graub and Milton Graub. Courtesy of Dr. Milton Graub.*

tific program, and especially for the scientific leadership of Robert Beall, Ph.D., who garnered the scientists who identified the abnormal gene (Figure 11.3) and the biochemical abnormality.

By 1970, I had been President for six years, my practice ever more demanding, and our medical problems at home were difficult. I was also getting very tired and I felt I had made my best contribution to the CF cause and so decided to pass the baton. Every person has a different contribution to make for a cause and I felt that I had made mine and it was time for someone else to make his or her contribution. My first vice-president all these years had been Ray Mulford from Toledo, Ohio. Ray was an exceptionally able executive who had graduated from Stanford University and was now President and CEO of Owens-Illinois Glass Co. He had a 20 year old son with CF and had been a conscientious member of our Board of Trustees. Ray was my logical successor and I had asked to meet with him at the Corporate Offices in New York City to discuss him succeeding me as President. He had fantastic credentials, i.e., a member of President Eisenhower's task force on economics, a Board member of many National Corporations, and a close friend of the Bromfmans of Canada. During our conversation, I was especially impressed that he invited me to be his guest at the Augusta National Golf Course in Georgia. I was also tremendously impressed with his humbleness and humility. I asked him what his children thought of him, a father who had accomplished so much and was noted throughout the land? He looked at me and quietly said, "They think I'm a schnook." How characteristic of teenagers.

I finally posed the important question. Would he accept the presidency, which he was in line for? I stressed how much more he could contribute as President of CF than anyone else, and we needed him. After much discussion, he stated that in his judgment he would do the cause a disservice, as he would not be able to spend the necessary time. He was honest and most sincere, and he was right. The leadership we needed would require time and attention.

Epilogue

It has now been 50 years that Evelyn and I have been part of the CF struggle and the Foundation and the White House also have acknowledged Evelyn's contributions (Figure 11.4). Those early years were indeed a struggle. The trauma of the initial diagnosis, the loneliness when it was made, the inadequacy of the early treatment, and the hopelessness of the prognosis all came into focus. But when we made that crucial decision to not look inward to our own CF problems, but to embrace the overwhelming challenge to obtain control for the disease, we suddenly had a focus, a driving force which turned our outlook from a negative one to a positive one. Now we had a beautiful goal, which has lasted to this day. With this perspective, we were able to inspire other parents and other people to work for Cystic Fibrosis and help us to reach this exciting day.

Of course, there were many depressing moments, as we saw our own and so many other children pass away. But, there were so many beautiful moments to cherish and be thankful for, such as:

> To observe the loving, competent, and dedicated care that all the CF physicians gave. I have always contended that CF physicians were a special breed unto themselves who were attracted to this cause because of their basic goodness.

> To observe the beautiful partnership with the NIH in the past years, which started with the tenure of Doris Tulcin and resulted in the elucidation of the abnormal gene and identification of the biochemical abnormality.

> To see the creative partnership with industry developed under the leadership of Bob Dresing, which enabled our Foundation to support the explosion of scientific data that developed.

> To fortuitously obtain Bob Beall as our scientific guru, to coordinate and direct the mass of scientific data that became available.

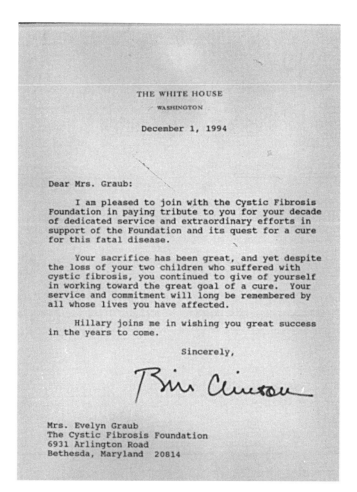

THE WHITE HOUSE

WASHINGTON

December 1, 1994

Dear Mrs. Graub:

I am pleased to join with the Cystic Fibrosis Foundation in paying tribute to you for your decade of dedicated service and extraordinary efforts in support of the Foundation and its quest for a cure for this fatal disease.

Your sacrifice has been great, and yet despite the loss of your two children who suffered with cystic fibrosis, you continued to give of yourself in working toward the great goal of a cure. Your service and commitment will long be remembered by all whose lives you have affected.

Hillary joins me in wishing you great success in the years to come.

Sincerely,

Bill Clinton

Mrs. Evelyn Graub
The Cystic Fibrosis Foundation
6931 Arlington Road
Bethesda, Maryland 20814

Figure 11.4. *Letter to Evelyn Graub from President Bill Clinton, 1994. Courtesy of Dr. Milton Graub.*

To see our CF Foundation under the leadership of Frank Deford become one of the most respected health agencies in the country.

And finally to be thankful that my loving wife Evelyn had the optimism, faith, and strength to support us both through the early trying years and now to share the joy of the many accomplishments of our Foundation in these recent years.

12

One Family's Special Mission

Doris F. Tulcin

It all began 46 years ago, when a most beautiful baby girl was born into our family. Ann was our second child, just 22 months younger than her brother Roger. She was born at the Doctors Hospital in New York City in June 1953. We did not know then that she was born with a blocked intestine that cleared spontaneously. The diagnosis of cystic fibrosis (CF) was not made at that time. She was a very small baby weighing only 5 pounds and 6 ounces. When I came home from the hospital, I had to leave her because her weight went below 5 pounds. The first 3 months of her life was very difficult. She was a very good baby, but was a typical failure to thrive infant. She suffered many bowel movements, ate voraciously, and could not gain weight. At the age of three months, she weighed only 8 pounds and had skin dried out like a crocodile. We had made the rounds of doctors to see how to help her, but to no avail. It was a mystery medically.

Finally, a trained nurse and a family friend, read an article in a medical journal by a Doctor Dorothy Andersen, who was a pathologist, about a strange disease called cystic fibrosis of the pancreas. At that time, we were so desperate that we called to make an appointment to see this doctor at Babies Hospital at the Columbia Presbyterian Medical Center. Dr. Andersen diagnosed her with CF. This diagnosis was made through the standard duodenal drainage procedure that measured the pancreatic enzymes in the digestive tract. Dr. Paul di Sant'Agnese had not perfected the sweat test for clinical use at that time. The diagnosis was a tremendous blow to our family. Dr. Andersen told us that there was not a great future for our daughter and possibly she might have a year to live. We were very heartbroken parents. We knew that we had to do everything that we could to keep her alive and keep her as well as possible. Dr. Andersen had discovered a banana formula, called Probana.[R] She had been working on a United Fruit Company grant and prescribed eating only bananas, strained meat out of a baby jar, and the formula for 1 year. Pancreatin[R] was added as the pancreatic enzyme replacement for digestion, vitamins, and Gantrisin as the antibiotic.

We were then directed to a wonderful pediatrician at Babies Hospital, Dr. Agnes Wilson, who worked with us to get this child on the right road. Unfortunately, Ann developed a severe virus infection soon after her diagnosis and had to be admitted to the hospital for intravenous therapy. She survived that and came home at age five months and started to thrive during the next few months. At the age of one year, she had "caught up" and although small, she was back to a fairly normal weight. She was doing everything and was as alert as any other one year old.

We really didn't know much about the disease in those early years, and when we would go for a checkup, Dr. Andersen would just feel her limbs, say she was doing very well, and that was about all.

My family really had a tough time in accepting the diagnosis of a mystery disease and the death penalty that went along with that diagnosis. We turned to my father, George Frankel, who had a long commitment to children and their medical needs. He was a very close friend of Basil O'Connor, President of the National Foundation for Infantile Paralysis (later called the March of Dimes Foundation), and former law partner of President Franklin D. Roosevelt. My father and I went to Mr. O'Connor to seek his advice on how to organize a national Foundation. We knew that we had to do something and find out more about CF. No one seemed to know anything about the disease, and even the physicians were stymied.

With O'Connor's advice, we set out looking for families around the country. We located families and physicians in Boston, Connecticut, Philadelphia, Washington, and California who had already organized and were raising funds to support research. These groups were giving small research grants to local doctors. It became apparent that the only way we could make an impact and raise any significant money was to form a national organization. This was accomplished in 1955, with incorporation in Delaware and with the first headquarters in Philadelphia. Dr. Wynne Sharples was elected as the first President. She was a pediatrician with two children with CF. The new Foundation was called the National Cystic Fibrosis Research Foundation (NCFRF). A charter was drawn and chapters were organized. Growth was slow, but in time, parents and physicians started to make progress. These small groups started events to raise money to focus on research. The first few grants were small, about $25,000 each, but they started to make a difference.

I would not have been able to make it through those early years without a wonderful, caring family, who pledged their complete support to me and this Foundation from the very beginning. I will always be grateful to my father because his guidance and leadership were crucial from the Foundation's inception. My parents were devoted to my daughter and to all the children who were struggling with this disease. As we watched my daughter, Ann, grow into a beautiful, healthy child, my family began its long history of commitment to educating the public and raising as much money as we could.

In June of 1956, I started my own chapter, called the Scarsdale Chapter, after the town where I lived. My younger sister, Geraldine, became the Treasurer and my eldest sister, Elizabeth and her husband, Norman, who lived in Houston, Texas, chartered the Houston Chapter. My father continued to work on the National Board, and after some years in Philadelphia, the headquarters moved to New York City. My father strongly believed that New York would provide more exposure and public support.

During the late 1950s and early 60s, we continued to call upon the Infantile Paralysis Foundation for guidance and advice. Dr. Kenneth Landauer was recruited from that Foundation to become our first Medical Director. He had been instrumental in developing the specialty Center-oriented program for people afflicted with polio and felt that the Center Program concept would be excellent for the NCFRF. It would provide centers of care for the children. There was very little significant treatment and few antibiotics and physicians were constantly struggling with new methods and new ideas. It was a hit and miss, trial and error approach. During this time, the Foundation continued to raise money for research and Professional Education, so this new program of delivery of specialized care was very audacious. George Barrie, another staff member from the Polio Foundation, joined our Foundation as the Executive Director. The chapter network was constantly expanding and as a result, the budget grew to provide more grants.

As stated previously, my own beginning with the Foundation was in 1956 as President and founder of the Scarsdale Chapter. Another mother from the area, who had a young teenager with CF, helped me as co-chair to form a local Board of friends. We started on a long road of many, many different fundraising projects from special events to door to door campaigns. We became officially chartered as the Westchester County Chapter in January of 1957. In 1959, we hired a professional staff person to guide us. Her name was Katherine Earnshaw and we moved the office from my home to an office in White Plains. In the first few years, we raised more than $60,000, which was a great deal of money for us and we felt that we were becoming increasingly successful. Unfortunately, my co-chair lost her 16 year old CF daughter from complications due to measles, which were deadly for CF children in those early years. Almost like the scare with polio, you felt that you had to stay out of crowds because of the threat posed by exposure to measles. This was our first experience with a devastating loss, and we became more determined than ever to make a success of our efforts.

We did experience some very special times. One, I recall in particular, was my first very important fund raiser. I planned a luncheon at my parents' home in Greenwich, Connecticut. We set up a tent and invited 300 to hear about CF and to meet the newly elected Governor of Connecticut, Abraham Ribicoff. He was a good friend of my Dad's and would be our guest speaker. The nightmare happened when the film broke down and the medical speaker, Dr. di Sant'Agnese, was not easily understood. I had to save the day and give an impromptu speech in order to save the program. This was my introduction to the world of fund raising speeches. It worked and we educated 300 people to CF. The Chapter then was accepted as an entity to deal with.

Another important milestone was the first declaration of CF Week in New York State in May of 1958. Governor Averill Harriman signed the Proclamation. I was aided with this event by William Carlebach, father of children with CF, and then Deputy Commissioner of the New York State Department of Commerce. Gary Moore, TV Personality and a local resident, became the County's first Honorary Chairman. For our tenth anniversary, we named Roberta Peters, along with Peter Lind Hayes and Mary Healy, as our Honorary Chairpersons. They were very good friends and local residents.

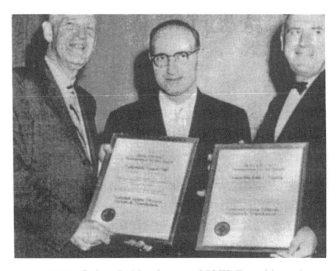

Figure 12.1. *Robert L. Natal, center, NCFRF president, shown with Senator Lister Hill of Alabama, right, and Congressman John E. Fogarty of Rhode Island, who were presented with the 1961 Cystic Fibrosis Distinguished Service Award. Courtesy of Mrs. Doris Tulcin.*

My father continued to wield his influence through the Governor, who went on to be elected Senator and finally Secretary of HEW (now Health and Human Services). Through Senator Ribicoff, we enlisted the help and interest of the two most powerful health people in the Congress, Senator Lister Hill and Congressman William Fogarty (Figure 12.1). Together, they were able to help us design language that would create more interest for government investment in CF research.

The Chapter that I worked so hard with forged ahead with many large events. Some of these included luncheons in New York City that honored such well known people as Mary Lasker, Dr. Leona Baumgartner, Dr. Dorothy Andersen, Mrs. Bernard Gimble, and Edward Bernays, just to name a few. A great deal of money was raised and the New York Times ran features on the Chapter and its events.

House and Garden Tours of wealthy individuals with magnificent art and sculpture were the rage in those years. The popularity of these tours brought great publicity and allowed us the greatest experience of touring the famous sculpture gardens of Joseph Hirshhorn. We were fortunate in having his home and art collection to show also. This tour attracted over 1,000 visitors and we were able to show this estate for 2 years, raising many thousands of dollars. His collection is now housed at the Hirshhorn Museum as part of the Smithsonian in Washington.

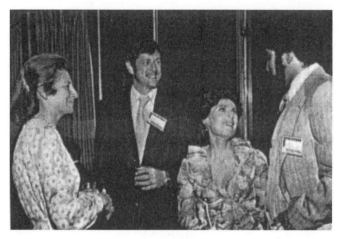

Figure 12.2. *At a banquet reception in 1975 from left to right,
President Doris Tulcin, Frank Deford, Roberta Peters, and
Franco Harris. Courtesy of Mrs. Doris Tulcin.*

On the personal side, another child with CF was born into our family. My
husband's brother and his wife gave birth to a baby girl who was just four years
younger than Ann. This family moved to California when the child was small
where she struggled with a very severe case of the disease. Despite all efforts, she
died at the age of 17 years from complications from CF. This was a very difficult
time for all of us and especially for my daughter. Ann was a junior in College and
this was her first experience with a death from CF of someone so close to us. However, her college years were fruitful and she continued to flourish and grow into a
beautiful and productive young woman. We, as a family, made many trips and she
led a very normal life, starting with school, camp and sports. She became an excellent tennis player, coached and tutored by the famous coach, Nick Bollettieri. This
relationship with Nick continued throughout all my work with the Association of
Tennis Professionals (ATP) and their many years of support for CF. During the
early 1970s, the ATP became affiliated with the CFF through Frank Deford, sports
writer for Sports Illustrated, and father of a young daughter, Alex, with CF. I met
Frank when CF became the official charity of the ATP through the Aetna World
Cup in Hartford, Connecticut. Many of the players were friends of Frank and they
were, at that time, the top players in the world with such famous names as Arthur
Ashe, John Newcombe, Jimmy Connors, Don Drysdale, Bob Lutz and Stan
Smith, to name a few. This relationship strengthened over the years through an
annual dinner named after Jack Kramer called the JAKS dinner. JAKS was the
academy awards of tennis and brought together all the tennis greats, as well as
major corporate tennis buffs. This event was held annually in New York City and
the Cystic Fibrosis Foundation was the beneficiary (Figure 12.2). This wonderful
exposure as well as the thousands of dollars raised really lifted awareness in New
York to a very high level.

"Sixty-Five Roses" (for cystic fibrosis) was a phrase coined by a young child in Florida in trying to describe his disease. The phrase became a symbol for the Foundation and the launching of Sixty-Five Roses events nationwide was in full swing. Baseball Clubs called Sixty-Five Roses Clubs were started by Don Baylor, baseball legend, and soon many cities followed, as we did in New York with the New York Yankees and New York Mets. Sports really brought out the best in everyone. The young players, bursting with good health and energy, could identify with young people who were struggling with a disease. Some of these relationships with baseball remain today.

We were blessed with the best medical supervision for Ann. She was treated by Dr. Harry Shwachman of Boston Children's Hospital and Dr. Carolyn Denning of Columbia University, and later St. Vincent's Hospital. Because of this excellent care, I wanted to provide local CF care for families who found it a tremendous burden to travel from Westchester County to New York City. I approached the Westchester County Medical Center, then called Grasslands, to see if they would be interested in setting up a clinic for care of CF. They agreed and I immediately set in motion a search for a Director. Dr. Tom Anderson was our first Director. Two years later, the kindest, gentlest physician ever known, Dr. Armand Mascia became the Center Director. This Center, founded in 1966, is still a thriving facility with hundreds of patients and an excellent staff. The Center is named in memory of Dr. Mascia who served it for 20 years. I worked as a clinic coordinator in that Center for 10 years, ably assisted by two wonderful mothers, Kay Finnegan and Marge Kennard. Both of these noble and brave women continued to work and support the Center, although they each lost their CF child during that time. I met so many wonderful families and many of them have remained my friends over these many years.

Serving the Foundation

During the late 1960s, Dr. Billy Graub, then President of the Foundation, approached my father to see if he would support a program focused on research. The idea was to bring together young researchers so that they would have an opportunity to meet with one another, explore the disease of CF, and help us move forward. This new program, called the GAP (Guidance, Action, and Projection) program was initiated and funded by my family. It lasted many years attracting wonderful, bright, young people. Many of them, who came as young potential stars, are now the shining lights of our medical world.

Unfortunately, my father died in 1971 and never really saw the great success of this very imaginative and innovative program. My mother had died in 1963 of cancer. I missed them both, as they were always there for both my child and me (Figure 12.3). They would be very proud to see the tremendous growth and vitality of this Foundation as we look at it today. They played such a crucial role in those early years.

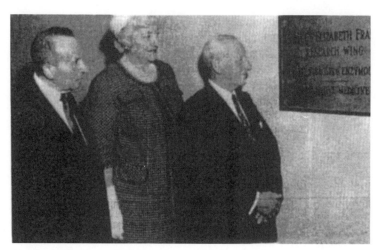

Figure 12.3. *Dean Marcus Kogel on left showing Elizabeth and George Frankel the plaque in their honor for support of research at the Albert Einstein College of Medicine in 1959. Courtesy of Mrs. Doris Tulcin.*

In 1971, I was elected to the National Board as a Regional Trustee from New York and in 1972, became a Vice President of the National CF Foundation. This responsibility allowed me to focus more on national business and I knew that my local chapter with a competent staff would keep business going on as usual. I still remained very active locally. My first assignment as a Vice President was to negotiate a situation between the Cleveland Chapter (Rainbow) and the National Board. There was heated disagreement over Chapter affairs with volunteers, many of them CF parents, who expressed frustration and some anger. This was my first meeting with Bob Dresing, who was the leader of the Cleveland group. It all ended very amicably and was my first arbitration with volunteers from other chapters. It was also the beginning of my long partnership and friendship with Bob whose leadership and strength would partner with me throughout my years of leadership for the Foundation.

As a Vice President, I became interested in the problems of the young adult with CF. My own daughter was approaching this time of development and I felt that we had to focus on adults who were forging on to college, work, marriage, children, and all the normal problems of just growing up. They had to face the problems of insurance coverage, work discrimination, and hospitalizations. This was a tremendous challenge. We put together many conferences and seminars on the problems of the young adult (for a time we had a "Young Adult Committee") and to this day I feel that these activities were a major step forward in establishing the fact that young people were living with CF, not dying.

I had served as a Vice President for President Bob McCreery for 4 years, and in 1975, I was asked if I would consider being elected as National President. After careful consideration of my personal needs at home, I accepted the responsibility, but I had to set the wheels in motion to find a President for the Westchester

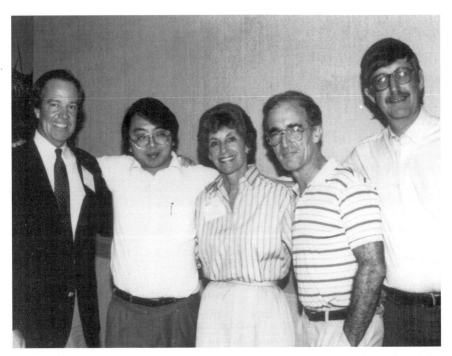

Figure 12.4. *Robert Dresing, on left, and Doris Tulcin, center, with the leaders of the researcher teams that discovered the CF gene. From the left, Lap-Chee Tsui, John Riordan, and Francis Collins. Courtesy of Mrs. Doris Tulcin.*

Chapter. I had served in that capacity for 20 years. Bob Dresing helped me to persuade my brother, David Frankel, to fill my shoes, which he did reluctantly but extremely well for another 20 years. My family continued to share the burden and take up the leadership role whenever called upon. In addition, my sister Geraldine continued to work as Treasurer with the local chapter as did Elizabeth and Norman in Houston. They continued to be the best family and never stopped showing their support for me and for Ann.

I was elected National President in April of 1976. My first assignment from the Board was to give early retirement to the National Director, Welch Boyer. He had served the Foundation well for 10 years, but it was felt that it was time for a change. The National headquarters were in Atlanta, so the trip back and forth for me from New York was a weekly requirement. Dr. Amoz Chernoff became our Medical Director. After a year of my presidency in Atlanta, Bob Dresing and I felt it would serve the Foundation well to move our headquarters from Atlanta to the Washington D.C. area. We needed greater recognition for support at the National Institutes of Health (NIH) so with final Board approval, we moved to Rockville, Maryland in January 1978.

The move set in motion our request for Congressional support. We received a mandate from that body to produce a report on "Future Directions of

Research for Cystic Fibrosis" and the report was to be returned to the Congress within one year. This report was called "A Plea for a Future." The study amassed hundreds of volunteers to address all the important issues related to our patients, to our physicians, and to our researchers. It was reported back to the Congress in 1979 and was the single most important step into the research future for the Cystic Fibrosis Foundation.

In 1979, Dr. Robert Beall was approached to become our Medical Director. Bob was at the NIH, serving at the National Institute for Diabetes Digestive and Kidney Disease (NIDDK), and directing the Diabetes and CF programs. Bob accepted the offer and came on board in 1980. Through his guidance and foresight, the study submitted to the Congress was analyzed and the Research Development Program (RDP) was developed. There are many wonderful stories in the development of this effort, but that story is another history. In 1982, my Presidency ended and Bob Dresing became the National President. I went on to chair the newly designed Research Development Campaign, a campaign to raise $25 million over 7 years to support the Research Development Program. This campaign was the first capital campaign ever undertaken by a voluntary health agency. It was a tremendous challenge, but with the help of some wonderful volunteers, the money was raised.

During those years of the campaign, I received two federal appointments of four years each to the National Heart Lung and Blood (NHLBI) Advisory Council of the NIH. This was a very important appointment for me because it taught me how grants were awarded. It also gave us additional exposure at this Institute and stood me well in my lobbying efforts with the Congress for additional research support.

In 1987, my husband died. During that year, I decided that my volunteer efforts could now take on a more demanding role. I joined the staff of the Cystic Fibrosis Foundation and learned how well the staff worked with the thousands of volunteers nationwide. It has been a wonderful experience and one that I feel proud to have undertaken. Since that time, I have worked in the New York area as Executive Director of the Greater New York Chapter. It is a wonderful feeling that I can continue to serve the children and adults to whom I have dedicated my life. My daughter, Ann, now 48 years old, has been married for 25 years, and has 2 children, the eldest now in college. Ann is a teacher and still a great tennis player. A highlight for all of us was the finding of the CF gene in 1989 and being present along with Bob Dresing at the awards ceremony later (Figure 9.4).

Although we have suffered many personal losses, life for my family has been fulfilled in many ways. We continue to count our blessings. The greatest blessing of all in my life has been the support of the most wonderful family. They have never turned me down in any request that I have made to them. Starting from the beginning my parents, my husband, my sisters, my brother, my brother in law, my nieces and nephews, all have joined together to serve the children. We all share this labor of love and will continue to be there until we are not needed any longer in this fight. We want to bring this disease to closure. We want to know that our mission to cure this disease has been accomplished.

13

An Impossible Dream

Henry I. and Madeline C. Bernbaum

Our son Willard Alan was diagnosed with cystic fibrosis (CF) in 1953, an event that had a major impact on our lives and that of our other children and family members, but especially on Will's life. Over the course of his 35 years of living, Will ultimately embodied the thoughts and words of "The Impossible Dream" by Joe Darion. The thoughts relevant to fighting an unbeatable foe, bearing his burden with unbearable sorrow, fighting for the right to live without question or pause, and striving with his last ounce of courage to reach his goals came to have very personal meaning to Will. He ultimately lived by these words and thoughts and hoped the world would be better for his struggle.

Of our four children, only our second son, Will, had a health problem. Despite a normal feeding regimen, he had loose stools and lost weight. Our pediatrician, Dr. Earle Smith, recommended goat's milk, which was not easy to find and did not help. We became more and more concerned until a boiled skim milk and karo syrup formula was successful and he finally did gain weight. Throughout the ensuing months there was concern about his health since he wasn't a robust or healthy looking infant, developed a cough, and continued with the loose stools. Despite the efforts of our dedicated pediatrician, this was an unsolved mystery.

At 21 months of age, Will became almost comatose and was hospitalized at the then Babies and Children's Hospital (B&C Hospital), with a diagnosis of mumps encephalitis. During the ensuing days of recovery, Dr. Smith brought in a consultant specialist, Dr. Samuel Spector, who was on the staff of the hospital and a highly respected diagnostician. He ordered a duodenal drainage test. On the basis of the results and the continuing cough and stool symptoms, he told us the diagnosis was CF and that there was no effective treatment.

The full impact of this diagnosis did not hit us until Madeline, who had trained as a Speech and Hearing therapist and was knowledgeable about medical libraries, researched the subject and found only autopsy reports, no research papers, and that it was a fatal disease.

We were devastated. This was 1953, when the state of the art was a big zero, there was no on going treatment available, and the advice was essentially to take him home to die. There was no place to turn to and nothing to be done for our Will. At this time, fortunately for us, we were not aware of the genetic heritage aspect of the disease so the fact that Madeline was pregnant with our third child was not a worry. Soon after, our daughter Marla was born and there were no problems! Time passed and we raised our family with Will continuing to cough and experience loose stools. In this interim he did not have any serious illness, but as typical parents, we lived under that constant threat.

At the beginning of 1956, sparks began to fly for CF in Cleveland. The sparks were generated by a family group, the Jaffe Cousins Club. One of the member couples, Sam and Henrietta Trott, had a living child with CF and had already lost another child to CF. The Club members decided to establish an agency dedicated to initiating support of CF medical research, then virtually non-existent. They authorized their lawyer member, Robert Jaffe, to secure from the State of Ohio, the necessary non-profit Articles of Incorporation. These Articles, approved and issued by the State on December 10, 1955, created THE CYSTIC FIBROSIS FOUNDATION, CLEVELAND CHAPTER. Bob Jaffe, a very capable attorney (subsequently to become solicitor for the City of South Euclid and later appointed to a Federal judgeship) knew of no other organization devoted to the CF cause so, with great foresight, he provided for a multi-chaptered agency within the State.

Prior to this and to the best of anyone's knowledge, no family in the Cleveland area with a CF child was aware of another such family. Each set of parents walked alone with their burden, lacking any benefit of mutual sympathy and comfort. Each new family, when told the fateful diagnosis, had minimal information and a suggestion of perhaps a four year average survival. It was very depressing, but now this first step by the Cousins Club ignited a small flame that would bring parents in the locality together.

Through several efforts, the names of five more families thought to have children with CF were obtained. In February 1956, the Chapter formation meeting was held in the home of the Jaffes and was attended by Phyllis and Lawson Anderson, Jeanne and Robert Horn, Rita and Walter Mikulitz, Lois and Daniel Obloy, the Trotts, and us. The Jaffes and Alice and Lou Cherko represented the Jaffe Cousins Club. Along with an explanation of the purpose of the meeting, they presented us the Articles of Incorporation and a check. In retrospect, this check was the first contribution to local medical research for CF and constituted the entire contents of the Jaffe Cousins Club treasury. It was slightly in excess of $200.

The original incorporators were Robert Michne, Ethel Rallis, and Robert Jaffe. The pre-organization meeting trustees named were Robert Jaffe and Samuel and Henrietta Trott. The officers elected that night were: Phyllis Anderson, President; Robert Horn, Vice President; Jeanne Horn, Secretary; and Lawson Anderson, Treasurer. The first Board of Trustees consisted of these officers plus: Henry Bernbaum, William Wallace, M.D., Walter Mikulitz, Samuel Spector, M.D., Lois Obloy, Robert Jaffe, and Henrietta Trott.

Subsequently, the first General Membership Meeting was held in April 1956 at the South Euclid City Hall. CF parents, relatives, and friends from greater Cleveland and northeastern Ohio attended. Thereafter meetings were held monthly in the Amphitheater of the B&C Hospital for the General Membership. Board Meetings were also held monthly in the homes of the various CF family members.

The next episode in Cleveland, one that had lasting significance, was a meeting between a number of the Cleveland CF parents and Dr. William Wallace, Director of the Department of Pediatrics at the B&C Hospital, concerning the start of research on CF at that facility. The bottom line was an offer by Dr. Wallace to put a doctor to work on CF if we could raise $2,500 as seed money and then provide on going financial support. He also indicated considerable doubt that we would be successful, based on his past experience with other similar situations. We left that meeting determined to raise the funds. In the ensuing effort, there were salami sales, rummage sales, and a whole litany of all kinds of other money raising events. We did raise a good bit of the money but in all honesty the credit for a major portion goes to a neighbor of Bob Jaffe, contractor Ben Wakser, who took our cause to heart and solicited all of his suppliers. He is owed a large debt of gratitude for that was indeed a most critical time for us.

At the first Annual Concert of the Suburban Orchestra fund raiser for CF on December 12, 1956, that first grant of $2,500 was presented to Dr. Samuel Spector, who represented the Department of Pediatrics.

In the fall of 1956 between the time of our meeting with Dr. Wallace and the check presentation, Dr. LeRoy Matthews, an Assistant Professor of Pediatrics, was appointed to direct the research program and the CF treatment clinic then being planned. As committed, the opening of a weekly CF clinic began in July 1957, along with the beginning of the clinical and basic research program. This was the humble beginning of what was to become a nationally and internationally acclaimed Center for the treatment of CF. In addition, under Dr. Matthews' guidance, this Center went on to attract millions of dollars of private and federal support for its basic and clinical research and its treatment programs over the years.

The initial general meeting was attended by several new CF families including Sal and Sally Maritt. Sal and Sally immediately became totally involved and part of the leadership of the Chapter. Their participation was critical in those early years. The Gayneau family came to one of the early general meetings and became mainstays. They were grandparents of two CF children. In the Chapter history, Bill Gayneau served as mist tent maker, President, and Regional President, and was involved along with Harriet in virtually every fund raising event. One of our big annual fund raising efforts was the summer carnival held on the parking lot of the Cedar Center shopping strip in South Euclid. Bill and friends of similar maturity would arrive with a truck loaded down with small gauge railroad track and several little kid sized push cars. They would install the track and spend the day and evening running the loop and pushing the cars. It was a popular ride and gave those mature folks lots of exercise.

The Jaffe Cousins Club provided continuing help in those early years through Alice and Lou Cherko (Sam Trott's sister and brother-in-law), Sam's father Mr. Trottsky, Joan Jaffe providing our early secretarial services, and Dorothy and Morris Stoller. In due course, Dorothy handled the secretarial load followed by Wilda Casarona, a close friend of the Maritts, and also Jeanne Horn. These capable volunteers were a vital support when we had no office and could not afford to hire services. Morris Stoller was a great help with free service from his printing company.

The need for legal services and advice were generously provided gratis first by Robert Jaffe, our incorporator and subsequently for many years by Edward Klein. Ed and his wife Anne were grandparents of a CF child. They were also among our most devoted volunteers. Anne for many, many years spent several days a week providing clerical assistance in the chapter office. Their children, Henry and Lois Goodman, were very generous also in their support and were a key family in solving a number of major local needs. In the final years of our continuing development, Paul Downs, who served many other roles as well, was our legal support.

The Bernbaum family as originally planned was to have four children and Madeline was again pregnant. The possibility that CF was a genetic disease was still an uncertainty. But in the ensuing months, it became much more clear that CF was genetic in origin and that we were at risk. We worried a lot during the pregnancy, but Lawrence, along with Marla and Steven, also proved to be without CF! We were the typical Mendelian theory family, with a one out of four ratio with CF, but there was no knowledge as to which of the non-involved children might be carriers of the gene.

In the late spring of 1957 Will came down with a severe Friedlander's bacterial lung infection, was hospitalized, and placed in what was referred to as the "wet room." This room was all white tile, floor to ceiling, and was clouded with moisture which condensed on and dripped on the contents of the room, patient, hospital personnel, and parents. We were advised to be prepared for the worst as Will's condition was considered to very possibly be terminal. He proved to be stronger and more resilient than expected, recovered, and in due course returned home.

As a result of this admission and treatment, we believe Will was the first CF patient cared for by the new clinic, as it began in 1957. If not, he was most certainly among the very first few to be seen there. For the rest of his life, over thirty more additional years, Will and B&C Hospital would see a great deal of each other. In his childhood and early teens he was on the regimen of being seen for history and examination, other testing, and respiratory culture on a regular basis about every four weeks. All too frequently hospitalization was necessary for intravenous antibiotic treatment and what became termed a "cleanout." The comprehensive treatment program developed by Dr. Matthews for aggressive care of the disease initially included continuing home aerosol antibiotic administered two to three times daily, pancreatic enzymes with each meal to aid digestion, often oral antibiotics, daily physical therapy to remove as much mucus as possible from the lungs, and sleeping in a mist tent at night.

The aerosol procedure started in a rudimentary fashion and fortunately improved over a period of time. At first, we started with a rubber bulb, hand squeezed "pump." Each treatment of aerosol meant approximately 30 to 40 minutes of squeezing the bulb until the receptacle was empty. Somewhat later we heard about a small medical compressor that had just reached the market. With some difficulty we obtained one of these pumps and found it to be a godsend. Not only did it relieve us parents of the physical squeezing burden but it also reduced the treatment time for the patient.

The aerosol treatment was universally followed by the physical therapy component of the Matthews' regimen and was variously referred to as clapping, thumping, or pounding. The parents had to be trained to be their child's lung therapist, learning how to cup the hands and rhythmically clap the twelve positions on the front, sides, and back of the chest. That was the easier part of the training. Each of the clapped positions was followed by applying the hands to the chest and vibrating as the child exhaled slowly following a learned pattern and then coughed and expectorated as much mucus as possible. Learning to do the vibrating seemed to be much more difficult for us. Dr. Matthews' standard explanation of the physical therapy to loosen and remove the mucus was the example of "getting the Ketchup out of the bottle." Everybody seemed to understand that explanation.

Postural drainage in the home initially was a makeshift kind of arrangement to position the child's head down in a sloped position to facilitate the flow of the mucus for expectoration during the treatment. Household furniture and sofa pillows were utilized to try for the proper body angle. It usually meant that the therapist parent was awkwardly crouching on the floor and very uncomfortable. Very quickly it became obvious that a postural drainage table needed to be developed and made available. After some experimentation, medical staff and therapy technicians developed and approved an upholstered tabletop hinged to a base with an adjustable steel rack at the opposite end, to provide adjustable angularity. The tabletop also had shoulder pads located to prevent the child from sliding off. One of our Board members, George Maden, had the parts for the first few batches fabricated and did a great deal of the assembly work himself in his garage business shop. This item was in great demand as word of the availability got around and then the volume of tables requested became a problem. We charged on a cost, non-profit, basis and were shipping them around the country. Fortunately our product came to the attention of the South Euclid-Lyndhurst Kiwanis Club, who decided to undertake the assembly as a community service project. We ordered the frames, while they scrounged donation of the rest of the material needed and produced the tables in batches of fifty several times a year. Originally the Kiwanis leaders were Robert Gillespy, Justin Baum, James Black, and Dr. Mailman, to name those we personally knew and dealt with on the project. Over the years, they produced in excess of 1000 postural drainage tables. Since the need was across the entire country, other similarly motivated groups, such as the Knights of Pythias, produced variations of our table design for their local families.

When Will was hospitalized for more intensive treatment of the pulmonary infection, it involved intravenous (IV) antibiotics. The IV bags were mounted on a steel pole and a base with wheels for mobility. There were always a number of children on the CF floor interacting with each other and it was an interesting sight to see them moving through the hall or in the cafeteria rolling the IV poles along. None of them thought it unusual as it was part of their existence in the hospital, but for visitors it was a strange sight. Later, Dr. Robert Stern's "heparin lock device" permitted discontinuous IV therapy and forever freed the patients from their IV poles.

Before long, the Board decided that "bumper stickers" would be a great help in popularizing the words, CYSTIC FIBROSIS, and making our existence known in the community. We investigated commercial sources and found it expensive beyond our means. However, being employed by American Greetings Corporation, which had a large silk screening operation, it didn't take me too long to figure out that we could do this on our own at a fraction of the cost. We got the screens and artwork donated, bought the materials, and set about to print 5000 bumper stickers. Walter Mikulitz volunteered his basement and one Saturday the Board members became printers. Unfortunately it was a warm humid day unsuitable for drying ink and Walter's basement soon was festooned with hanging strips, as was his yard and garage. It was a late night when they all were finally dried and packed. Fortunately we never had to do that project again as, after we joined the National organization, it provided all the public relations materials except for our local brochure.

Madeline and I became totally engrossed in the CF activities, along with the other original families—the myriad details of meetings, fund raising, correspondence, and overall planning were a daily diet. Between taking care of our family and the CF chapter we were extremely busy. We dropped our other professional organization roles and activities and concentrated on CF. I became the second President of the Chapter and devoted my efforts to the organization. We formed what came to be lifetime friendships with the original founding families and a number of families that came along in ensuing years, including those of our lead medical people.

A sidelight on relationships was that we both had prior contact with members of two of the other founding families. Phyllis Anderson and Madeline had been high school classmates at Glenville High School. Sam Trott's drugstore was located on the corner of Lakeview Road and Earle Avenue in the Glenville district. We knew him by sight. As a teenager I had many a chocolate milkshake at his soda fountain. Our later close association provided one of the strange quirks of fate that arrange our lives.

Joining the National Organization

Concurrently with and initially largely unknown to the early Cleveland group, other organizations of a similar nature were forming in Philadelphia, New York, the State of Connecticut, Boston, and Los Angeles. Also at that time, Dr. Wynne Sharples, the mother of two CF children, and others formed the National Cystic Fibrosis Research Foundation (NCFRF).

These new groups elsewhere in the United States gradually came to our attention and contact was initiated and maintained through the medium of personal letters and exchange of newsletters. I was designated as point person for much of this activity and we had correspondence with Dr. Sharples in Philadelphia because we were interested in becoming part of the national effort through the NCFRF. However, this developed into an impasse that could not be surmounted as the NCFRF position was to take 90% of funds raised by a Chapter (later reduced to 85%) and that it would have sole control of how the funds would be used. We could not agree to do this since we had total faith in what was rapidly developing into an obviously vital and successful local program and could not place it at risk through the judgment of "outsiders."

In 1958, after continuing contact with NCFRF proved fruitless, we hosted a meeting in Cleveland of representatives of five other CF groups from northern Ohio and Michigan. By this time Dr. Matthews' clinic was well established and was attracting patients from a larger general area. It was decided that those in attendance would author a letter directed to the officers and the trustees of NCFRF suggesting that they change their policies to make affiliation possible without endangering the research and treatment program at Babies and Children's Hospital. We received letters of agreement from a few of the NCFRF Trustees and I received a phone call of agreement and support from a Dr. Milton Graub. One letter agreeing most strongly with our position was written by a Mr. Birenbaum. We remember his comments in particular because of the similarity of our names and because not too much later we met his daughter, Mrs. Evelyn Graub.

Contact continued between the Cleveland lay group and the NCFRF leadership from time to time during the next year as we strongly felt that unity under a national banner would in the long term provide the best possibility for progress. In early 1960 we learned that a major change had taken place at NCFRF. Dr. Sharples had resigned after five years as President, was replaced by Robert Natal, and that the National organization had moved its headquarters from Philadelphia to New York City.

Subsequently in 1960, George Barrie, NCFRF Executive Director, who was empowered to negotiate with us, contacted us. A contract was written which basically met our local requirements. It guaranteed that our Chapter would retain 75% of local funds raised and NCFRF would receive 25%. Also if we failed for some reason to reach our budgeted minimum support level of $47,000 for the B&C Hospital research program, NCFRF would make up the difference. This was quite a concession on their part and recognition that the program had great merit under the leadership of LeRoy Matthews. The remaining requirement was that one member of our Board would be appointed to serve as a Trustee at Large on the National Board. It was agreed that we would submit two names and that NCFRF would make the choice. They chose my name. This imposed another burden on our family life involving, for my fifteen years tenure at National, five to six trips a year to New York City then later Atlanta for Executive Committee and Board Meetings. This activity also included special Board committee participation and chairmanships, all creating time demands that had to be satisfied. Through all the years Madeline met with much more of the home and family challenges and did it all with great success.

At the time of my appointment, the Board of Trustees of NCFRF was composed of regional and at-large members. The country was divided geographically into eleven regions. Regional Trustees were elected by popular vote of the chartered chapters, one from each region normally at a Regional Conference meeting. Almost without exception these trustees were parents of CF children. At large Trustees were appointed by Board election usually because of their interest and hopefully their elevated position, wealth or influence. Nothing derogatory was meant by these criteria since all of these people were selfless, dedicated, and totally empathetic in their service to the struggle against CF. If they were ever referred to as "do gooders" it was out of respect and acknowledgment that they served without the special and more selfish incentive that drove us parents. The best possible example of such a person was our cherished second NCFRF President, Bob Natal, a non-CF parent, under whose guidance and devotion major organizational strides were made between 1960 and 1966.

Over many of the years following the 1960 Cleveland merger into NCFRF our local percentage retention rankled many of the other major Chapter leaders and their related physicians since Cleveland was "different." On any number of occasions I had to defend our contract terms, and I believe in almost all cases successfully, due to the preeminence of the program and its statistical results. For those who understood the circumstances and appreciated the contribution of the Matthews/B&C Hospital program, it was not as much of a problem. Directors of the new CF Centers around the country came to B&C Hospital in 1961 to be introduced to the program of care and treatment pioneered by LeRoy.

During the merger negotiations, we also came to know and respect the NCFRF Medical Director, Dr. Kenneth Landauer. Like George Barrie, Ken was another Infantile Paralysis Foundation (Polio Foundation) alumnus fresh from the conquering of polio and an extremely articulate and well organized medical leader. His major recommendation for the medical program was to initiate and complete the installation of a national system of "Care, Teaching and Research (CTR) Centers." These would be similar to those so successfully established for polio at the major medical schools/hospitals around the country, which almost automatically insured a whole host of benefits, including more uniform and improved treatment, interconnected research relationships for medical and scientific personnel, and the accumulation of current statistics. Beginning in 1961 and within a brief span of time, Ken established thirty four Centers spread throughout the United States.

In Cleveland, concurrently with the events of the 1957-1960 period, we had major developments transpire on the fund raising front. In 1957 there was a housewives uprising against the parade of door to door solicitations by a proliferation of health agencies. Their demand to consolidate fund raising was led by several prominent Cleveland area women, in particular by Mrs. George J. Urban, the wife of the mayor of the City of South Euclid. In the first drive in May 1957, five of the smaller agencies, including CF, joined together and conducted a Combined Health

Collection in 16 suburbs that approved the concept. Our Chapter members enthusiastically supported this in every community where they resided, usually in leadership roles. In our community of University Heights, Madeline volunteered for years as the community co-chairwoman. It was an added burden on the families but it provided desperately needed money for our cause and there was no other way. Earlier we had investigated possible membership in United Way and been rejected.

In late 1959, community leaders headed by Paul Sprague, brought into life the Health Fund of Greater Cleveland which replaced the Combined Health Collection. The concept was a drive for health agencies in the spring and a drive for welfare (United Way) in the fall and it gained the support of the community at all levels. However, the major health agencies did not come into the fold despite many efforts to convince them. The first Health Fund drive was held in 1960 and provided $16,133 for CF. Each year the Health Fund increased its fund raising capability and in 1974 provided $157,000 for CF. Despite this successful Health Fund operation, a serious problem in fund raising arose in Cleveland. United Way (United Appeal) was finding difficulty in welfare fund raising and decided to absorb Health Fund and use it to augment its faltering appeal. Their pressure was irresistible, and despite every effort to protect research when compared to the needs of welfare, the Health Fund disappeared into United Appeal (later called United Way). Thus, an era of major growth in research funding through that vehicle ended. Thereafter the United Appeal share of our annual budget continued to grow modestly each year. This was not in proportion to our research program needs and meant increased emphasis on special event fund raising, which United Appeal encouraged. It also meant that on a long term planning basis, fund raising outside of Cleveland would have to make up the difference in support of the basic and clinical research programs now sited both at the hospital and at the Western Reserve University School of Medicine.

The Pharmacy Program

From the inception of the clinic when real treatment began, the CF children required expensive antibiotics, in relatively massive amounts. At the first organizational meeting, Sam Trott offered to provide all CF pharmaceuticals at cost to all Chapter members. As the membership roll increased, Sam's patient volume increased. At one point the Board learned that Sam was personally absorbing losses from a number of truly indigent families. This obviously could not be allowed to continue. Steps were taken to adjust our incorporation from strictly research to include limited care and to establish an impartial committee to create and administer a confidential care program for drugs, supplies, and equipment. This program stayed in effect for many years and was a low budget item, but provided drugs for the few children not covered otherwise. Then the societal unrest of the times stepped in and impacted adversely on our pharmacist, Sam Trott.

The day of the infamous Lakeview Avenue riot, brought to a boil by the death of the Reverend Klunder under the tracks of an earthmover, was the end of an era for Sam. His drugstore, a successful business for decades, was completely vandalized and stripped of everything. Radio newscasts all that day told of the destruction going on, the police sealing off and barricading the area, and the life threatening hazard to all in the area. This included Sam! Madeline and I, and the Maritts, early key members and close friends of ours and the Trotts, rushed to Sam's home to comfort and be with his wife and to wait for Sam who was trapped in the store. After many hours of trepidation, Sam drove his wagon into their drive-way. There was, of course, great relief that he had escaped unscathed. The only items salvaged from his store and allowed to be removed by the rioters were CF drugs and materials, which we unloaded and stored in his recreation room tempo-rarily. Sam immediately arranged with a pharmacist friend to utilize his pharmacy to service the CF children without any disruption of service. In the following weeks Sam concluded that he would not open a new store. This was a true crisis since Sam's pharmacy was the sole source of reasonably priced drugs for the entire CF clinic population.

The Board met and developed a new concept. With Sam's agreement, we would employ his services and open our own non-profit CF pharmacy. This phar-macy program came to pass. Initially the volume was insufficient to meet expenses and required a modest subsidy from the general fund. As the patient load grew at the Center and the volume grew at the pharmacy, we established policies for con-stant price revisions to insure we did not exceed a 6% profit. This was necessary since our budget was closely monitored by the Health Fund and we were not allowed to continue any subsidy. In order to operate the pharmacy in the "black" we were forced to be nominally profitable, hence the 6% rule. Each year, financial planning volunteers determined the amount of money that could be removed from the pharmacy operation account and transferred to the research account. As the volume increased, that portion of the 6% transferred also grew. In recent years when the National CF organization decided to open its pharmacy modeled on the Cleve-land operation, the latter was thereafter closed down. At that time, the Cleveland pharmacy, at cost, had sales in excess of a million dollars per year. Without a Sam Trott there would never have been the unique Cleveland CF pharmacy, or the sub-sequent National CF pharmacy program. Sam ran the operation like his own busi-ness with his heart and soul, a gruff man with a soft heart of gold.

Over the years, we benefited greatly from the executive talents of Jon Martin who served in many roles including that of Chapter President. Jon was the uncle of the two CF daughters of his brother James. Initially Jim Martin was the active member along with his wife Sally and her mother until Jim's business career led him to Texas. Jon became a leading member undertaking many roles, including representing our agency with Health Fund and United Way. His position as an officer of the Cleveland Trust Bank (later Society and now Key Bank) as well as President of the Heart Association provided great credibility for our agency.

After a few years it was apparent that, for indigent families, coverage from the Crippled Children's Program was desperately needed. Pioneering work opening this service to eligible CF patients had already occurred in Pennsylvania. Three courses were open to us, the short route through the Attorney General of Ohio, the long route through the legislature, and the improbable route of influencing the medical people who controlled the Crippled Children's Committee. An informal lunch meeting was arranged for three of us to meet with the Attorney General. We received a negative lesson about politics. Going via the legislature would take years. Dr. Matthews undertook personally to convince the medical people that it was wiser to open the policy than to stonewall the inevitable. He succeeded and our indigent patients were quickly eligible. However, it became an almost unending battle to accomplish two other objectives, adequate funding increases in the budget and acceptance of patients over twenty one years of age. The Columbus, Dayton, and Cincinnati Chapters joined us in these efforts, but the leadership role for CF in the state became the willing responsibility of Richard Shaltens. He and his family were among our early members and were at the forefront of the effort in all phases. His mother, Mary, was an extremely talented craftsperson and her products were a significant source of chapter revenue. Largely through his persistence there was success in the "over 21" program and budget improvements.

I was fortunate to work with Bob Natal on National affairs from 1960 to 1966 until he developed cancer and died in April 1967. It was a sad time indeed. Although he was not a CF parent, he was completely dedicated to the philosophy of the Foundation and put endless hours into its activities. Dr. Milton "Billy" Graub succeeded Bob in the leadership role, performing with equal fervor to 1970. For Billy, it was much more difficult for he had to commute from Philadelphia to New York whereas Bob commuted across the street from his business office to the NCFRF offices in Manhattan. As a member of the Executive Committee from 1961 on, it was my pleasure to work closely with them and enjoy their friendship. By this time our Executive Director, George Barrie, had resigned to operate his own private business and had been replaced by Welch Boyer. Both of these men were graduates of the Polio Foundation, which produced a generation of skilled health agency professionals. Since George had shepherded our Cleveland Chapter entry into NCFRF and maintained close and friendly relations with us, we saw him depart with sincere regret and reluctance. George was honest and forthright in his dealings and statements to a fault.

During the early years, CF groups separately and independently started up in Ohio, almost wherever one or more CF families lived. Publicity generated both locally and nationally stimulated awareness of clinics and children came to B&C Hospital mostly from northern Ohio, but also in large numbers from adjacent states. These families participated in our pharmacy program, attended our meeting, received our newsletters, organized local fund raising groups, and forwarded funds either to the Cleveland Chapter or directly to the research program. We became partners with these northern Ohio groups and formally joined together in 1962 as the Northern Ohio Federation of Cystic Fibrosis Chapters, NOFCFC. Each of these member groups continued to raise funds in their own locality and provided support to the research programs. In some instances, to broaden the base and increase support, when invited we traveled to the communities and encouraged the initiation of group or chapter activity. Most often these efforts were undertaken by several of us for each such trip, most frequently by Donald Davis and Dan Obloy and/or me. Don and his wife Barbara were early members of our Cleveland group and extremely active in all phases of the development of the Chapter. They lost their daughter, Valerie, at an early age which, if anything, served to increase their dedication to the cause. Valerie, wearing her aerosol mask, was the subject of a painting gracing the front page of our second published piece of local literature. Don was the major fund raiser of our Chapter and did yeoman service over the years as President and later as NCFRF Ohio Regional President.

The next phase of development converted the NOCFCF into the Cystic Fibrosis Chapter Federation, CFCF, which became a chartered National Chapter independent of the originally chartered Cleveland Chapter. The two Chapters continued to operate in this configuration until 1978 when, for a multitude of reasons, it became advisable to merge into one Chapter with one National charter covering the 21 Northeastern Ohio counties. On December 5, 1977 the National Board voted to approve the formation of the merger as the Rainbow Chapter. On March 1, 1978, the Rainbow Chapter began operations. The first slate of officers was Hank Bernbaum, President; Wilton Workman, Vice President; Mary Ann Blosser, Secretary; and Mike Meredith, Treasurer.

Will's Progress

Meanwhile our family pattern continued. With the support of the care program, Will grew and matured as a happy youngster who was into everything wholeheartedly. He played very actively to the point that he could fall asleep at the supper table. Playtime was constrained by treatments and he intensely disliked sleeping in the mist tent. He had a number of hospitalizations, losing school time but always doing quite well academically. Such was the routine of our family life, getting along pretty well despite occasional setbacks. One morale breaker occurred when Will was in his eighth year and had been ill and hospitalized for an increase in pulmonary symptoms. In a serious discussion with LeRoy, who by then was a pretty close friend and collaborator on Chapter affairs, I felt comfortable about asking him what he thought about Will's survival chances. I know it was with great emotional regret that he told us that the chances of him seeing a twelfth birthday seemed slim to none. That was a difficult time for us.

When Will was sixteen and hospitalized at B&C Hospital for a two week stay, he was one of five CF patients at the time. Typically they socialized and shared experiences and concerns. Unfortunately, one youngster passed away during Will's stay. This event impacted adversely on everyone, patients, staff, and parents. A few days later Will was discharged. Within a few months through the communication grapevine that linked us all together, my wife and I learned that the three others had passed away as well. You have to know that this kind of news depresses everyone. It was always devastating, with sympathy for the families and concern for the impact on the survivors. We tried to shield Will from learning about these deaths out of concern for the psychological impact. He learned about it anyway. This kind of event played a part in shaping these youngsters. Finding out about mortality so early discouraged a few of them in the families that we knew and this knowledge messed up their lives. However, despite the grim awareness of the fatal nature of their disease and the lack of predictability of their health and life, the great majority of the children we knew coped quite well. If anything they were stronger and went about the serious business of life with some disregard for pessimism. Those that we knew who survived into adulthood included two nursing graduates, teachers, accountant, pharmacist, nightclub singer, priest, lawyers, finance expert, and many in technical and business positions, and our son, a medical internist. Sadly quite a few of those listed are no longer with us. Nevertheless optimism prevailed as each year research in drugs and treatment regimens lengthened life and improved its quality.

In 1967, an opportunity arose for Madeline and me to enjoy a week of vacation in Florida. We had been away together at the same time only one other time since we had started our family. We were only gone a day and a half when we received a call that Will was in the hospital after an episode of hemorrhaging from the lungs, called hemoptysis. This had never happened before and was absolutely frightening for all involved. We immediately returned home. This was the first of a fair number of these lung hemorhages that Will would endure during the balance of his life. Each one was, of course, life threatening and therefore most upsetting. I'm sure that it would be difficult for most people to fully understand how this threat always weighed on him and us after this first event. On three occasions after such events, he underwent an operative procedure to block a blood vessel to the lung to stop the bleeding. Each time he underwent this delicate procedure it was with the additional threat of possible procedure associated injury, such as paralysis.

Will's life continued rather typically as a teenager despite the medications, treatments, and extra demands of his disease. He seemed in good general physical condition and played sandlot baseball. His teammates kidded him about his slow speed on the base paths, but his power and coordination at bat were a more than equal offset. He hated the high school gym requirement of swimming, because the water was always too cold for him. In a somewhat humorous way he managed to get excused from swimming on the basis of CF. He managed this despite the fact that he was an experienced swimmer having spent parts of every summer at his grandfather's cottage on a small lake in southern Michigan. Will was a reasonably good student in high school but did not excel, spending as much time as possible socializing with friends and enjoying life rather than hitting the books. He graduated from Cleveland Heights High School and was accepted at Ohio State University in 1969. We made special arrangements for his living facility rather than the normally required dormitory arrangement. He had a small refrigerator for his medications and he resided in an apartment with a friend. After another bad hemoptysis episode, he had to rush back to Cleveland.

Until this time in 1971, we and Will had been under the impression that he had suffered significant lung damage. During this hospitalization, Dr. Matthews had a bronchogram performed and to everyone's surprise, there was much less lung damage discernible by this test than anyone had expected. This was a critical time of decision for Will, as previously he had made no long term career plan but lived for the good times of the moment. This life style was based on his acceptance of the fatal nature of CF, knowledge of the mortality statistics, and his desire to enjoy those few years. The surprising lung report gave him a new lease on life and he decided he wanted to be a medical doctor.

Thus began the dream that carried with him through the rest of his life.

From that date forward nothing but this dream of being a medical doctor mattered. He endured the scars of unfair rejection and extra years of academic preparation in pursuing his dream. He never gave up and pursued it relentlessly, but each rejection hurt. To fulfill his dream, he switched to a premedical curriculum and crammed courses to make up the lost ground, graduating on schedule in 1974 with a degree in psychology.

The Foundation

As a National organization in the early 1970s, we were always dissatisfied with our fund raising growth rate and thereby in our ability to support and augment our research programs. Among persistent efforts to examine ourselves and break out to new levels of support, the administration and the then President, Robert McCreery, a Cleveland Chapter member, set up an advisory committee comprised of essentially Madison Avenue advertising people. The essence of their report was that the term "Cystic Fibrosis" was too difficult for the public to understand and not really marketable. Their recommendation was that the name be changed to some acronym based on "Lungs" since the vast majority of CF children succumbed from destruction of lung function and also because there were many other lung diseases with huge numbers of victims to enlarge our market. This report was presented at a Board meeting with favorable representation by professional staff and was likewise greeted with favor by a significant number of the NCFRF Board members. The meeting then became the scene of dissent by a small group of CF parent trustees who felt totally opposed to any name that did not include the words "Cystic Fibrosis." A motion was made to this effect but defeated by majority vote. As we left New York, the concerned group of parent trustees discussed possible Chapter secession from the National organization given the obvious intent to proceed with an acronym. With the total agreement and collaboration of Bob Dresing, who at that time was a first term Regional Trustee, we partnered in long distance phone conversations with other like minded trustees and major Chapter Presidents. The National office was aware of what was happening and, as momentum gathered, elected to back off. Through the medium of Dr. Graub, we were contacted and asked if we would accept a compromise name change to "Cystic Fibrosis Foundation." We were delighted with the offer and in due course the new name went into effect. This was a very significant action in that it perpetuated and forced into common usage the words "Cystic Fibrosis," which might otherwise have remained purely a term used only by medical people, such as the term "mucoviscidosis."

I continued to be active in my roles, locally and at the national level. As new local cases were diagnosed the parents, almost without exception, attended our meetings and became, to a greater or lesser degree active members. In the late 1960s, one family stood out particularly in their desire and efforts to participate and make a difference. Robert and Sarah Dresing brought their enthusiasm and became extremely active in all phases of our activities. We provided every opportunity for more work in the cause and ultimately sponsored Bob as a Regional Trustee of the NCFRF. He was elected and served until 1976. Upon my resignation, by prearrangement and in recognition of his obvious capability, he was appointed a Trustee at Large and no longer was at risk of the Regional Trustee popularity election process.

Bob went on ultimately to serve several very distinguished terms as the National President and CEO. During his watch, national fund raising grew spectacularly, research burgeoned, and the CF gene was discovered. The Cleveland Chapter contribution to National lay leadership through that interval had included two of the six top level leaders, McCreery and Dresing, and provided four occupants of the top medical position; Drs. LeRoy Matthews, Carl Doershuk, Thomas Boat, and Pamela Davis. All aspects considered, the Cleveland impact was significant, if not vital, to the progress of the CF struggle.

As the years passed, our survivors became adults and some became volunteers in the cause which was great! Paul Downs served as our legal advisor, Board Member, President of the Rainbow Chapter, National Board Trustee, and in other National roles. Others who served on the Rainbow Chapter Board included Gary Schilling, Joseph Kester, Douglas Cramner, Charles Shifman, Betty Berlin, Charlene Openo-Lucha, and Willard Bernbaum. Any inadvertently omitted names are truly regretted for this was a monumental victory in itself in view of the dire life forecasts of their childhood.

Medical School and Beyond

In 1974, Will had applied to ten medical schools and was rejected by all, despite good Medcat test scores. He was a social worker for Cuyahoga County while attending Cleveland State University night classes. In due course he earned a Masters degree in biology in expectation of enhancing his qualifications for medical school acceptance. He again applied to the schools and again was rejected. This was a period of dejection for him. He changed jobs and was a research lab worker at Western Reserve University and an instructor in Pharmacology at Cleveland State University for the nursing curriculum. In 1977, he decided to apply one more time, but only to Ohio medical schools. One reply of rejection from the Toledo School of Medicine was surprisingly frank in saying that the rejection was based entirely on his CF. Since this type of discrimination was completely illegal, there was consideration by our National organization to pursue the matter in court. However, shortly thereafter, Will was accepted by the Western Reserve University School of Medicine and we elected not to pursue the matter with Toledo. I always suspected that the doctor who wrote the Toledo letter did so deliberately to encourage a suit; otherwise his frankness in disclosing discrimination made no sense. Will received his

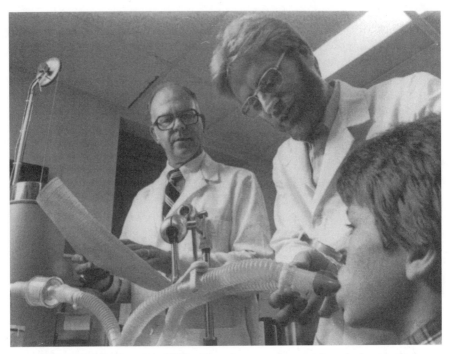

Figure 13.1. *Medical student, Willard Bernbaum, assists a patient during a pulmonary function test in 1984 with Dr. Carl Doershuk in background. Note the more simple set up compared to Figure 5.1. Courtesy of Mr. Henry Bernbaum.*

letter of acceptance at our home and opened it in our presence expecting another rejection. I never saw my son happier than at that moment in his life.

Will's medical school years were full (Figure 13.1) but not uneventful. He had a number of hemoptyses and several related blockage procedures. Unfortunately he also was a victim of the Guillian-Barre syndrome, believed to be associated with that year's flu vaccine. This experience for Will and our family was a horror story of its own, as the paralysis crept up his legs and body. Happily the paralysis stopped advancing before affecting his ability to breathe. He spent many weeks in the hospital and later at home in recovery. For some time he continued to wear leg supports but finally recovered about 95% of the use of his legs and discarded the supports. The result was one more challenge passed and one more obstacle surmounted. Between this illness and the hemoptyses, he lost a lot of time in his medical school career but made it all up and graduated with his medical school class in April 1982 in his 31st year of life.

As a sidelight to our family story, probably because of our constant and close involvement with CF and the medical profession, three of our four children became doctors.

After graduation from medical school, Will decided to train for the internal medicine specialty and was accepted as an intern at the Mt. Sinai Medical Center in Cleveland. The next three years were again complicated by hemoptyses, hospitalizations, embolism procedures, and gradually more breathing difficulty. He asked no favors and received none. He completed the Internal Medicine residency three months late in 1985, as he needed extra time to complete his rotations as a result of a life threatening lengthy hospitalization. He applied for and received appointment to the staff of St. Vincent's Charity Hospital and worked there until shortly before his death.

Aside from his school and training career, Will led a very active life for as long as he could. In the post high school years, he took up paddleball and played a good game through college until he became too short of breath to continue such a fast paced sport. Whenever summers permitted, he took trips to the national parks with friends and family to backpack, camp out, and hike in the wilderness areas. His camera was always ready for the next beautiful scene or wild animal. He did Yellowstone in the winter and in summer, the Tetons, and the Beartooth Mountains. Glacier National Park was his favorite and he returned there several times. His favorite color prints were enlarged, personally framed, and mounted in his home. In Cleveland, he hiked all the park areas in the Emerald Necklace, the chain of preserved natural parklands surrounding the city. The National Park phase ended during his medical school years when he no longer could handle this activity.

During his residency, Will met Geralyn Kraft, a nurse at Mt. Sinai Hospital. They fell in love and in July 1985 they were married. Life was beautiful, Will's health was fairly stable, and work was interposed by vacations with Geri to Canada, England, and Alaska. Geri quickly acquired the physical therapy skills and became a major player on Will's treatment team. However, his state of health was declining. It was more and more difficult to keep up the pace. In September 1986, he celebrated his 35th birthday with all his friends and extended family at a surprise party arranged by Geri. He continued his internist role with increasing difficulty through the last day of March 1987 without missing a day. During the latter days of this period he administered IV antibiotics to himself as directed by his physician, while refusing to be hospitalized. Geri convinced him to go on oxygen but he continued to refuse to enter the hospital, although he did request a family friend and lawyer to arrange his last will and testament. These were hard moments for wife, parents, and siblings to handle. Each of us spent as much time with him as possible.

Heart/lung transplant programs had been performed with some success in England and were being started in the US. Will was doubtful initially but it was apparent that the present course held no hope, so he accepted transfer to Temple University Hospital in Philadelphia for a heart-lung transplant. But his time was too short and he passed away on the morning of May 1, 1987.

At his wish, Will was cremated and his ashes were taken by the family to the Beartooth Mountains Wilderness. After a simple ceremony that included family contributions and a reading of The Impossible Dream, his ashes were scattered near one of his campsites in a place that he loved.

His life was memorialized by the creation of an annual award, initiated by the staff of Mt. Sinai Hospital. The award was made to a member of each graduating class of residents from 1987 through 1999 when Mt. Sinai Hospital closed and the award was transferred to University Hospitals. In its first year there as part of the residency graduating program of the new millennium, the award was presented by Dr. Darryl Miller, a departing chief resident who had been the 1997 recipient of the award at Mt. Sinai. It is appropriate that UH will remember Will each year, both as a medical school, and RB&C and University Hospitals alumnus. In 1988, the National CFF honored his memory by establishing The Willard A. Bernbaum, M.D. Cystic Fibrosis Research Laboratory now located on the eighth floor of the Celeste Research Building on the Case Western Reserve University campus. Every year on May 1st we visit the lab.

During his final time, Will told the family that he didn't want to be forgotten "as if I had never lived." We each remember a multitude of all types of incidents and mental images of an unforgettable personage who graced our lives with his presence. We will not forget him. We also wish to express our appreciation to the physicians who cared for Will, contributed to the quality of his life, and were his mentors and friends during all of those years; Drs. Earle Smith, Sam Spector, Lee Matthews, Tom Boat, and Bob Stern. Also we wish to express the same warmth of feeling for the nursing and therapy staffs at Rainbow Babies and Children's Hospital whose caring dedication to the patients over the years has been no less than phenomenal.

We knew so many wonderful devoted people over so very many years that worked so hard making their contributions to this cause that we feel guilty for not being able to list them with their own paragraph of accomplishments. Some are mentioned because they fit into this abbreviated history, but many will not be named and for this we must apologize. We are faced with recollections, now over a 50 year span, dealing with what turns out, in retrospect, to be a complex local and national health agency development. For those not mentioned, their comfort is that they know what they achieved in their part in the success of the Foundation. They played a part in improving the quality of life for these children, extending their lives far beyond the less than four year average when we started and indeed well into adult life and experience. We endorse this position for ourselves as well.

One couple, our friends the Andersons, deserve special comment. No one has been more devoted to the CF cause in Cleveland than Phyllis and Lawson Anderson from the very beginning, throughout the developmental years, and on into the current era. Very early on, they learned that their child did not have CF and fortunately had been misdiagnosed. Nevertheless they functioned for CF with the same intensity as those of us with CF children. During the earlier days of the Cleveland Chapter, the office of President was quite time consuming with all the growth, fund raising activities, organizational development in the northern Ohio area, etc. The Chapter was particularly blessed by the Andersons. Despite the change in diagnosis of their daughter, Cheryl, from CF to Celiac Disease, they

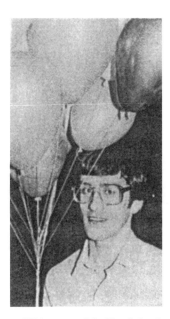

Figure 13.2. *"Volunteer of the Year" for the Cleveland Chapter in 1980, future Dr. Michael Konstan, chaired the annual "Bucks for Breathing" for CF by his fraternity at Case Western Reserve University. Courtesy of Mr. Henry Bernbaum.*

maintained their interest. Each served as President, as well as in many other capacities.

The Chapter was additionally favored by three gentlemen without a family relationship to CF, who devoted many years of service on our Board of Trustees and also served leadership terms as President. These were William "Bill" Clauss, a local bank manager, and Robert Burkhart and Paul Shreck, industry executives, who, despite their exceedingly active business lives, provided that leadership. It is indeed fortunate that such public spirited people step forward and volunteer their talents to worthy causes.

The current Director of the LeRoy Matthews Cystic Fibrosis Center, Dr. Michael Konstan, succeeded Carl Doershuk upon his retirement in 1998. Dr. Konstan is another who has a long standing and unique history of involvement with CF. He attended Case Western Reserve University in the late 1970s and, among his many activities, organized and successfully ran an annual campus carnival type fund raiser for the benefit of CF (Figure 13.2). His interest in CF does go back a long way! In addition, he went on to medical school and was a classmate of Will's, graduating with him in May 1982.

In retrospect, the original gift of $203 from the Jaffe Cousins Club stimulated the first $2,500 Chapter check to Babies and Children's Hospital and thereafter a spiraling annual support for clinical and basic science research. In 1990, the Chapter was selected for the Isaiah Award for Human Relations given annually by the American Jewish Committee, Cleveland Chapter, to the local organization deemed to have made a genuine community contribution worthy of this award. As part of our submission, we did a 34 year historical report on our Chapter activities. This included a tally of total net funds raised and distributed, which amounted to $7,387,442.

In final comment we wish, of course, that each of our children had been born and remained healthy, but the roll of the genetic dice deemed otherwise. Under these circumstances, we feel rewarded for our efforts because our son and many other CF youngsters lived and are living longer and better quality lives because we, and all the others like us, did our best to help. We watch for each advance and still await a cure for Cystic Fibrosis.

14

Early Years

Phyllis S. and Lawson S. Anderson

We became involved with cystic fibrosis (CF) in the early 1950s following the birth of our second child. In August of that year, Phyllis, being seven months pregnant, resigned her position as a nurse in the Maternity Outpatient Department, University Hospitals of Cleveland. The following day, her husband, Lawson (Andy) received a telegram with "greetings from the President" recalling him to active duty in the Air Force at the time of the Korean conflict. Instead of beginning his third year as an accounting major at Fenn College, now Cleveland State University, he ended up assigned to Tinker Air Force Base, in Oklahoma.

We, along with our three year old daughter, Cindi, arrived at the base in late September and immediately went to a local obstetrician as I was having toxemia with the pregnancy. The weekend before the baby was born, I was admitted to the base hospital by a different doctor who proceeded to induce labor, and we learned that my first doctor also had been called back to active military duty. After two days of no progress, the flight surgeon in charge of the hospital told me that, in the interim, the second doctor had been called to another duty post. The flight surgeon contacted a private physician in Oklahoma City, an anesthesiologist, who was the one that finally delivered our baby, Cheryl, on October 24, weighing just under 6 pounds. Due to the toxemia, I was heavily sedated and could not take care of her. Normal procedure was for the mother to care for her child 24 hours a day. Our hospital stay lasted ten days, whereas normally mother and child would be discharged three days after delivery. Cheryl began having 18–20 loose, foul-smelling bowel movements a day. Her weight went down to well below 5 pounds. The doctors were concerned and told us they thought she had "Sprue," which they stated was uncommon in the United States. By two months of age, she was being fed mashed bananas, had been on 13 different formulas, and was being treated with antibiotics for pneumonia and cough.

After seeing various doctors concerning her continuing symptoms, we were told they were not sure what she had and that we should return her to Cleveland to die, as she was critically ill. We could not accept that because I was a graduate from Frances Payne Bolton School of Nursing at Western Reserve University and knew of the reputation of University Hospitals of Cleveland and Babies and Children's Hospital (B&C Hospital). When we returned home, we contacted Dr. LeRoy W. Matthews, a personal friend, whose wife Blanche (Rock) had worked with me in Maternity OPD at MacDonald House. Cheryl was just five months old when admitted to B&C Hospital for diagnosis and treatment. With her symptoms of frequent loose bowel movements, cough, and recurring pneumonia along with the other tests that had been performed, it was felt that she could possibly have cystic fibrosis of the pancreas (also known then as pancreatic fibrosis, mucoviscidosis, or fibrocystic disease of the pancreas). She was started on pancreatic enzymes to be mixed with the bananas and other food. Her bowel movements did decrease and she continued on this regimen until the sweat test procedure became available there in 1953.

The sweat test consisted of my changing to a gown and taking the then three year old Cheryl into a small heavily moisturized room containing numerous humidifiers. She was in a hospital bed and wrapped in many blankets to make her sweat. She was obviously unhappy and irritable, but after an hour sweat was collected wherever the technician could find it by drawing it up into a pipette and the sweat was then tested for salt content. Needless to say, this made for a "bad hair day" for me, and a very unhappy child. It was a great relief to us when the test came back negative and she was no longer considered as having CF. Ultimately, she was diagnosed as having celiac disease and she gradually improved. In 1957, an improved method was available to do the sweat test and Dr. Matthews asked us to have another one done. This time, we were in a regular hospital room with no humidifiers. A pilocarpine patch was put on the underside of her arm. After a period of time, the technician removed the patch to test for salt concentration. This test was much easier on both Cheryl and me. It was a marked improvement and again we were relieved and grateful that the results were negative.

In 1955, a family group known as the Jaffe Cousins Club met socially each month. It was recognized that one family, that of Sam and Henrietta Trott, who had already lost one child to CF and now had a son with the disease, could not attend club functions because of the child's illnesses. The members decided to have a rummage sale to raise money to fight this disease. In December 1955 with funds totaling $206, a non-profit corporation was established to provide funds to be used for research into the cause and cure of CF. This organization was known as the Cystic Fibrosis Foundation, Cleveland Chapter and was incorporated in the State of Ohio.

Early in 1956, a meeting was held by a few of the CF families with Dr. William Wallace and Dr. Samuel Spector at B&C Hospital to discuss the idea of starting a CF organization to raise funds for research. They were very understanding and supportive and recommended a meeting with known CF families. This meeting was held in February 1956, at the home of Robert and Joan Jaffe. In attendance were six families representing CF involvement (Henry and Madeline Bernbaum, Bob and Jean Horn, Walt and Rita Mikulitz, Dan and Lois Obloy, the Trotts, and ourselves), and two families from the Cousins Club, Bob and Joan Jaffe and Lou and Alice Cherko. The purpose of this group was to raise the funds necessary to begin to support research on CF.

At the meeting, after discussion of what might be accomplished we stated that, even though it now had been determined that Cheryl did not have CF, we would provide any help that we possibly could to fight this disease. As a result, the following officers were elected and our long term commitment to CF began: President, Phyllis Anderson; Vice-President, Robert Horn; Secretary, Jean Horn; and Treasurer, Andy Anderson (since by now he was a certified public accountant).

The first Board of Trustees consisted of the above named officers along with Drs. Wallace and Spector, Robert Jaffe, Walter Mikulitz, Mrs. Dan Obloy, Mrs. Sam Trott, and Henry Bernbaum. Our first mailing address was in the Hippodrome Building in downtown Cleveland, and our first public meeting was held in the South Euclid City Hall in April 1956. This was publicized in a local suburban newspaper and was attended by over 60 people. Drs. Wallace and Spector were elected to the Board of Trustees and spoke about the funds required to start research. They also recommended having a Medical Advisory Committee. They were then the first elected to that Committee.

Subsequently, the monthly meetings of the Board of Trustees were held in the homes of individual Board members. This helped to create a closeness among us and a determination to raise funds. Most of these meetings lasted well beyond the midnight hour. A monthly newsletter was started and written by the Bernbaums and mailed out to all members and friends by the Horns and Andersons.

We also had public meetings where programs were presented. One of these was by Mrs. Lloyd Block from the Detroit Chapter, who presented a film produced by the Los Angeles Chapter entitled "That They May Live," which portrayed the life of the afflicted children, the very limited treatment available, and the urgent need for medical research. It indicated the growing awareness of the general public and was an excellent educational medium.

Throughout the year, we participated in numerous fundraising projects such as collecting state sales tax stamps for revenue, selling Christmas cards and salami for one dollar, and kosher wieners for $.79 per pound. We also sold foam covered hangers and found that rummage sales were the most profitable, netting three to seven hundred dollars per day for a two or three day period even back then. We had wonderful cooperation from members and friends on all of these projects, especially from Mariana and Herman Treu, Mary and Al Brodberg, the George Madens, the Bernbaums, Trotts, Obloys, Mary Shaltens, and Don Dewey.

There was so much to do and all of us worked hard, but we also had a lot of fun. One episode occurred when a woman with a two year old and a Taylor Tot (stroller) came to our rummage sale at West 45th and Detroit Avenues. We had so much merchandise that some of it was displayed on the sidewalk. The lady had taken her child into the building to shop and left the stroller outside. A customer bought it for one dollar and the lady was quite indignant on returning and said that it should have been sold for more than that. Fortunately, Andy was able to run down the street, catch up to the purchaser, retrieve the Taylor Tot, and refund the money, thereby returning the stroller to the owner.

At our September general meeting, it was announced that, through the generosity of one of our members, Sam Trott, a pharmacist, and CF parent, a pharmacy program to provide pharmaceuticals and prescription medicines was being made available to CF patients at a nominal cost. Somewhat later, this was adjusted to cost plus 10%, which included mailing if required. This very giving gesture would have a significant impact on keeping cost of prescriptions as low as possible for our CF families and later stimulate a similar program at the National level for all CF families.

All the proceeds from the fundraising projects were needed to fund a treatment and research program, which was to be started in July 1957. Dr. Wallace had indicated that if we could raise $2,500 as seed money by the end of 1956, the program would be started at B&C Hospital. Our major fundraising effort to meet this goal was a benefit concert by the Suburban Symphony under the direction of Robert Weiskopf. This was held in a large auditorium at East 50th and Euclid Ave. in December and was sold out. The feature presentation was by Carol Sindell, an eight year old child prodigy violin soloist. Along with the other funds we had raised, the proceeds from this concert made it possible to present Dr. Wallace a check for $2,500 for the beginning of the research project.

The Medical Advisory Board was approved and consisted of Drs. Wallace and Spector, Dr. Richard Hodges, and Dr. Robert McEvoy pediatricians, Dr. E.A. Mortimer a Pediatric Professor from City Hospital (now MetroHealth Medical Center), CF parent Dr. Keith Noble from Alliance, Ohio, and Dr. Arthur Steinberg, Professor of Biology at Western Reserve University, who was interested in human genetics.

By early 1957, we had 83 paid members and had raised a total of $6,700 since inception. The Medical Advisory Board recommended a medical program to fund a research doctor to establish a CF treatment clinic at B&C Hospital and to start an investigative research program and the Chapter Board approved a total grant of $7,500 for the research year July 1957 to July 1958. Dr. LeRoy Matthews, who had been our consultant in research right along, accepted this assignment. He established the Clinic which was to evaluate methods of treatment in use at that time, to develop newer ones, and to closely observe the condition of each patient through regular monthly checkups. Joy Lemm started working part time in the new mucus research laboratory.

The membership grew rapidly to 120 by midyear. Our first brochure was composed by Aaron Mercer, the grandfather of a CF child, with the first year production totaling 5,000 units. The amount increased each year, creating an inventory of over 120,000 units by 1960 for the Health Fund drives. Little public information was available in 1956, so this was a significant accomplishment enabling us to publicize the disease and the need for research. Members, working in a basement workshop, set up a silk screening operation and produced thousands of bumper stickers. The logo used on these bumper stickers and other printed material was a picture of a child who was using an inhalation mask for therapy, with the letters "CF" imprinted.

Our first anniversary ball fund raiser was held at the Midday Club in the Union Commerce Building at East 9th Street and Euclid Avenue. The cost seemed unbelievable at $5.00 per couple. To save the expense of a decorated cake so that more money would be raised for the research project, several members decorated a hatbox as a cake for the occasion. Cleveland Chapter members who lived in surrounding communities started chapters in Lorain, Summit, and Stark counties. Members of these chapters also began fundraising activities, including selling orchids and plants in Lorain and Elyria by Norma Leatherman and Adrienne Kerr selling candy and Christmas cards, in the Akron area by the Eliot, Gertz, and Reynolds families, and in the Youngstown area by the Allison, Hicken, and Shilling families. Various other families sponsored street carnivals by CF children and their playmates.

The Cleveland Chapter continued to add new fundraising projects in addition to our lucrative rummage sales. These included kiddie carnivals held in a parking lot at Cedar and Warrensville Center Roads and bowling contests. Numerous people worked on these projects, including the Pattersons, Florence Mercer, Molly Dise, Morrey and Dottie Stollar, Edith West, Barbara and Don Davis, Sally and Sal Maritt, the Horns, and many CF children who were old enough to help along with their families.

Our first big break with publicity came when Josephine Robertson, medical editor of the Cleveland Plain Dealer, interviewed Dr. Matthews and me on the research project, the opening of the CF clinic, and on the operation and aims of the Foundation. At a general meeting, Dr. Matthews spoke on the sweat test and agar plate test, which was used then as a screening method. In the agar plate test, the child put the palm of the hand on the plate to collect sweat. If there was excess salt, the chocolate colored plate turned yellowish. This screening test was soon abandoned, as it proved best to do the actual sweat test to screen and diagnose suspected children.

Fundraising continued to be successful and the projects approved for the current year were fully funded. Some additional funds were used to purchase pulmonary function equipment for testing of the CF children. At a general meeting, Dr. Steinberg, who had just joined Western Reserve University as Professor of Biology and was involved in the field of Genetics, spoke about CF as a genetic disease. He had received a grant of $14,000 from the US Public Health Service for a two year study to conduct a genetic survey relative to the incidence of CF throughout the State of Ohio from 1950 through 1953. Families were requested to supply data and assist with laboratory experiments. The study hoped to determine the incidence of CF in the general population, to conduct blood studies to determine other genetic similarities or differences among CF patients, and to investigate the increase in patient numbers in this previously "100% fatal disease."

About this time, negotiations were being held with United Way, an agency started many years earlier to collect funds for charitable organizations, in an effort for CF to be included in its annual drive. Their recommendation was that a combined Health Fund be started to raise funds for research by charitable health related organizations rather than having a single health drive by each agency. Some of the health agencies that eventually joined together were the Kidney, Diabetes, Muscular Dystrophy, Arthritis, Hemophilia, and Cystic Fibrosis Foundations.

Dr. Harry Shwachman came to Cleveland in November. He was from Children's Hospital, Boston, and an Assistant Professor of Pediatrics at Harvard University School of Medicine. He talked about the medical history of CF, diagnostic methods, treatment, and prognosis. His presentation in the amphitheater of B&C was very well attended; one reason being the desire of our families for more information, as little was printed at that time. He reported that by the end of 1957 there were 28 Chapters in the National Cystic Fibrosis Foundation and ten independent Chapters. Cleveland Chapter was one of the independents and did not join National then as we felt that money raised here would be better utilized at B&C Hospital, as the clinic and research programs were already making good progress.

Hank Bernbaum was elected president in January 1958, and in June we welcomed Dr. Melvin Wise from Montreal, Canada as our first research fellow. He was to work in the newly established pulmonary function laboratory. The lab was used for the testing of pulmonary function in children with CF, to permit objective evaluation of the various forms of therapy (aerosol therapy and mucolytic enzymes administered by aerosol), and to determine the rate of progression of the disease.

Since the proposed combined Health Fund drive was not yet officially organized, the Cleveland Chapter initiated a limited house-to-house solicitation in various suburbs throughout Cuyahoga County. Some members involved were Mrs. Matthews known as "Rock", Wilda Casarona, Sally Maritt, Rudy Pfieffer, Jean Horn, Henrietta Trott, Sandy Gaw, Rita Mikulitz, Mal Bernbaum, and Joan Raggets. In an effort to publicize CF, one of our more aggressive members placed the bumper stickers on many stop signs in one of the suburbs where we were soliciting. I received a call from the police chief of that city who politely requested that they be removed quickly. The member was notified and he proceeded to remove the stickers. This drive in addition to other projects raised over $14,000 and our membership continued to grow to 286 by the end of 1958.

Throughout the year, we had excellent speakers at our monthly meetings and these included a psychologist, dietician, physical therapist, pediatric surgeon, and the various doctors involved in our CF research effort. These meetings were all heavily attended, averaging 75 to 100 people, and added significantly to our success.

In January 1959, Andy was elected as the third president. At that meeting Dr. Steinberg presented the results of his two year genetic survey. This was the broadest study to date and accurately predicted the later generally accepted incidence of CF for this population. The study revealed that CF patients and normal carriers of the CF gene did not appear to have other similar genetic characteristics. At that time, there was no accurate clinical method of recognizing a healthy individual who carried the recessive CF gene, and from this aspect, CF posed a constantly growing threat to society. We were pleased to learn that Dr. Steinberg received an award from Case Western Reserve University in 1999 in recognition of this and his other significant contributions to the field of genetics.

Dr. Matthews, who was continuing to serve as our research consultant as well as providing care and evaluating the results, was invited to the first International research conference on CF sponsored jointly by the National Institutes of Health, the Public Health Service, and the National Cystic Fibrosis Research Foundation. This was held in Washington, D.C. in 1959. He reported that 35 physicians and scientists were working in the field of CF and an additional 35 basic scientists well versed in allied basic research fields attended. The clinical picture and present status of research progress was presented for the benefit of the basic scientists who critically discussed this research and suggested new methods and research projects. At the next meeting, Dr. Matthews presented his first annual research and clinic report in which he reviewed the description and effects of CF, diagnostic procedures and tests, treatment practice at the clinic and in the home, as well as demonstrating equipment used in the home. He reported that 54 cases showed rather uniformly remarkable progress, benefiting from the full comprehensive treatment program. He further announced that over the past 13 months not one patient had expired, even though a number of new cases brought in would have normally been considered in terminal stages.

In 1958, we were fortunate to have the Hon. Judge Daniel Wasserman join us as an honorary member of the Board of Trustees. In an important step, he then worked with us to create a Civic Advisory Board of 32 interested civic-minded citizens to advise and provide assistance to CF in areas of public relations and fund raising. We had to change the location of Board meetings to the B&C Hospital amphitheater where our general meetings were also held because the size of the Board had outgrown our member's homes. The first Advisory Board, appointed in 1959, covered a broad spectrum of the Cleveland community and greatly extended our efforts.

We continued to be successful in fundraising and a grant of $15,000 was presented to Dr. Matthews for the year July 1958 to July 1959 for research purposes. Total contributions since 1956 reached $53,500. Dr. Wise, our research fellow who was completing his year with us, spoke on the disturbances of pulmonary function in CF. We welcomed Dr. George Eddy, our second clinical fellow in CF and Dr. Joseph Potter, Ph.D. in Biochemistry to work with Dr. Matthews in the mucus research program, who were appointed for the year 1959-1960. We continued to have the kiddie carnivals, which raised over $1,000. The two favorite concessions were a kiddie train with Bill Gayneau as conductor, and a dunk the dolly operated by Roger Leininger and his friends. Many other members participated in these activities. Fortunately, one of them, electrician Al Baskin, who was entertaining as a clown, also did double duty by fixing many blown fuses.

In September, it was reported that Dr. Spector had been granted $110,000 from the National Institutes of Health for five years of CF research. As far as was known at that time, this represented the largest federal or private grant ever made to fund research in CF. We were able to distribute a new brochure on CF during our house-to-house Health Fund drive which was held in Chagrin Falls, Hunting Valley, Middleburg Heights, Brookpark, and Independence, and was chaired by Frieda Corcoran and Cynthia Leininger. Two additional new chapters were started, one in Youngstown by the John Hickens, the George Shillings, and the John Stephens, and the other in Loudenville by Mrs. Glenn Reynolds.

In October 1959, we attended the annual meeting of the National Cystic Fibrosis Research Foundation (NCFRF) in Philadelphia as invited guests. Representatives from 36 states and the Washington, D.C. Chapter attended. Other guests were representatives from Toronto and Montreal, Canada and ourselves who were not members of the National organization. It was reported that NCFRF had 90 chapters with 18 applications pending. This represented a significant growth in the four year period since the National Foundation was started. The requirement for affiliation with NCFRF that 85% of funds raised needed to be forwarded to them seemed excessive to us. We could not meet that requirement because of our commitment to Western Reserve University and Babies and Children's Hospital. In part, this was due to the recommendation by the Cleveland Chamber of Commerce that most of the funds raised should be spent in Cleveland. The speakers at the Conference at the technical sessions included Dr. Dorothy Andersen from New York, and Dr. Shwachman, along with Dr. Matthews.

In 1960, we were approved as a member of the Special Health Agencies of the Welfare Federation, which was known as Health Fund of Greater Cleveland. The first solicitation by this organization totaled approximately $375,000, of which CF received approximately $28,000, which represented a significant increase over our individual drive. We then received an increasing amount each year and by the mid 1960's, it amounted to over $70,000. The Health Fund was absorbed into the United Way and our annual share increased to approximately $250,000.

Drs. Leon Dembo and Earle Smith, private pediatricians well known in the community, joined the Medical Advisory Board. We had grown so much that we had to open our own office and were fortunate that one of our members, William West, was able to locate one at 1715 Euclid Avenue in downtown Cleveland. At this time, we also hired our first employee, John Baird, as administrative secretary.

In 1960, we served as hosts for the 2nd Annual Regional Conference held at B&C Hospital for Chapters from Northern Ohio, Pennsylvania, Indiana, and Michigan. Ideas were exchanged regarding fund raising (93.7% of each dollar of total income was used for research in Cleveland). It was reported that the mortality rate of CF patients seen at the Cleveland Center was 1% annually compared to 10% nationally. In 1957, prior to the start of our treatment program, there were 16 known deaths due to CF. From 1957 to 1961, there were only 3 deaths of patients in the program.

Dr. Eddy demonstrated the pulmonary function equipment and Dr. Potter demonstrated his basic research equipment and its use in the mucus studies. Mrs. Lee Johnson, research technician, demonstrated the sweat test and the latest equipment for inhalation and mist therapy treatments. Mrs. Norma Leatherman, Lorain Chapter, presented a check for $10,000, funds raised by them to be used for the research program. Dr. Harry Nudelman joined us as a research fellow in 1960. Additional progress was made in 1961 with Sal J. Marrit being elected president.

Dr. Carl Doershuk completed his residency at City Hospital and B&C Hospital in 1961 and was welcomed as the first two year fellow having been awarded a pulmonary disease training grant from the US Public Health Service.

After extensive negotiation with NCFRF covering many months, it was mutually agreed that we would become a Chapter of the National organization in 1961. A great deal of credit for our joining NCFRF was due to the tireless efforts of our President, Sal Maritt and Hank Bernbaum. We were able to maintain our affiliation with the Health Fund of Greater Cleveland and Hank was elected a trustee-at-large of NCFRF. We were proud that Cleveland was considered one of the leading research, treatment, and teaching Centers in the country.

Our Chapter has provided outstanding medical and lay personnel to NCFRF over the years. These include Drs. Matthews, Doershuk, Thomas Boat, and Pamela Davis, each of whom have chaired many committees at National; Robert McCreery, who served as President of the National Foundation and subsequently the International CF Association; Robert Dresing, who also served as President of the National Foundation; Hank Bernbaum, who served as Vice President and on many other committees; and Bruce Baskin, current member of the National Board of Trustees.

In 1964, the first Conference of newly formed Region VI of NCFRF was held in Columbus. This conference and subsequent ones were well attended and brought together those lay and professional workers who were dedicated to furthering the CF cause. They were held for the exchange of ideas concerning progress in the research and treatment programs along with ways to improve fund raising and public relations. The stimulus to improve the Crippled Children's Programs in the various states, and later to add CF adults to these programs, came from the personal interactions afforded at these meetings. The member chapters of Region VI were Cleveland, Dayton, Columbus, Cincinnati, Kentuckyana (Louisville), Blue Grass (Harrodsburg), and Wheeling, West Virginia.

During that year, a significant change occurred when the drugstore owned by our pharmacist, Sam Trott, was destroyed overnight during the Glenville riots. His thoughts were with CF children and he was able to flee the area taking medications for them with the help of an employee. This created an opportunity for us to move the Chapter offices to larger facilities, include the pharmacy program, and maintain the overall Chapter program at Mayfield and Lee Roads in Cleveland Heights.

Also in 1964, Dr. Matthews was awarded a 7 year grant from the National Institutes of Health (NIH) for $648,000 to conduct more extensive research studies in CF and related obstructive lung diseases. This was one of the largest grants awarded by the NIH at that time.

We have been very fortunate to have had dedicated Presidents and their Boards. These include in order of service: Phyllis Anderson, Henry Bernbaum, Lawson (Andy) Anderson, John Maritt, Paul Schreck, John Neilson, William Clauss, Jr., William Beyer, Donald Davis, William Gayneau, Jon Martin, Robert

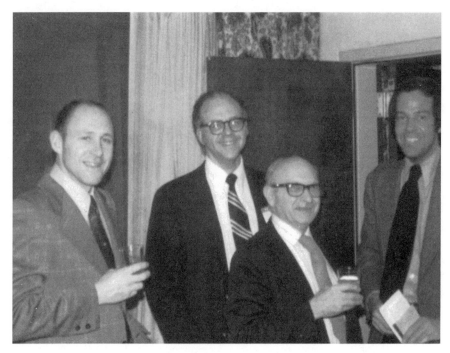

Figure 14.1. *Samuel Trott, third from left, was honored as the first Man of the Year by the Cleveland Chapter. Others from the left, Cleveland Chapter President, William Beyer, Dr. Carl Doershuk, and Regional Trustee, Robert Dresing. Courtesy of Mr. and Mrs. Lawson Anderson.*

Burkhart, Paul Downs, Michael Mudler, Arthur Bacon, Ralph Dise, and John Suffron.

Additional pulmonary fellows working in the CF and pulmonary disease program up to about 1980 were Drs. Terry Gillespie, Suzanne Miller, Susan Pittman, Robert Stern, Thomas Boat, Robert Wood, and David Orenstein. We are proud that all have remained active in CF care and projects.

Throughout this period of time, the education of the public was especially accomplished by members and doctors speaking about the various aspects of CF on radio and television and in articles appearing in magazines and newspapers. The Chapter honored Sam Trott in 1964, as the first recipient of the Man of the Year award at a banquet (Figure 14.1). Subsequent honors were bestowed on Dr. LeRoy Matthews in 1966 with joint honors to Dr. Doershuk and Hank Bernbaum in 1970.

A big debt of gratitude goes to all people involved in the growth of the CF Foundation for the many hours of time, talent, and money donated unselfishly, including but not limited to the following: the production and sale of Christmas cards; the many carnivals and symphony concerts; the Holly and Ivy Balls for over

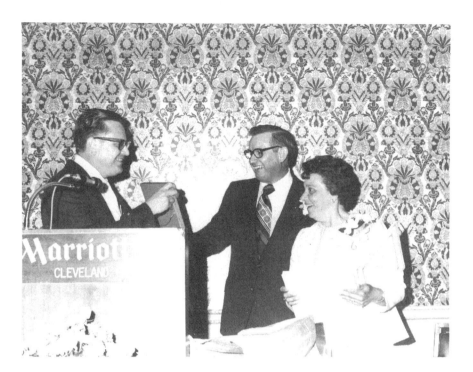

Figure 14.2. *President of the Cleveland Chapter, Don Davis, presents the "Man of the Year" awards to Lawson and Phyllis Anderson, both past presidents of the chapter. Courtesy of Mr. and Mrs. Lawson Anderson.*

10 years; and the donation at cost for the mist tents assembled by Bill Gayneau and friends, and the postural drainage tables produced by George Maden and the Kiwanis Club of South Euclid-Lyndhurst. These projects raised many thousands of dollars, which provided funds for the growing basic and clinical research programs.

Our daughter, Cheryl, who along with her older sister, Cindi, was well aware of the problems of CF children while growing up, and was inspired to enter nursing school. Upon graduation, Cheryl began to work at B&C Hospital (now Rainbow Babies and Children's Hospital) and this included working with the CF children. She became a certified respiratory therapist and, during the past almost two decades, has administered aerosols and taught about all the various newer forms of mucus clearance treatments that have become available for both CF children and adults. Also we had been blessed with the birth of a healthy child, Tom, who was born one night shortly after we attended a general membership meeting at B&C Hospital.

And finally, we have been honored to play a role in the beginning of the Cystic Fibrosis Foundation in Cleveland, helping to finance research into the cause and cure of CF, and to be recipients of the Man of the Year award in 1974 (Figure 14.2). Now 45 years later, we rejoice at the growth and success of fundraising projects by CF families and the National organization and the increase in people involved in research and treatment. It was a wonderful experience working with CF families and doctors, and we are thankful for the valued friendships that were developed during that time. Our special thanks go to our dear friend, the late Dr. LeRoy W. Matthews for all his foresight and success in the research and treatment of CF patients, in making Cleveland an outstanding CF Center, and with a debt of gratitude to his wife, "Rock," and their entire family.

15

Experiences as President: Making Progress

Robert D. McCreery, Sr.

Soon after the September 17, 1952 birth of Frankie's and my son in Cleveland, he displayed severe breathing problems not controlled by various medications. As problems continued, we were referred to Dr. LeRoy Matthews, a young Babies and Childrens Hospital pediatrician interested in cystic fibrosis (CF). When Doug was hospitalized, Frankie spent many hours with him in their mist room. He did not have cystic fibrosis (CF), however studies showed him subject to severe allergic breathing reactions from eggs, cow's milk, and multiple other items. Doug's health was under better control by 1956 when Lee asked me to join a group of CF parents organized as The Cystic Fibrosis Foundation, Cleveland Chapter. My early participation was largely to show appreciation for Lee's significant help with Doug. Little did I then realize how the relationship would involve my future.

In 1955, the Cleveland Chamber of Commerce solicitations committee issued a policy statement regarding the many money appeals being promoted in the area by health groups that suggested the public would soon react unfavorably to the more than 100 national health organizations expanding their organized appeals throughout the United States. Fifteen of these organizations were then active in Cleveland, of which ten were holding general money solicitations annually. The recommendation that health agencies, in particular, should combine their efforts into a joint Spring fund raising effort had merit but no organization existed to develop such a combined drive. With this encouragement, by 1958 women from sixteen Greater Cleveland suburbs developed a campaign known as the "Women's Revolt." This effort was so successful that the Chamber of Commerce organized help to promote a Combined Health Fund dedicated to raising money from residential areas, corporations, and employees previously plagued by multiple health drives.

Because of Doug's problems, Frankie became involved in the Brecksville Health Fund concept on behalf of CF. Brecksville quickly joined other communities in the combined solicitation for health needs. With about 100 supporting members, The Health Fund launched its first drive in 1960. An Allocations Committee was appointed of physicians and civic leaders to review budgets, agency programs, and recommendations which, when totaled, became the Health Fund goal for the year. I

To obtain a book with details and pictures beyond the scope of this chapter, contact Mr. McCreery at 3190 Roundwood Road, Cleveland, Ohio 44022

became Secretary of the Health Fund in 1962, followed by being elected President for 1965-66, then Board Chairman for 1967–68. At first, the National Cancer Society and American Heart Association elected independence from the combined Health Fund relying on appeals directed to victims and public concerns posed by their disease interests. However, as the Health Fund achieved success, solicitation conflicts between the three groups led to the formation of the Cleveland Plan, and I then served as a Cleveland Plan Trustee representing the Health Fund from 1968 to 1970. The concept successfully demonstrated Greater Cleveland's financial support for organizations dedicated to health research and patient needs.

In 1961, the Cleveland CF Chapter joined the Foundation as the Cleveland Chapter. Then in 1964, as a result of my activities in chapter affairs and fund raising, the Region VI Chapters (Cleveland, Columbus and Toledo chapters in Ohio, and the Wheeling, West Virginia chapter) joined in electing me their Regional Trustee to the New York based Board of Trustees of the NCFRF. When I arrived there, the Foundation was administered by Director George Barrie, who reported to the Executive Committee and ultimately to all National Trustees. As a Trustee, I first became a member of the finance committee and later the executive committee. From these groups, new and lasting friendships were established with David Baker, a senior New York banker, Ray Mulford, CEO of Owens Corning Corporation, Paul Etchepare, owner of the Wyoming Warren Ranch, Henry Rathert, special IRS fraud investigator, and several research and medical providers.

About a year after I was elected a National Trustee, Dr. Graub became President. He was excellent in resolving issues raised at Trustee meetings. As new chapters were created, differences arose with some Chapters wanting to fund local doctors with local raised money without regard to quality review and priority evaluation from the National organization's committees. As the Foundation grew, the problem became less severe.

Following the Foundation's 1969 New York meeting, I was asked to consider being a candidate for President during the three year term beginning April 1970. I respectfully declined and returned to my Cleveland activities. By then, George Barrie had departed and the new National Director, Welch Boyer, began encouraging me to reconsider. Dr. Graub then visited Frankie and me in our Brecksville, Ohio home to express his support and explain how my leadership would be helpful as CF National President.

With limited forward vision, I finally agreed to be a candidate and was elected President by the National Trustees for the 1970 to 1973 years. Upon becoming President, I determined to devote all possible time and effort to the position. The fund raising group and medical committees were advised that I expected to be included in their various meetings. As President I needed to know all aspects of Foundation efforts to be an effective leader. Fund raising people welcomed my willingness to appear at functions and deliver speeches. The medical persons were less willing to accept my participation as they were to meet, discuss, and make recommendations, without my non-professional involvement. The issue was resolved when it became known I would attend their meetings, refrain from discussion of professional matters but retain options to voice thoughts on overall Foundation matters. I was soon accepted by the medical group and often contributed in discussions that were more about medical politics than patient or science matters. Such meetings confirmed views of several individuals that more basic science research was needed beyond that provided by the dedicated patient care doctors who sometimes viewed themselves as basic research persons.

While Billy Graub was President, a basic science advisory committee made recommendations for specific research; however limited funding precluded serious execution of their proposals. During a chance discussion with Merck's research director, he suggested I visit Dr. Richard Sidman, Bullard Professor of Neuropathology at Harvard Medical School for his thoughts on how to achieve more attention to the basic science needs of the Foundation. I arranged to meet Dick and found him most willing to assist. He agreed to recruit other basic scientists to join a Presidential Research Advisory Committee reporting to me as the NCFRF President. Dr. William Rutter of the University of California, San Francisco, and Dr. Joel Rosenbaum, Department of Biology, Yale University soon augmented the advisory group (Figure 15.1). Their recommendations included allocating stated amounts of Foundation money to fund a limited number of outstanding young research scientist oriented persons. These grants would provide salary, travel, and other costs to those selected, conditioned on their total commitment to do CF basic research during a specified time.

I presented the proposal to the NCFRF Medical Council and received a very mixed response. Dick Sidman followed me by responding to their questions. A few of the older physicians took extreme exception of my creating the committee and for basic science persons assuming input into a disease far from their expertise. In the end, it was my decision to proceed with the committee's recommendations. The first Research Scientist recipients were Dr. Paul Quinton, a Los Angeles Ph.D. physiologist; Dr. Ricardo Martinez, a Columbia Missouri pediatrician and physiologist; and Dr. William Shearer, a St. Louis pediatrician and immunologist.

Luke Quinn, a retired military officer, was retained by the Foundation prior to 1970 as a part time lobbyist to assist the CF organization's relationships with Washington and the National Institutes of Health (NIH). Through his and others efforts, the NIH organized a Conference on Genetic Disease Control in October 1970 that I attended as NCFRF President along with Ray Mulford, CEO of Owens Illinois, Toledo, Ohio, and a number of scientists. That meeting was among the early efforts of NIH to address CF genetics.

The NCFRF had agreed to host the Sixth International Cystic Fibrosis Congress to be held in Washington D.C. in 1973. When held, attendance far exceeded earlier meetings. This was a most comprehensive program in comparison to previous meetings; the 1964 Paris steering meeting, the 1965 first ICF[M]A (International CF Mucoviscidosis Association) meeting also in Paris, the Berne, Switzerland (1966) and Cambridge, England (1969) meetings. Numbering the meetings identified as a Congress became unclear; however the Cambridge, UK meeting was definitely number five and the Washington D.C. Congress number

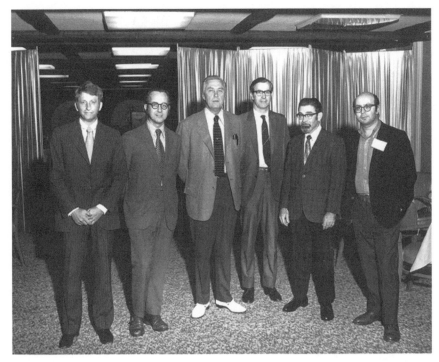

Figure 15.1. *A GAP Conference in 1972 brought together the Scientific Advisory Committee. Left to right, Drs. William Rutter, Richard Sidman, President Robert McCreery, and Drs. Eric Shooter, LeRoy Matthews and Joel Rosenbaum. Courtesy of Mr. Robert McCreery.*

six. Planning programs and committee assignments for our 1973 meeting became very complex and time consuming. Soon, the early registration increased to more than 1,000 people coming from multiple nations. Mrs. Pat Nixon, the wife of President Nixon, members of Congress, and various leaders from the NIH agreed to participate. The conference was most successful and resulted in expanded Cystic Fibrosis awareness in the US and around the World.

When I became President, the National CF offices were in leased space in an older New York building at 202 East 44th Street. In 1971, we learned that American Home Products desired the location for a new office building and had obtained control of all space except that held by the Foundation. It then became my responsibility to negotiate with executives of American Home Products a monetary amount for canceling our lease that would more than compensate our relocation costs. After multiple meetings, a most favorable settlement allowed the Foundation to consider new locations in New York and other cities such as Dallas, Washington D.C., and Atlanta. After a careful review of all factors, Atlanta was selected and the Foundation relocated to Atlanta's Lenox Square in late 1972. Some Board and staff members at the time are pictured in Figure 15.2.

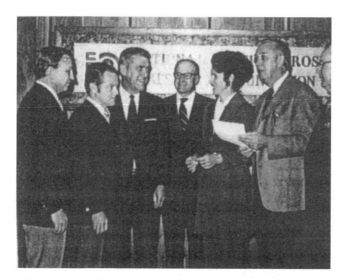

Figure 15.2. *Headquarters staff and Board members in 1972.*
From the left, Lt. Col. James Watkins, Dr. John Herndon, Welch
Boyer, Paul Etchepare, Mrs. Walter Burry, Robert McCreery,
and Grover Angel. Courtesy of Mr. Robert McCreery.

Before Luke Quinn's death, I spent numerous evenings at his Watergate apartment as he entertained various members of Congress. From those introductions and other contacts, opportunities developed for myself and others to appear before House and Senate committees on behalf of CF. Through my Washington CF exposure, I received a Presidential appointment to the twelve member General Medical Science Advisory Council of NIH for 1973 through 1976. Being a Council member gave access to other Institute Directors and departments where my voice for CF basic research was often heard.

If time had permitted, CF fund raising would have consumed all my time participating in various events across the US. Each appearance expanded public awareness and money raised for the Foundation. Hollywood events were special and exciting, yet complicated because of pressures exerted by a few for special funding. Additional time was required to participate in medical meetings and interaction with NIH and government leaders. As my three year CF Foundation Presidency ended, I was elected to further serve from 1973 to 1976. Fortunately those years did not involve challenges of the type faced earlier. Travel, meetings, and speeches, continued with increased visits to NIH and Congressional offices and income to the National office continued to increase.

As pediatric pulmonary medicine became an outgrowth of the CF Center program, some of the specialists were treating increasing numbers and diversity of patients. Many suggested the Foundation's purpose should be expanded to "Cystic Fibrosis and other Pediatric Pulmonary Diseases." The suggestion produced per-

sonality and purpose conflicts that led some pulmonary specialists to later form
their own organization named The Association of Pediatric Pulmonary Centers.
The National Cystic Fibrosis Research Foundation name was cumbersome as compared to other health organizations. During my second term, and after extensive
discussion, the Trustees agreed to a change that was accomplished by adopting
"The Cystic Fibrosis Foundation" (CFF) as the organization's new name.

Dr. John Herndon was Medical Vice President for medical affairs and
Welch Boyer National Director of the Foundation when I became President in
1970. Relations between John and Welch were strained and often negative to the
organization. During my second term, it was determined the Foundation would be
better served if John departed. After his termination, an extended search produced
Dr. Amoz Chernoff as a qualified candidate. It was apparent to me and others that
his talents were ideal to be the Foundation's Medical Director. I negotiated an
employment agreement with Amoz that served the Foundation well throughout the
remainder of my Presidency.

My second and final three year term as American CF President ended at
the May 10, 1976 Atlanta, Georgia annual meeting. Frankie and I were given gifts
followed by this presentation that defined my six years as CF President:

"Traveled more than 20,000 miles a year for Foundation business.

Spent an average of 20 weekends a year away from his home and
family.

Who has helped you and your chapters increase shareable income
to National from 2½ million when he started to more than 4½
million in six years with equal additional income retained by
chapters for local programs.

Who has gone up and down the halls of Congress, The National
Institutes of Health and other official agencies to stimulate
increased funding for our programs.

Who has been the guiding force behind implementation of our
research and medical care programs.

Who has led your National Board of Trustees in the refinement
of policy, programs, and procedures, which have eased pressure
for all of us.

Who has responded to invitations to represent and speak for us at
countless Foundation special events.

Who has often times assured volunteers and staff to stay cool and
keep our sights on the real business as to why we are in business.

And all of this, plus the stimulation, excitement, and influence of
his special personality has been done for the privilege of serving
without any Foundation compensation."

My history with CF covers more than forty years of leadership roles in Cleveland, the National Foundation, and International Association activities stemming from LeRoy Matthews asking me to join the Cystic Fibrosis Foundation, Cleveland Chapter. Each involvement generated new friends throughout much of the world and a multitude of good memories. Like life, the organizations have grown and accomplished many wonderful things while building new leaders, each of whom endeavors to reach ever greater goals based on past discoveries and events.

It is a proud pleasure to recall my part in each group mentioned in this history of CF-related health organizations in which I have been involved.

The past six years are now history. I look forward to participation in the American Foundation's future and want to be helpful as you move ahead in addressing the many CF problems needing better solutions.

I take with me the experiences and friendships of being your President as I assume leadership of the International CF organization. I will need to draw heavily on your expertise and assistance to increase CF awareness, medical support, and growth of CF programs among the International community of Nations.

The membership of the International Association is symbolic of cystic fibrosis itself. There are few geographical, economic, and sociological boundaries to the disease and the organization created to enhance awareness, understanding, and solutions.

I ask that you move with me into this role in spirit and commitment. Accept my thanks for everything you have done and will do for the CF Foundation while accepting my challenge to do yet more.

16

Organizing the Foundation's Medical Program: Collaboration from the Beginning

Paul A. di Sant'Agnese, M.D.

In the early and middle 1950s, it became evident that it was not only the cystic fibrosis (CF) patients who needed help, but also their parents. They felt bewildered, sometimes desperate, abandoned and alone with their child (often more than one) suffering and frequently dying of a strange, mysterious almost unknown disease for which there did not seem to be a cure. In most cases, they had difficulty getting help because most physicians did not know much about CF or how to cope with it.

In an effort to alleviate some of these problems, I thought it might be helpful to get the parents of CF children together, have group sessions, have them share their concerns, help each other discuss their experiences with physicians and hospitals, where to go, and where to get help. So the motivation at the time was not an attempt to raise funds for research, but to try to help the parents and patients in their time of need. I discussed this problem with Dr. Harry Shwachman from Boston Children's Hospital, the other medical center where a large number of patients with CF were being followed. He agreed with me as to the need for action.

The first person I talked to early in 1955 was a Mr. Blitzer, the father of an affected child. He quickly went to work and within a few weeks many of the parents had gotten together. They were functioning as a group, sharing experiences and, with their interaction, fulfilling a great need to vocalize their concerns, release their emotions, realize that they were not alone, and exchange experiences as to the medical care and where to get it. Indeed, it was a teaching experience not only for CF parents, but for their physicians as well.

Dr. Dorothy Andersen was against such an effort on our part as perhaps she felt physicians should not be involved in matters that did not directly concern the care of patients. Both Dr. Rustin MacIntosh, the Chairman of Pediatrics at Babies Hospital and I tried many times to convince her, but she steadfastly refused to participate directly in any group activities. There were many parents' meetings at which I actively participated. A local chapter was formed giving more substance to the fledging organization. And there were several TV shows in which I took part as the doctor, together with the parents and the head of the New York CF Association. This effort was in order to increase the understanding of the public and indeed make people aware there was such a disease as CF that needed their help and appeal to their generosity.

The endeavor was started as a humanitarian effort to try to help the parents and patients with CF. It was a great surprise when a few months after the beginning, a check for $5,000 was presented to Dorothy Andersen and me by a sergeant in the Air Force and father of two CF children in the name of the New York CF Association. Thus fundraising, primarily for research, quickly became one of the most important goals.

Also in the mid 1950s, Dr. Wynne Sharples, a pediatrician from Philadelphia and mother of two CF children, led the formation of the aptly called National Cystic Fibrosis Research Foundation (NCFRF) and became the first President. The goal was to promote research and raise funds. Dr. Sharples was very well connected socially and politically and succeeded in getting some of the powerful members of Congress interested in the problem. This eventually resulted in my recruitment in 1960 by the National Institutes of Health (NIH) and the creation of a branch of the NIH dedicated in large measure to the study of CF.

With Dr. Sharples' retirement, also in 1960, the organization moved from Philadelphia to New York City. Mr. Robert Natal, a New York attorney, and not a parent, was a moving spirit of the New York lay group and became the second President of the NCFRF. New Chapters were formed in various cities, medically we began to coordinate our activities, and the Foundation became better known.

In addition to the activities in New York and Boston, there was increasing medical activity and interest in Philadelphia, Cleveland, and other places. More and more, we were in touch with each other and began to have regular meetings, usually chaired by Harry Shwachman or myself, to discuss medical and organizational problems. Dr. Giulio Barbero representing Philadelphia, Dr. LeRoy Matthews from Cleveland, Dr. Paul Patterson from Boston and then Albany, and others were among those present.

The Medical Program

From the beginning, it was decided that the Foundation would be organized in two separate, but cooperating units:

A lay Board of Trustees charged with the administrative and the fund raising responsibilities and

A General Medical and Scientific Advisory Council (GMSAC), which, in Washington lingo, was to "advise and consent."

The goal was to improve the care of patients, spread and increase the knowledge of CF among the lay and medical public, and eventually to recommend the dispersing of any funds available for research and the care of patients. It was also important to train additional physicians for the care of CF patients.

In addition to myself and Harry Shwachman, Paul Patterson, LeRoy Matthews, Giulio Barbero, Will Waring, and others were among the first members of the GMSAC. Harry Shwachman and I alternately chaired the medical sessions. The two groups, lay and medical, worked harmoniously together to fulfill the goals of the Foundation. Almost all the lay trustees were parents of CF patients and thus highly motivated. I cannot think of any instances during the many years I was active in the CF Foundation in which there was any major disagreement between the medical and lay groups.

In the first years, I used to go to the CF Foundation headquarters in New York City from Bethesda, Maryland every two or three weeks and, of course, when there were meetings of the Medical Council and often of the Board of Trustees. The staff at the CF headquarters, led by Mrs. Katherine Earnshaw, was always very cooperative and helpful in every way, and there was always a pleasant and productive relationship with the medical group.

In 1960, Dr. Kenneth Landauer, a physician previously with the National Infantile Paralysis Foundation (later Polio Foundation), became the first Medical/Scientific Director of the NCFRF. The structure of the Medical Council was formalized, a structure that has remained essentially the same for almost 40 years to the present time. It was decided that there be a Chairman and Vice Chairman of the GMSAC, each elected for a non renewable term of two years, with the vice-chairman automatically succeeding the chairman. Harry Shwachman was the first chairman. I was the first vice-chairman and then the second chairman, and then, Patterson, Matthews, Barbero, Doershuk, Denning, and others. The Chairman and Vice-Chairman of the Advisory Council, together or separately, were to attend the meetings of the Board of Trustees, thus assuring liaison between the two groups who were working so well together towards a common goal.

Various committees were established: Professional Education Committee, Research Committee, and, at the suggestion of Dr. Landauer who had seen this work well at the Polio Foundation, a Center Committee. The mandate of the latter was to establish CF Centers throughout the country for the care of CF patients, training of physicians, and stimulate research in the disease. Other committees were added later.

This structure of the medical arm of the CF Foundation proved extremely effective. For the parents and patients, the establishing of the CF Centers, which now blanket the nation, was a great boon. The parents now knew where to get specialized care for their children, where to find physicians who were familiar with the disease and at the same time to be able to commune with other parents who faced the same problems. For the patients, the medical care and treatment improved dramatically over time as shown by the increasing rate of survival from a few years of life to the present median of 32 or more years. For the physicians, there was an increasingly successful effort to clarify the nature, diagnosis and treatment of CF, and eventually an orderly coordination and distribution of the funds raised for pursuing research projects.

An example of the work of the Professional Education Committee is the "*Guide to Diagnosis and Management of Cystic Fibrosis*: a syllabus for physicians," first published in 1963. Several editions followed. There were other publications for physicians covering various topics including how to perform and interpret properly the sweat test. A number of conferences and meetings devoted to CF also were sponsored and organized.

Unfortunately, President Natal became ill and had to retire. Dr. Milton Graub, a Philadelphia pediatrician and CF parent, became the third President in 1963 and continued the successful growth and development of the Foundation.

At first, very little money was raised for research in CF, but eventually the funds available gradually increased. The process of judging and awarding research grants at first was quite disorderly. In the late 1960s when my tenure as Chairman of the Medical Advisory Council was ended, I became Chairman of the Research Committee and reorganized the process along the lines of the procedures followed by the NIH. The evaluation of each application for a research grant was assigned to a group of experts, not necessarily members of the CF Foundation. One member was to submit a written report to a meeting of the group, the other members having read and evaluated the application would then vote as to whether the application for the grants was approved or disapproved, and if approved would assign it a priority number. The grant would then be funded according to its priority and the funds on hand. As more funds became available, the training of physicians to staff the CF Centers became a major concern. Some of the money was allotted on a competitive basis to grants for qualified physicians to spend one or two years at a qualified CF Center to become familiar with the diagnosis and care of CF patients. Several other committees were formed later to meet the increasing needs.

The headquarters of the CF Foundation were in New York City for several years. In 1972 they moved to Atlanta, Georgia and then to Bethesda, Maryland in 1978, where they are still sited. Ken Landauer was succeeded as Medical/Scientific Director by Dr. John Herndon after a long search conducted mostly by myself, as the then Chairman of the Medical Council. At that time, I realized how difficult it was to find and attract qualified people for the job. I was in touch with several medical foundations and to my surprise found that in many instances the post of Medical Director was vacant. After the move to Bethesda, we were lucky to get Dr. Robert Beall to accept the post of Medical/Scientific Director. At first, he was very reluctant to accept this position and I worked quite hard to persuade him to make up his mind. I felt he was the best qualified for this position with his background at the NIH extramural programs and therefore was knowledgeable about grants and had contact with many people. He later became Vice President in charge of medical affairs and then the President and CEO of the Foundation. Under the present leadership and with the discovery of the gene for CF and of its innumerable mutations, which helped propel CF into the limelight, the CF Foundation has become one of the best organized and most successful medical and health related Foundations in the United States. I am proud that several of my former clinical associates at the NIH have or have had key positions on the Medical Advisory Council and have greatly helped the medical/scientific program to its accomplishments and to fulfill its goals. At a meeting in the middle 1960s, Harry Shwachman, Paul Patterson, and myself were named "Founding Fathers" of the CF Foundation in recognition of our pioneering and continued efforts in setting up and organizing it.

The CF Club

This is another success story for CF. For sometime, Dorothy Andersen and I had been discussing the possibility of getting a few interested investigators together and forming a "working group" in CF. Finally, in the spring of 1959, Dorothy invited a few involved physicians to a two day meeting to discuss CF and make plans for a forum to present and discuss problems and investigations related to this disease.

About ten or 15 of us met at Buckhill Falls in the Poconos area of Pennsylvania in very friendly and pleasant surroundings. In addition to Dr. Andersen and myself, Barbero, Shwachman, Matthews, Patterson, Nancy Huang and a few others were present. Under the Chairmanship of Dorothy, there was a free discussion ranging from organizational problems to more specific detail of research and treatment of CF. It was decided to call this fledging organization the "CF Club" which would meet once a year with the intention of creating a forum for the presentation of papers relating to the various aspects of CF in a friendly, informal atmosphere. This would allow free discussion and, divorced from the usual goal of scientific meetings, publication of the data presented was not required.

The second meeting of the CF Club was in1960 in Rockport, Massachusetts, again chaired by Dorothy Andersen. Twenty or thirty people attended the two day meeting. There were informal presentations and discussions. It was decided to meet once a year with a different chairman each year: Giulio Barbero was elected chairman for the next year and later I followed as the chairman, then Harry Shwachman, and down the line. There was not to be any stated membership except for the chairman and secretary, although a record of the people in attendance was kept for correspondence purposes. At the Rockport meeting, I suggested that the CF Club meet each year in conjunction with the meetings of the Society for Pediatric Research (SPR) and American Pediatric Society (APS), thus avoiding travel to two different meetings by the attendees. And it would afford the opportunity for other pediatricians attending the meetings of the Pediatric Societies to drift in to the CF Club meetings and become more conversant with the problems of this disease. I also did not think the CF Club would be very successful as a "stand alone" organization at that time and would severely limit attendance. This suggestion was accepted and the CF Club met with increasing success and attendance by physicians and some basic researchers at the time and place of the meetings of the SPR-APS for the next 25 years.

However, starting in 1987 and following the breakthrough discovery of the CF gene in 1989, a great deal of publicity followed. With the widespread recognition of CF as a paradigm of recessive genetic disease that was frequently mentioned and discussed not only in scientific meetings, but also in the press and on TV, the CF Club format was changed. A hugely successful new annual meeting, called the North American Cystic Fibrosis Conference, was organized by the CF Foundation and held each year in different sites and with an attendance increasing to several thousand people. The 14th annual meeting of this organization was held in late 2000 with an attendance of over 3000 people, a tribute to its organizers its growing success, and its impact on research and treatment progress.

With the passage of time, many of the details of those early years of the Medical Council have escaped me and I no longer have records of those days. Certainly many of the other contributors will have interesting details to offer.

17

Growth of the Foundation's Medical Program

Carl F. Doershuk, M.D.

I began my pulmonary training fellowship in 1961,and found that Dr. LeRoy Matthews loved to relate past events and how things developed. It was not long before I learned much from him about the early development of the Foundation's medical program in the late 1950s. Unfortunately, there are few of the remaining participants to relate those early organization efforts and of the events which followed. I will contribute what I learned from him, from various newsletters and reports, and from my own experiences. Chapters 11, 16, 25, and 26, relate other early medical developments. My involvement began with the lay members of the Cleveland CF chapter in 1961. By 1964, my first exposure with the National medical program was as a member of the Fellowship Committee reviewing applications for training. This position led to the Education Committee and then a multi-decades leadership involvement with the National medical program, including Chairman of the Medical Advisory Council, and then with the Board of Trustees, as a Vice President and member of the Executive Committee.

The early medical leaders had a two-fold activity in the world of CF. One, they were interested in organizing a format which would permit, at minimum, an annual meeting for the exchange of information and ideas. The second activity was to work with the lay members to develop a strong and viable nationwide medical program within the Foundation structure.

On the meeting side, Dr. Matthews related that in 1959 Dr. Dorothy Andersen organized the first annual meeting of what came to be called "The CF Club" that was held near New York City, perhaps in Buckhill Falls. In subsequent years they met in conjunction with the annual Pediatric Research Society meetings that the CF interested physicians would also be attending. Drs. di Sant'Agnese, Shwachman, Patterson, Barbero, Harrison, Huang, and Matthews, among others, attended. From old newsletter reports and other bits of filed information, by the 3rd annual meeting in 1961, more than 100 physicians attended the CF Club meeting and 20 papers were presented and discussed. By the 10th annual meeting in 1969 in Atlantic City, 43 papers were submitted, but there was time for only 24 to be presented. It was of interest to read that the evening before the Club meeting in 1969 a panel presented "Testing of Newborns and Screening for Cystic Fibrosis." This is a topic that continues in discussion even now.

In their other role, the leading physicians had been meeting with the Foundation Board of Trustees about developing a medical advisory group and a research and care program within the Foundation. Dr. Graub, one of the original founders of the Foundation in December 1955, and Doris Tulcin have described the establishment of the Foundation and identified the founding members and other major early participants. At some point, a General Medical and Scientific Advisory Council (known as GMSAC) was formed. Fortunately, but much later, the name was shortened to Medical Advisory Council (MAC). Each Chairman was to serve for a two-year period. Dr. Harry Shwachman from Boston was the first chairman, followed by Drs. Paul di Sant'Agnese from Bethesda, Paul Patterson from Albany, LeRoy Matthews from Cleveland, Giulio Barbero from Philadelphia, myself, and then Dr. Carolyn Denning from New York. The major task during Carolyn's tenure was to lead the medical group through the move from Atlanta to Washington, D.C. in 1978. Unfortunately, she was not able to be a contributor to this book. I do not have the record of the many other MAC chairpersons who followed. Other than Paul di Sant'Agnese, who was one of the founding members of the medical program, I am the only surviving MAC Chairman through my time in office in 1976 who can report on some of the events.

There is indication that the first medical committee was concerned primarily with medical education. Of course there were extensive lay education publications and programs developed as well. Soon Research and Care Committees were added with a Chairman for each. Dr. Matthews was an active participant in the early GMSAC and provided regular progress reports about his treatment program to the committee. He was an active participant in the CF Club too. These sessions provided continuing opportunity for him to present his comprehensive treatment approach and the early results he obtained, since he had the foresight to set up ongoing clinical evaluation of the patients from the beginning of the program in 1957. Thus he had continuing data and results to report at each meeting about the survival and improved status of the patients being treated. At the Foundation level, Dr. Sharples, from Philadelphia, led the incorporation of the Foundation in 1955 and had been President since then. Her correspondence with Dr. Matthews included comments about her resignation indicating concerns about the direction of support for research, content of medical and general CF education, and other directions pulling the Foundation leadership. She resigned effective January 1, 1960 after serving for five years as the organizing stimulus and first President of the NCFRF. Robert Natal became President and the Board moved the Foundation headquarters from Philadelphia to New York City.

Dr. Kenneth Landauer was recruited in 1959 from the National Infantile Paralysis (Polio) Foundation to be Medical Director. This was about the time that the nationwide polio vaccine immunization program was effectively eliminating new cases of polio. The polio care centers had proved to be very effective but were now needed less and less and being closed. At the November 1960 meeting of the NCFRF, the Board approved and announced the initiation of a Regional Cystic Fibrosis Research and Teaching Centers concept, stating that it was the "basis of the new NCFRF research program." The release further indicated that "the program was designed to give the Foundation and its affiliated Chapters a leading and unifying role in expanding and intensifying research in cystic fibrosis, and in making better care available to children afflicted with this disease."

The new emphasis would be on grants to medical schools and teaching hospitals, to help create a national network. This plan followed Dr. Landauer's recommendation to use the Polio Foundation model, which had established care centers at major medical institutions across the country. The CF goals would be similar; the first goal was to increase the number of patients and provide exemplary care, and the second goal was to provide the nucleus and stimulus for the clinical and basic research that was needed. It was noted that the CF Foundation and its Chapters had been effective in obtaining Congressional support, which led to the appropriation of more than one million dollars for CF research in 1958, with additional funding support in 1959 and 1960 (see Chapter 11). The leadership of the Foundation felt that the availability of these funds would free up sufficient Foundation dollars for the new program.

Once this plan was accepted, the first meeting for potential leaders of the planned new CF Centers was scheduled to be in Cleveland in late 1961. The choice of location was apparently due to Dr. Matthews' presentations of the improving patient outcomes and the marked decrease in annual mortality to about 2% per year following the start of his "comprehensive approach to care." As a beginning trainee in July 1961, I had but little awareness of the coming event, let alone its significance. On reflection, it is my opinion that the success and outcome of this meeting marked the beginning of one of the most effective, exemplary, and outstanding combined lay and medical programs conducted by a voluntary health agency at the national level that the country has ever experienced. In this case, the problem was a relatively unknown genetic disease with high early mortality, CF. The challenge was enormous.

The meeting was held in Cleveland at the Wade Park Manor, an impressive nearby residential hotel, and at the old Babies and Children's Hospital. I remember that Dr. Matthews presented many of the CF patients, all looking quite healthy, to the group. Among other presentations, the basic requirements for a pediatric pulmonary function laboratory and the special microbiology lab techniques needed to accurately deal with CF respiratory cultures were described. Meeting the approximately 100 leading physicians from the nation's major medical centers, many who were already recognized for their involvement in and contributions to CF, was a special occasion for me and provided the opportunity to learn of their experiences. Little else is recalled other than remembering that the Foundation put on an impressive meeting.

The development of the new Centers and their care staffs, the improved education of clinicians and trainees, and the utilization of the comprehensive treatment approach all contributed to a steadily increasing survival for CF patients. In tandem, the close relationship of the Chapters and Centers facilitated greater general awareness of the disease, the Foundation's ability to raise funds, and support of the research that was needed. However, many years would pass before the discovery of the CF gene truly permitted the focus of research needed to lead toward a better understanding of the disease, the anticipation of improved control measures, and possibly even the frequently mentioned control or cure.

Up to 1961, there were two medical committees advising the Board. One was the Medical Education Committee and the other was the Scientific Advisory Board. Before long these committees were combined into one, the GMSAC. In addition a Research Committee and a Care Committee, soon renamed the Center Committee, were added to the Advisory Council. Within the GMSAC, Dr. Matthews became the first Chairman of the Center Committee. Its purpose was to recruit and accredit the new Centers and establish appropriate standards. He and a few others, including Dr. Gunyon Harrison from Houston, invested many hours traveling to recruit new Center Directors. Dr. Matthews soon developed the basic forms used to establish uniform data collection from patient visits and initiated the annual reporting mechanism to the MAC and the Foundation by the Centers.

The first annual Center Committee report to the Advisory Council and the NCFRF Board of Trustees occurred in 1963. There were 2,085 patients reported under care in 1962 with 62 physicians involved. In just four years, by the end of 1966, there were 5,116 patients reported, 128 physicians involved, and at least 32 Centers reporting. It was anticipated that 7 to 8 more Centers would be added in the next year. Foundation support of the Centers had increased from $650,000 in 1962 to $817,000 per year in 1966. The growth in patient numbers was excellent, the settings for patient care were improving, and the educational efforts were thriving. But the potential for significant research progress was still well in the future, as there was no real understanding of what the basic defect was or what research direction would be most useful or important to support. Until Dr. Paul Quinton's description of the chloride sweat defect in 1983 and the discovery of the CF gene in 1989, no one had a clue. However, with the attention generated by the increasing number of Centers and the number of identified patients under care, more hypotheses about etiology were developed and there was increased public awareness of CF.

There was a major meeting of the Center Directors, led by the members of GMSAC (Figure 17.1), for two and one half days in Denver in September 1963. Dr. Jack Docter thoughtfully sent me some of the CF Medical Notes sections of the National News Bulletin from around that time. The September issue reported an interview of Dr. Harrison, Director of the Houston Center, commenting on progress achieved by early diagnosis. He was quoted, "During the program's first few years the patient was not diagnosed until the disease was full blown. Now, with physicians more aware of the systemic effects of the disease, children are referred early with lung disease or gastrointestinal irritability of minimal nature. Until two years ago, patients were from one to three years old at time of referral, whereas now they are between three and 18 months old." He added, "The results of early diagnosis are also reflected in increased longevity and reduced mortality. Better management has definitely prolonged lives." However, it is recognized that even today when infants diagnosed early by the presence of meconium ileus or a positive family

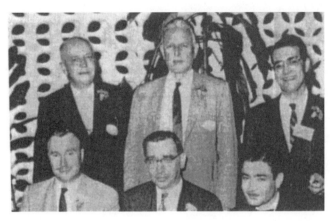

Figure 17.1. *The NCFRF General Medical and Scientific Advisory Council met in Denver in June 1963. Seated, left to right, Drs. Paul Patterson, Harry Shwachman, chairman, and LeRoy Matthews. Standing: Drs. Kenneth Landauer, Vice-President for Medical Affairs, Joseph Stokes, Jr., and Giulio Barbero. Not present, Drs. Paul di Sant'Agnese, vice-chairman; Milton Graub; and Gunyon Harrison. Courtesy of Dr. Carl Doershuk.*

history are excluded, it is disappointing that many children still are not diagnosed until beyond one year of age. The later the diagnosis, the greater the possibility of significant and irreversible lung damage and/or nutritional deprivation occurring. In the article, Dr. Matthews was quoted also, "the key to therapy is treatment of all three principal changes which interfere with normal pulmonary hygiene: accumulation of secretions, inflammation and edema, and spasm."

The following day, over 200 general practitioners attended a full day course sponsored by the Foundation concerning the recognition, diagnosis, and latest events in CF, with the goal of greater awareness and earlier diagnosis. A sidebar note in the September 1963 Medical Notes from the Foundation contained a bit of humor. During the Conference, Dr. Alex Spock, and Dr. Jack Docter agreed to be interviewed by a local radio station. When the NCFRF representative introduced them to the announcer, that gentleman shook his head in disbelief saying, "Dr. Spock and Dr. Docter? You're kidding!"

There was a down side to the greater awareness of the continuing fairly bleak survival prospects. This information had a negative impact for many patients, especially those reaching teenage years, which was upsetting for almost everyone involved. The information that served to provide effective public relations purposes in support of the raising of funds also had the potential for a negative effect on families, caregivers, and especially patients. At issue was the publicity to increase public awareness of the severity of CF (early death) versus the negative impact on the patients and the Center personnel caring for them on a daily basis. There was also resistance to the often overstated implication of a possible near-term cure (which was attractive but much too optimistic). I recall Dr. Harry Shwachman, then chairman of the GMSAC, speaking out strongly against publicizing optimism about an early cure. This issue led to vigorous and emotional discussions among the lay and medical volunteers in the Foundation. It is still somewhat of a dilemma of balancing the story of continued clinical and research successes while effectively drawing public attention to the continuing very life threatening seriousness of the disease.

The negative impact on one individual patient regarding the publicity of a limited CF life span in public reports was recently related to me. A now thirty some year old patient told me of his many days of absence during high school by complaining of not feeling well, even though he could have easily attended school. He did poorly in his classes, with the exception of being a straight A student in physics. This should have attracted school attention that he had more potential than just being an average student. He misunderstood the publicity about the projection of average survival to 18 to 20 years at best (at that time), and his misunderstanding had a strong negative influence (understandable) when he was a teenager. In this regard he probably was not very different from many, many other CF individuals who did not realize that the age, about 18 years when he was growing up, was the average prediction of survival and that many patients lived much longer. Also, he missed that the survival age was improving yearly. Later on, when he came to the realization that his health was remaining stable and he better understood his potential for fairly long term survival, he was motivated to finish his college education and then a undertook a demanding MBA program. He completed the college work and the MBA with straight A grades in all his courses. Unfortunately, this significant accomplishment on his part had been delayed by quite a few years. He was not alone in having carried a negative view of his survival chances for too long a period of time.

Also, it is unfortunate that CF, with its over 900 different mutations, is still very difficult to understand and study, even today, making longevity predictions tenuous at best. The hope that the discovery of the gene in 1989 would have led, by now, to fully unraveling the basic pathophysiological mechanisms, and its secrets and faults has yet to be realized.

There was rapid growth in the number of CF patients cared for at our Center from 24 in 1957, to 82 in 1960, and to 147 patients by 1962, with only 4 deaths, still well less than 2% per year over that time span, despite the many advanced cases referred. This continuing decreased mortality rate was a marked change from the earlier experience. Our Center's average of almost one new patient per week was exceeded in 1962 when new patient admissions increased to 72 and the total number of patients under care was around 200. Obviously the plan to collect patients in Centers was working well in Cleveland and, from the 1963 National Centers data presented above, the plan was working well elsewhere too. Our census increased to 374 in 1970 and peaked at nearly 500 in 1975 as the Ohio Centers in Akron, Dayton, Columbus, Cincinnati, and Toledo, and nearby Pittsburgh became fully established and attracted patients.

In addition to improving the situation for CF patients, the Foundation's Center program deserves considerable credit for providing the stimulus for improved care for many other children with pulmonary conditions. The reports of rapid increases in the CF patient census at the Centers did not include the even greater number of non-CF pulmonary patients that were referred for sweat testing, but who had a negative sweat test and were fortunate to not have CF. However, most of these children still had significant pulmonary problems, and some had gastrointestinal diseases. Both conditions required further diagnostic measures and expertise in care to be developed at the Centers. These referrals resulted in virtually every CF Center becoming the focus for patients with severe asthma or other pulmonary disease. The patient volume in the Centers increased markedly requiring more staff and faculty members, along with the further training needed to provide effective medical services.

Thus the secondary and largely unheralded benefit from the CF Center program, the development of Divisions of Pediatric Pulmonology at the same locations, followed from the increasing numbers of pulmonary patients referred to the Foundation supported CF Centers. Initiation of the new Pulmonary Division occurred at our institution in 1969 and at almost every medical center during the decade of the 1970s.

An additional development stemming from the Foundation Center program was the creation of a group of federally supported Pediatric Pulmonary Centers, whose role was to train the ancillary personnel needed at every institution. This concept was probably the brainchild of Dr. John Herndon, the Medical-Scientific Director of the Foundation at the time. The start of Pediatric Pulmonary Centers and the Pediatric Pulmonary Training Centers, were another tangible and beneficial byproduct for pulmonary patients that came from the successful growth of the CF Center movement. Now, there are more than 110 CF Centers, an increasing number of Adult Pulmonary Centers, and an untold number of Pulmonology Divisions at academic medical centers.

The Patient Registry

Dr. Warren Warwick had the foresight to propose collection of patient demographic information and mortality/survival data from the Centers at the meeting of Center Directors in Seattle in 1964. In view of the usefulness of demographic and outcomes databases in other diseases, the Center Directors initially subscribed to this project with some enthusiasm. When increasing questions arose, especially around the reporting of mortality experience by the Centers and how the data might be used, the General Medical and Scientific Advisory Council (GMSAC) approved a Data Registry GAP Conference that was held in Philadelphia, October 28–29, 1971. Representing the Centers and the Advisory Council were physicians who had database experience and/or had reported survival data. These included Drs. Paul di Sant'Agnese, Douglas Holsclaw, Nancy Huang, Kon-Taik Khaw, Harry Shwachman, and myself.

The other invited individuals had expertise in statistics, use of life tables, and/or other registry experience. They included Shirley Braverman, Temple University Health and Science Center, Arthur Littell, Ph.D., University of Texas, Cecil Nesbitt Ph.D., University of Michigan, Richard Pogue, Ph.D., Medical College of Georgia, and Calvin Zippin, Sc.D., University of California, San Francisco. Dr. Warwick, as originator of the database and the analysis used, served both a Center and an expert role. John Herndon, Ph.D., Medical-Scientific Director, represented the Foundation. Robert Greenfield, M.D., Associate Director for Planning and Evaluation, National Institute of General Medical Sciences, provided additional experience and support. I served as Conference Chairman and Frank Primiano, Jr., Ph.D., Case Western Reserve University, was both participant and recorder.

The initial session addressed the understanding of the methodology useful for analyzing the collected data and the second session provided considerable discussion of the application of this methodology. The final session dealt with recommendations to the GMSAC and potential future goals. In summary, the consensus of the Conference was that the NCFRF Patient Registry System was a model system for morbidity and mortality collection and reporting. The completion of the, then active, phase of the Registry was urged. The expectation was that it would result in a consistent approach to data collection and analysis, use techniques acceptable to all participants in the Registry, yield definite objectives, and determine what could be feasibly accomplished with the funding available. This significant conclusion and recommendation for continuing the registry has had a long-term beneficial impact for both the care and research programs. Both Dr. Graub and Dr. Davis comment on the continuing importance of the patient registry, especially as it efficiently supports both the clinical and basic research efforts.

The GMSAC and the Board of Trustees subsequently recommended continuation of the registry under the direction of a new committee comprised of Drs. Barbero, Greenfield, Nesbitt, Pogue, Will Waring, and Warwick. These decisions and conclusions were another example of the lay, medical, and research participants working together within the Foundation structure to develop the elements for long term successes.

There is an unfortunate footnote to this story. Dr. Warwick continued to provide most of the support for the patient registry through the Minnesota Center until the Foundation took over the entire operation. To complete the transition, he forwarded all of his data and registry materials to the Foundation office in Atlanta. The misfortune occurred during the move of the Foundation's headquarters from Atlanta to Washington, D.C., in 1976 when all of the tapes containing the Registry data collected to that time were included in a shipment of Foundation archives that were lost perhaps in a truck accident. The detailed raw data found in the existing registry now go back twenty some years, while the collected information on the natural history of the disease between the 1950s and 1980s is available only in summary reports and papers published earlier.

My Experiences

My initial exposure to the lay part of the Foundation and the intensity of the input of the parents and family members was compelling for me. In September 1961, Dr. Matthews asked me to attend a Chapter meeting. He generally appeared about the middle of the meeting, so we had time for hamburgers at Hatton's deli on Euclid Avenue near downtown (still in business today). We then walked into a small office that was crowded with parents, including a number whom I recognized from clinic visits. I was immediately impressed by the intensity of involvement and commitment by everyone there. Fund raising was the major topic along with the latest progress report. Dr. Matthews was clearly held in great respect for what was being accomplished. From then on, I became an active volunteer.

I was aware of the annual CF Club meeting and of the 1959 International Meeting held in Washington at the Woodner Hotel. The NIH and NCFRF sponsored the latter meeting with at least 70 noted clinical and research participants and was very successful. So I was looking forward to my first CF Club meeting in Atlantic City in 1962. In those days, we enjoyed the archaic but wonderful examples of the late 1890s hotel architecture overlooking the Boardwalk and the Atlantic Ocean and beach. It was an unforgettable experience to return there annually for a number of years. The Foundation headquarters were now in New York City, George Barrie (also recruited from the Polio Foundation) was the National Director, Katherine Earnshaw was the secretary and later the medical program coordinator, and Paul Nathan was the Public Relations Director and Science Editor.

The annual CF Club meeting in 1964 in Philadelphia was especially memorable. A large number of us were invited to the home of National CF President, Dr. Milton (known universally as Billy) Graub for a buffet dinner. The dinner was followed by an introductory presentation of a new concept and initiative by President Graub and the introduction of Dr. Giulio Barbero, who was an excellent and stimulating speaker. He proceeded to introduce the new approach that was another example of NCFRF's and Dr. Graub's imaginative thrust against the disease. The concept was called the Guidance, Action, and Projection program (GAP for short). The idea itself was developed by Dr. Graub and he secured the initial extensive funding support from Mr. George Frankel, Doris Tulcin's father, and continuing support came from the Frankel family's foundation. The goal was to identify strategic areas where there was lack of knowledge (GAP) and bring together the proper scientific experts whose meeting assignment would be to recommend a plan of action for each identified area. As with many new ideas, the concept was met with reluctant acceptance by some of those in attendance. However, this novel and effective approach developed by Dr. Graub proved successful. It was another example of the innovative and creative capability of the lay and medical/scientific members working together to add strength to the medical programs and provide awareness of problem areas or situations that could be of advantage to the Foundation's goals. It also provided a broader identity for the Foundation as an effective organization in the health agency field.

At my first CF Club meeting, there was a request for volunteers for various committees. I joined the Fellowship Committee in 1964 and served as chair in 1965. This was the beginning of my satisfying leadership role within the medical program at the National level to 1978 and with the Board of Trustees beginning in 1977.

In 1966, I was recruited to the Professional Education Committee. The original leaders were the participants in the first Education Committee, chaired by Dr. Barbero. They had produced the first *Guide to Diagnosis and Management of Cystic Fibrosis* published in 1963, with reprints in 1965 and 1968. As part of accepting the Chair position in 1969, I requested that the committee be authorized to produce a new version of the Guide. The other committee members were Richard Dooley, Bettina Hilman, Douglas Holsclaw, Lucas Kulczycki, and Harry Shwachman, with staff support by Paul Nathan. We met on a number of occasions, finding Paul's New York apartment a quiet meeting place. We frequently worked from early morning until late evening to achieve consensus for the new edition. Not wanting to waste time eating out, we usually prepared and enjoyed our own dinners, as several were good cooks, Bettina especially. The new version of the "Guide" was published in 1971.

About the same time, Dr. Herndon, the Medical-Scientific Director, had requested Dr. Nancy Huang to chair a committee of 25 knowledgeable contributors to produce *The Guide to Drug Therapy in Patients with Cystic Fibrosis*, published in 1972. These two complementary "Guides" proved very useful for everyone, especially for the many new physicians and other trainees coming into CF care at the rapidly growing number of CF Centers.

Over the years, I have felt very fortunate to meet and to know the first National Director, George Barrie, and also all of the Presidents who followed Wynne Sharples. President Robert Natal, a non-CF parent, was an outstanding individual and Foundation leader who died at all too young an age. Ray Mulford from Toledo and Henry Bernbaum from Cleveland were also outstanding individuals who, for personal and family reasons, were unable to accept nomination for presidency of the Foundation. Both were CF parents and were possible successors, but had to decline due to business and family commitments. The Foundation continued to grow during the Presidency of Dr. Graub, who also had children with CF. During that time the Foundation actively added more chapters, increased public awareness, and was increasingly successful in the effort to obtain congressional support of funding for CF research.

Robert McCreery, another from Cleveland, had a son with very severe asthma. As was somewhat typical for such a patient at that time, the asthma specialists recommended admission to a residential asthma center in Denver for a one to two year period. Instead, Bob heard about the success Dr. Matthews was having treating non-CF pulmonary patients and sought out his help. Grateful that his son's improvement was sufficient to permit him to remain at home, Bob accepted joining the Cleveland CF Chapter and became very involved. He subsequently was elected President of the National organization, following Dr. Graub's tenure. Welch Boyer succeeded George Barrie as the National Director with Bob as President and John Herndon was the first Medical-Scientific Director. Catherine Earnshaw was the medical department coordinator from 1964 to 1971. When the Foundation moved to Atlanta, she remained in New York to become the Executive Director of another health related organization.

With the move, staffing was expanded to support the medical programs and committees, along with additional personnel for chapter support and fund development. We medical volunteers were privileged to work with the excellent and supportive medical program people. We greatly appreciated the long hours they put in and their total dedication to the cause. It was a very difficult time for the medical volunteers when the Foundation decision to move to the Washington, D.C. area was implemented, as most of the staff did not or could not leave the Atlanta area for personal reasons. We later came to appreciate that this loss of staff was, fortuitously, soon well compensated. The consultant firm assisting the Foundation move added a person to specifically assure a smooth new start in Washington. That person was Caroline McPherson. Caroline did a great job and soon joined the Foundation as the Conferences Coordinator, later adding the Medical Program Coordinator position to her responsibilities. She has been a key individual for the Foundation and for all who have subsequently been involved. We have greatly benefited from her wise counsel and excellent support over the years.

As incoming Chairman of the Education Committee in 1969, I became a member of the General Medical and Scientific Advisory Council (GMSAC, pronounced GUMSAC by many, and not necessarily with great respect) which reported to the Board of Trustees. This position offered a new area of personal growth, as I found myself working directly with the early leaders and knowledgeable physicians who had been guiding the medical program and there were increasing opportunities to meet and work with the many impressive members of the Board of Trustees. This was truly an unexpected and new challenge for me. Sometime around 1976, the GMSAC title was finally accepted to be much too cumbersome and we finally shortened it to Medical Advisory Council, or MAC.

The Research and Center Committees were the two other major committees of the MAC. When Dr. Charles Lobeck was the Chairman of the Research Committee, he not only dealt with the research applications but also with fellowship applications which had either a clinical or basic research focus. One of the big issues his committee had to deal with was the evaluation and funding of clinical research as opposed to more basic or fundamental research. There were occasional unhappy responses about the committee recommendations and considerable discussion occurred at Council meetings around this issue, but Chuck was firm in presenting his and the committee's philosophy. Their recommendations stood the test of time and added to the maturation of the Foundation.

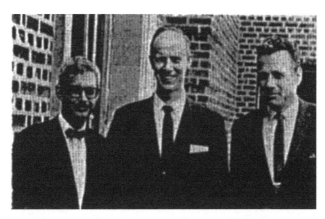

Figure 17.2. *Officers of the Cystic Fibrosis Club 1968-69, from left, Drs. William Waring, of New Orleans, president; Warren Warwick, of Minneapolis, secretary; and Jack Docter, of Seattle, vice-president. Courtesy of Dr. Carl Doershuk.*

For the Center Committee, there had been a rapid increase in the number of Centers and the supervisory role of the Committee was evolving. Drs. Jack Docter in 1965, and then Will Waring, Ralph Tiller, and others succeeded Dr. Matthews as Chairs of the Center Committee. Jack, Will, and also Warren Warwick later became CF Club Presidents (Figure 17.2). Since a number of the Centers were small and probably would never be able to meet the requirement for a Research designation, a decision was made to designate them as CT (Care and Teaching) Centers. The Council, and in particular Jack Docter, Ralph Tiller, and then Don Strominger, grappled with how to fairly evaluate the CT Centers in comparison with the full CTR (the "R" indicated research activity) Centers. With the rapid growth in numbers of centers, the financial support did not keep pace. The budget was tight and added to the problem of awarding funds. None of us envied them as they labored to work out an evaluation process that was generally acceptable. There were countless hours of discussion, even at the Council level. In 1969, a Care Committee chaired by Dr. Warwick drafted guidelines for the various clinical operations. At one time there was even a separate CT Committee established to evaluate, site visit, and rank those designated as CT Centers. This separation met with various criticisms and finally a single committee approach to evaluate all Centers was accepted. This process seemed to work equitably for all concerned and was later confirmed by National CF Board member, Doris Tulcin. Doris was serving as the liaison from the National Board to the Center Committee and reported to the Executive Committee and the President. I was pleased to find a copy of her letter to President Bob McCreery, reporting on her observation of the 1974 deliberations when Carolyn Denning was the Chairman of the Committee. Doris praised the care and professionalism exhibited by the committee members in their review of each Center and the funding recommendation for each Center. In her report, she stated that the funds were carefully and fairly expended. Her support of the Medical Advisory Council, and the Center Committee, was especially important to and very much appreciated by the medical volunteers.

Pseudomonas aeruginosa

My first contact with Doris was somewhat earlier when she had placed a telephone call to me as Chairman of the MAC. At that time, I had not previously met her but I knew that she and her family (the Frankels) were important supporters and leaders in the Foundation. The purpose of her call was to ask, "What is this thing called Pseudomonas?" I temporized my answer to learn of her CF daughter, Ann, then about 20 years of age, who recently had her first positive *Pseudomonas aeruginosa* respiratory culture. While I could provide general information, it was important that the family receive specific information in relation to their daughter's situation from her CF physician. However, from the general medical and overall Foundation viewpoint, it was embarrassing to me that a very informative response was not available in response to her very pointed questions about the Pseudomonas bacterial organism. The fact was that minimal research was being conducted or stimulated in this important area. Our conversation revealed another one of those CF knowledge "GAPs" that required attention. I felt prompted to organize a small conference on *Pseudomonas aeruginosa* held in Cleveland. This experience helped identify knowledgeable microbiologists and immunologists, among others, to provide the basis of a request for a larger Foundation supported GAP Conference held in San Diego. It was successful and led to a follow up conference a year or so later. The resulting stimulus and collection of information led to increasing interest in the unique chronic infection and damaging mechanisms of inflammation that are involved so specifically in the pulmonary disease of CF. More research projects resulted. Of note, this new activity occurred some twenty years after Dr. Charles May had stated in a monograph on CF in about 1953 that *Pseudomonas aeruginosa* was usually involved when persisting pulmonary infection was present. While we have now learned a great deal about this bacterium, it unfortunately remains the major agent of chronic persistent low grade infection that results in the progressive, irreversible lung damage in CF, even today. It remains difficult to treat effectively, let alone eradicate.

Toward the Strategic Plan

Giulio Barbero became the fifth Medical Council Chairman in 1971 and I became the Vice Chairman. Giulio summarized the developments of the previous decade in a presentation to the Board of Trustees. He commented on the status of research clues at the time. These included evidence for a circulating "CF factor," a generalized disturbance of membranes in secretory glands, some basic cellular abnormality evidenced by a staining pattern in cultured cells, and a problem in the electrolyte transport of sodium. He was quoted in the NCFRF CF News Bulletin. "As we look into the Seventies, … the major objective of the Foundation lies within its basic name – RESEARCH – and continues to be the primary objective which must be intensified!" With the Center program established, he and I shared the view that as we promoted the overall growth of the medical program, the need for more research and research funding from all sources, not just from the Foundation, needed to be a priority. Giulio was a good mentor, involving me in the planning processes and in the various issues that were important at the time. That made it easier to follow him as the sixth Chairman of the Medical Advisory Council in 1974. A number of important changes were occurring around that time. I soon realized that maintaining open lines of communication, not only among the diversifying number of medical committees and subcommittees but also with the various interest groups within the lay membership, would be an important part of my chairing role. I really enjoyed the experience of working with the Board officers for that two year period to 1976. They included Robert McCreery as President and Grover Angel and John Driscoll as Vice Presidents. The other officers and Executive Committee members were Alexander Maish, David Baker as Treasurer, Arthur Chamberlain, Robert DeBorde, B.G. Creemen, Robert Dresing, Paul Etchepare, Milton Graub, David Shapiro, Doris Tulcin and Jim Watkins. This was a stellar and dedicated group.

One request I had to deal with as Chairman of MAC made for a difficult position among Foundation members, Medical Council, and other volunteers. Some Chapters did not submit their full proportion of dollars they had committed, as they wanted to continue support of their local Center as they had done in the past, contrary to the formal agreement they had signed with National. As a result, for two successive years the Foundation approached the new budget year with a shortfall of incoming funds. Welch Boyer, the National Director, insisted that I join in a plea to all Chapters and their associated physicians, that all available funds be submitted urgently for budget commitments to be met. Without compliance, the position the National Director threatened was that funding would be decreased, but only for the Centers, a Foundation position that I found untenable. The draft of his statement took considerable modification for my agreement. As Council Chairman, I was the spokesperson for the membership of the Medical Council which annually had been expressing significant dissatisfaction over the lack of reasonable increases in funding for all of the medical programs. In my view, Council's perception was correct. Despite the annual increase in dollars raised, these amounts mostly went to hire ever more fund raising personnel and staff rather than for increases in program support for the research projects and the Center program. My concern was to keep the medical group, the administration, and Board working together for the long term goals of the Foundation. For the year 1975, total expenditures were planned for almost $4.5 million. The combined medical program budget (all aspects) was just over $2 million. Percentage wise, the medical budget had not increased in line with the reported 8% increase in dollars raised during the 1974 fiscal year. The Medical Advisory Council members, and I suspect most others, were relieved when, during Doris Tulcin's tenure as President, Bob Dresing became Vice President and instituted a new and effective management approach. There were a number of changes in staff around that time. Dr. Herndon left for a position at Mercer University in 1974 and a search committee was formed to search for his successor. His leaving was followed by that of Welch Boyer in 1976 and Hank Lione was appointed National Director. As Vice President, Bob Dresing relied on his previous experience to initiate and apply a systematic business plan and an over-all organizational management approach for the Foundation. Once his plan took effect, the annual crises no longer occurred. His effort marked the beginning of increasingly successful fund raising and the steady rise in medical program support that excels today.

As President, Dr. Graub initiated several creative efforts to improve the research focus on CF and Bob McCreery made further efforts. But research progress was slow, largely because no researcher had a real sense of direction. As a Foundation, there was an understandable difficulty in developing a philosophy about achieving a stronger research focus, although there were increasingly frequent discussions around long range planning. Any new research lead or finding was cause for considerable interest and excitement. The "Spock factor" was thought for a time to be a substance that inhibited the sweeping motion of the cilia (tiny hairs that help propel mucus along the airways) and there was a report of a fibroblast abnormality that was published in a prestigious medical journal. Unfortunately, it soon had to be retracted.

During his tenure as president, Bob McCreery continued the role of seek-ing ways to stimulate more basic research interest. A Scientific Advisory Commit-tee was formed including Drs. William Rutter, Richard Sidman, Eric Shooter, LeRoy Matthews, and Elizabeth Neufeld. At least one GAP Conference on "Developmental Biology" was formulated and held with Dr. Rutter serving as chairman.

Another hope was that the Centers would provide a focus for increasing basic research. However, it became obvious to me that, for the most part, the Cen-ters had not really been established or adequately funded for this purpose. As a result, many were receiving insufficient support to be able to increase research potential at their institutions. The fact that real research progress was not occurring at the Center level became very clear to me at the national meeting of Center Directors that I led as Chairman of MAC in 1974. To get a sense of the research status in the Centers, I asked for a show of hands from the 100 or so Center Direc-tors in attendance as to how many of the Centers had one or more NIH funded basic research grants at their institution. It was disappointing, to say the least, when only about six hands went up, including my own. This poll provided one estimate of the state of our NIH funded basic research then at our Centers and showed the difficulty the Centers had in fostering such research on their own, some 14 years after the Center concept had been initiated. However, the Center program was working quite well for the diagnosis and care purposes for which they had been established. The Centers were drawing together large numbers of patients and improving care and longevity. Patient, family, and general public education was improving steadily. Requests for federal funding had been successful for the cre-ation of a number of Pediatric Pulmonary Training Centers at some CF Centers. Their goal was to develop specialized education and training of the many other car-egivers needed to staff the growing number of centers. These personnel included nurses, respiratory therapists, nutritionists, social workers, and others with a special emphasis on the care of CF patients. But clearly these efforts were not attracting basic researchers to the CF cause.

On the clinical side though, the evidence of progress in improving survival was demonstrated by the holding of a GAP Conference on "Reproduction of Adolescents and Young Adults with Cystic Fibrosis" in February 1975. Bettina Hilman, then chairman of the Young Adult Committee, organized the conference that was attended by many scientists and physicians. In addition, there were nationally recognized experts in the fields of obstetrics, gynecology, and pulmonary physiology (especially as related to the changes during pregnancy) to focus on "this new generation" of individuals.

In regards to the research situation, however, I did have a better feeling as far as the future was concerned, in part because I was a member of the search committee for a new Medical Director. I was very supportive of the efforts to improve the research program and the long range planning and strategy talks. The search committee for a new Medical-Scientific Director was eminently successful when Amoz Chernoff, M.D. was attracted to the position. Dr. Chernoff was a research scientist and the leader of a large and well-funded research program at the University of Tennessee. He was looking for a new challenge, and felt he had found it with the CF Foundation. On the professional side, once he had examined and understood our structure, strengths, weaknesses and needs, he became a key individual in the successful planning of the Foundation's future. The leadership had developed increased awareness of and support for CF from the Congress and the concept of a joint project with the federal government was developed. The plan was to achieve an in-depth study to project forward all of the aspects and all of the needs of CF into the future. I was pleased because such a long range plan for the future would include strong recommendations for the support of research, as well as all the others issues faced by the CF community and how to achieve that support from all potential sources within and outside of the Foundation.

The result of this collaboration with the federal government was a milestone of progress for the Foundation. The initiation of the "Strategic Plan for CF" was ensured by President Doris Tulcin and led by Amoz Chernoff. This extensive effort included input from a large number of the Foundation family, lay, medical, and staff. One report was titled "Cystic Fibrosis: A Plea for a Future" and was presented to every member of Congress. Another report was titled "Cystic Fibrosis, State of the Art and Directions for Future Research Efforts" and submitted to the NIH. All of this effort established **The Plan for the Future** and has served the Foundation very well. As Medical-Scientific Director, Amoz served as the Principal Investigator and Giulio Barbero was Co-Principal Investigator.

The entire project was extremely well organized and included a Program Advisory Group and an Organizational Advisory Group (OAG) which was headed by J. Palmer Saunders, Ph.D., Dean of the Graduate School of Biomedical Sciences, University of Texas. I was only familiar with the OAG, which had five Working Groups. Dr. Carolyn Denning and I served as Co Chairs of the Clinical

Sciences Working Group. It was a privilege and pleasure to work with Carolyn. Our group alone had eleven members, including Paul di Sant'Agnese, M.D., Richard Erbe, M.D., Samuel Giammona, M.D., Millicent Higgins, M.D., Douglas Holsclaw, M.D., Charles Bluestone, M.D., Harvey Colten, M.D., Robert Wood, M.D.,Ph.D., James Pennington, M.D., Lynne Reid, M.D., and Barbara Underwood, Ph.D. There were thirteen additional contributors. The final report from all of the participating groups was in excess of five hundred pages. It took several publications to encompass all the recommendations and the supporting details needed to meet the requirements of the NIH, Congress, and other agencies. The result of these efforts made for an increasingly recognized and goal oriented voluntary health agency and a Foundation with clearly identified goals and specific aims. Participation in this project was very satisfying and the accelerating advances in research over the past 20 or so years attests to the excellence of the plan.

The increasing life span of those with CF led to a positive development that emerged from all of the Foundation activity. There was growing awareness of the increasing numbers of late adolescent and early 20 year old patients whose needs and issues were increasingly different from any encountered thus far. To meet this new (and welcome) challenge, President Doris Tulcin and the MAC recommended forming a new committee. There was initial disagreement about calling it the "Adult Committee" at that time and the compromise was "Young Adult/Consumer Services Committee." Soon the "young" would be dropped. The first Chairman was Dr. Hilman. Dr. Ivan Harwood was Chairman in 1978 and a memorandum from him indicated that two new members should be added to the Committee, a "consumer representative" and a Center physician. Paul Downs, a young lawyer active with young adults in his area, was nominated by Dr. Thomas Boat. After a thorough interview, Paul was appointed the "consumer representative," and was an excellent choice. He subsequently went on to be a Regional Representative to the Board of Trustees for a number of years, and also served as President of his own Cleveland Chapter for two years. The committee proved to be a successful addition for the times. In addition to Ivan and Paul, other members included Fay Smith, Jane Lowe, Bobbie Mackay, and Drs. Pam Davis, Bruce Axelrod, Tom Boat, Don Strominger, and Norman Lewiston. Tom Boat and Dr. Paul Quinton also served as Chairmen. Early on, the committee reviewed educational videotapes produced by psychiatrist, Dr. Cy Worby, conducted a survey on cost of care, and initiated legislative and lobbying efforts.

Another successful event "CF: Projections into the Future" was held in Jerusalem in 1976, thanks to the efforts of Dr. Graub. Over 100 scientists and physicians attended. A newsletter report by Dr. Chernoff, then Medical Director, noted that there was a large emphasis on the research aspects of CF. This conference was planned in conjunction with the 7th International Congress on CF which followed in Paris, France. This was an even larger meeting which emphasized more clinically related reports. It was definitely an international conference and the first that I attended where simultaneous translation in two languages was required.

Two concepts initiated in Cleveland deserve special comment because they eventually became significant components of the National medical program. The pharmacy program came from the contribution made by Sam and Henrietta Trott, a generous and thoughtful couple. Their family members comprised the "Cousins Club," which had resolved to raise money for CF research in support of the Trott's young CF son, who was quite ill. It was their plight with CF that led to the incorporation of the Cleveland Chapter in Ohio in 1955. Sam was a pharmacist with his own small pharmacy, so he was very much aware of the cost of medicines and knew that many parents were hard pressed to pay for them. He resolved to personally make all CF medications available to any CF patient at his cost, plus 10% for handling, which even included any additional cost for packaging and mailing. As the volume grew, he somehow managed to keep up with the extra workload and he also passed on the discounts that came as he developed greater purchasing volume. When his store was destroyed in a riot in 1964, he was inclined to retire. But the Chapter felt his work was much too valuable a resource for all of the families and did not let the program fail. An agreement was reached that the necessary space would be provided in the Chapter offices, which were relocating anyway. Every CF family continued to benefit. Sam's program was probably the first disease-specific mail order plan in the country. It avoided local pharmacy complaints because it was disease specific, covered a large area, and did not threaten them. After Dr. Robert Beall became the National Medical Director and became familiar with the enormous savings that were afforded families, Bob worked effectively to implement the pharmacy program on a nationwide basis through the Foundation. The hard work and generosity of the Trott's was typical of that of so many other volunteers and supporters everywhere over the years. The determination of the Cleveland Chapter to continue the cost saving mail order drug program ultimately led to the nationwide program for those with CF.

The second development from Cleveland had a significant impact on the establishing of the National research program. It stemmed from the Cleveland Center's CF Program Project research grant awarded and funded by NIH that began in 1964. This successful project was coupled with the insistence of the Cleveland United Way that any of its funds were required to remain locally. The Center had the support of the Cleveland Chapter and the close review and approval of research grant proposals by the local Medical Advisory Board. The Center policy was to consistently use these funds as "seed grants" to stimulate and encourage medical school faculty and others to start CF related research with the goal of them becoming successful in competing for NIH funding. CF Foundation and United Way funds were not used at the Center for patient care or services. Since each renewal of the Program Project grant by the NIH was competitive, we were very dependent upon strong new local grant proposals for the Project and were constantly encouraging them.

At the National level, the Research Committee and the Foundation had been funding individual research projects and basic science trainees with the expectation that this support would lead to more long term research interest and involvement by the laboratories involved. In support of this process, strong proposals by research fellows from the better laboratories were funded. Toward the end of their two years of work, these trainees were invited to present their results to Research

Committee members and Board representatives, so there would be a summary of their work. It was hoped these trainees, and importantly the labs in which they worked, would be stimulated to continue research in CF. Unfortunately, the conclusion had to be reached that this approach was proving neither effective nor productive.

By now, the Program Project concept of the NIH was being utilized by some other Centers as well, but for most Centers the competition for NIH research support was difficult. The NIH then introduced an additional funding concept, that of a Core Center Grant. In this arrangement, if there were sufficient NIH funded research projects around a central theme, such as CF, the program could apply for more funding in core support of the additional laboratories needed to further the progress of the funded research laboratories. The National organization, through its effective public policy advocacy program started by Doris Tulcin after her Presidency, encouraged Congress to appropriate funds for at least one Core Center for CF research. Our proposal from the Cleveland program was the first to be awarded a CF Core Center grant in the amount of $1.8 million covering a period of three years. This funding concept improved our local research productivity and was successfully extended under Dr. Pam Davis' leadership.

Dr. Beall and the Foundation leadership drew from the recommendations of the Strategic Plan, the productivity of relatively stable funding for the Cleveland program, and the potential for similar stable funding to enhance research elsewhere. Established research laboratories with the potential for good CF research were encouraged to compete for new and significant Foundation funding. With good progress, this support could be extended up to five years. Availability of stable funding attracted quality proposals and stimulated the interest of the best researchers and laboratories. This key to expansion of basic CF related research grew from the Strategic Plan and was called the Research and Development Program (RDP). The RDP plan would be very expensive and had never before been undertaken by an individual health agency such as the CFF. Its success was totally dependent on a significantly greater fund raising effort than ever undertaken before. Once again, the challenge was met by the determined, dedicated, and, in many cases, the very personal efforts of those who set out to raise the funds required. In addition to her other accomplishments, Doris Tulcin led this incredible and successful fund raising effort. The initial eight Centers included Baylor College of Medicine, Columbia University, UCLA, and the Universities of Alabama, Case Western Reserve, North Carolina at Chapel Hill, San Francisco, and Utah. Soon after, The Hospital for Sick Children in Toronto and the Universities of Chicago and Washington were added, building on the research focus that originated in Cleveland from the first Program Project Grant in CF in 1964. The innovative and successful RDP program, initiated and funded by the National CF Foundation, led to greater NIH recognition and support and has had a major impact on furthering CF research progress. The RDP strategy helped lead to the identification of the CF gene in a record period of time.

Dr. Charles Lobeck, Dean of the School of Medicine at the University of Missouri-Columbia and Vice Chairman of MAC, delivered the medical presentation to the Board of Trustees in November 1974 in Atlanta. With his usual clear insight, he noted two special strong points of the Foundation as reported in the CF Newsletter. "The Foundation has interrelationships of research, service, medical professionals and other kinds of health professionals, professional educators, laymen, patients, and their parents who are all working together toward one goal, and who are communicating with each other. Another outstanding aspect of the Foundation, is its Board of Trustees, which has both lay and medical representation. Also part of the team, is the professional staff, which responds to the goals of the Foundation. Almost no other system that I know of has this type of governing organization," he concluded. These aspects of the Foundation's governance were started early on, maintained, and improved upon. The continuing focus on the single enemy, CF, and the ultimate goal of success have served us well.

Success can be measured in a number of different ways. A recent report from the CFF notes that the care received through the network of 114 CF Centers has made a profound impact on the quality and length of life for people with CF. Over the past two decades the median survival age is reported to have increased from 18 to 32 years. Overall, there are about 9,000 CF adults. The percentage of adults has exceeded 35% and there are some 90 recognized adult centers in Pulmonary Divisions. These are measures of success which offer encouragement and of which we can be proud.

Another measure of success is in research progress. We now have an array of therapeutic approaches. These include gene therapy studies, interventions related to the abnormal CFTR protein, altered ion transport, and abnormal mucus secretion, and therapies against the infection and inflammation that leads to lung destruction. Basic science studies are being supported in each of these areas. The Drug Development and Approval Process is projected to take one half the time and one quarter of the usual cost for developing a new drug. The expertise developed in the eight Therapeutics Development Network of centers serves to significantly increase the efficiency of clinical trials. With these two mechanisms in place, there are some 20 new potential CF therapies in trial and in development while the cost of drug development should be greatly reduced and the time factor is also reduced. The technology of high-throughput screening, which greatly accelerated the drug discovery process for cancer and heart disease, has been adapted for CF drug discovery by the Foundation. This technique greatly speeds up the screening of potential compounds that might be useful in therapy. A third measure of success is the continued availability of funds to support these activities. The medical program grants budget has kept pace and has nearly doubled in the past three years with a report of over 50 million dollars in expenditures projected for 2000 and realistic planning for future years. By each measure, these programs are extremely successful and moving ahead with determination and clear leadership.

As with many of the other health and research related participants in this fight against CF, my usual daily professional activities generally blurred with those as a volunteer for the organization. It seemed that these opportunities and the interchanging of relationships added strength to the process and our endeavors. From a personal view, my relationship with the Cleveland Chapter from 1961 and the National organization from 1964 were the source of personal growth and continuing great satisfaction. Remembrances of friends, accomplishments, and wonderful memories surface frequently and are greatly treasured. But they are diminished in that, even with the finding of the CF gene in 1989, the pathophysiology underlying the basic defect still is not fully understood and still needs be the target of continuing intensive basic inquiry. Hope and the continuing determined efforts of the leadership of the Foundation and those dedicated to providing care and clinical research, along with a broad spectrum of insightful basic researchers, will bring us ever increasing longevity and a successful conclusion to this fight.

18

My Journey from "Sixty-Five Roses" to Dahlias: Creating the Strategic Plan

Amoz I. Chernoff, M.D.

> A young child with cystic fibrosis (CF) repeatedly, but mistakenly, said "sixty five roses" instead of "cystic fibrosis," when trying to describe his disease. "Sixty-Five Roses" became a symbol of CF and a popular and effective Cystic Fibrosis Foundation fund raising slogan.

I had heard the term "sixty five roses," but my first real contact with the Cystic Fibrosis Foundation (CFF) came about after seeing a "help wanted" advertisement in the journal *Science* in early 1975 for a Medical-Scientific Director. Having served as the Director of the University of Tennessee Memorial Research Center in Knoxville for over ten years, and beginning to feel the need for new challenges, the idea of applying for the post appealed to me. Nevertheless, after my initial interactions with the managing staff at the Foundation, I realized that this post would not mesh with my long range goals and I withdrew my application.

By May of 1975, following additional discussions with the search committee and with the gentle prodding of President Robert McCreery, National Director Welch Boyer, and members of the Executive Committee, a position description was framed which led to my acceptance of the role of Medical Director for one year during a sabbatical leave of absence from the University of Tennessee. During the later part of 1975, my role was carried out on a part time basis as a consulting member of the Foundation's management team, while during 1976 I served on a full time basis. During late summer of 1976, Doris Tulcin, by now the President of the Foundation, prevailed upon me to extend my tenure through June of the following year, with the request that I complete activities which were already underway and that I be available as a consultant when needed after that time.

During the initial phase of my tenure, I tried to learn as much as possible about CF and how the Foundation operated. Since my own scientific background was in the genetic, biochemical, and clinical aspects of the hereditary hemolytic anemias, such as sickle cell anemia and thalassemia, transferring this understanding to the new disease did not prove to be a daunting task. However, learning about the

Foundation turned out to be of a different order of magnitude. Even though I had developed and directed a large, multimillion dollar research group in Tennessee, the complexities of dealing with an organization so dependent on volunteer input and the need to satisfy the requirements and sensitivities of different constituencies proved to be more difficult.

Fortunately, the learning curve was fairly rapid and by the fall of 1975 I was beginning to understand the nature of the disease and to unravel the mysterious ways in which a health foundation must operate. I became more and more impressed with what progress had been made in understanding CF in the decades since it was first described and I thoroughly appreciated and respected the significant contributions made by many of the programs which had been instituted by the Foundation. I saw my role, however, not as being a cheerleader for the many good things which were going on, but rather as a prodder trying to improve the stature and operation of the scientific aspects of the Foundation. Therefore, many of my presentations, messages, reviews and talks given to staff and volunteers during the first portion of my tenure focused on what I saw as significant areas for improvement, and my hopes for what my office might accomplish in the future.

I was concerned about a number of areas of importance to the growth and health of the CFF. Communication among the scientific elements of the Foundation was often inadequate, long range planning beyond the need to find a cure for CF was limited, efforts to evaluate the programs already in place were not readily apparent, and little was being done to see whether the Foundation was making the best use of its limited financial resources. For example, in comments made to the Board of Trustees on December 8, 1975, I stated that, "While I recognize the central position occupied by the Centers program and of the Directors who run them, there seem to be few controlled studies underway and almost no measures in place to evaluate the effectiveness of the clinical programs in the delivery of health care. Regarding the research community, there is a need to rethink our goals and responsibilities in order to ensure support of the highest quality science and to make our limited research funds have as great an impact as possible on efforts of investigators committed to working on the CF problem."

Furthermore, the scientific aspects of the Foundation's staff structure, though not its volunteer scientific committees, were not highly regarded by the scientific community as a whole. In response to some of these concerns, my staff initiated a number of steps to improve communication, enhance scientific exchange, and begin to convert the Medical Director's office into a credible scientific resource and a focus for ideas and information. One such initiative was a "Newsletter from the Medical Director" which appeared irregularly during my stay with the Foundation. Another was an increasing involvement in the collection and statistical analysis of CF data. Other efforts emerged from my frequent interaction with early medical leaders, such as di Sant'Agnese, Shwachman, and Graub, and from the advice and guidance of numerous outstanding medical scientific contributors to our understanding of the clinical and psychosocial aspects of the disease.

The major outcome of these activities ultimately proved to be the development and carrying out of a proposal with the National Institutes of Health (NIH) to do an in depth study of CF and to develop a long range plan for the future. The plan was, in reality, an offer on the part of the Foundation to act as a technical resource for the NIH, which had been ordered to carry out an in depth study of CF. This was to include, "a compilation of CF research and treatment activities within the Public Health Service (PHS), including the NIH, and the outlook for future research breakthroughs." The Foundation's involvement in this activity came about because Congress, through the Foundation's efforts, had mandated that the Department of Health, Education, and Welfare (HEW) carry out such a study and report back to them on the needs for future effort and support in this field. The CFF had for some time, and for its own motives, wanted to examine this general question. The Board of Trustees, the elected leadership, various committee members, and the National staff had talked about a planning and goals effort for several years, but lacked the basis upon which to carry out a meaningful study. The contract, therefore, allowed the Foundation to collect such data and utilize them to make pertinent projections. The resulting document enabled the CFF to provide the Congress with an outline of needs for CF in the future and, at the same time, to utilize it to examine its own goals.

The approach used in carrying out the contract consisted of identifying a wide range of issues in CF that needed to be dealt with and then getting as much information about each of these issues as was possible. To carry out these tasks, we divided our committee structure into two sections. The first was the Program Advisory Group (PAG) which dealt with questions of basic research, clinical research, health care delivery, medical ethics, psychosocial support services, education and manpower needs, and the specific quality of life issues of interest to the patient and his or her family. The second was called the Organizational Advisory Group (OAG) which concerned itself with the various organizational groups which had an interest or involvement in CF, such as the NIH, other non-NIH Federal agencies (e.g., Maternal and Child Health, Federal Drug Administration, Social Security Agency, etc.), private health foundations (e.g., CFF, American Lung Association, National Foundation, etc.), professional medical and research societies (e.g., American Medical Association, American Nursing Association, Association of American Medical Colleges, etc.), and a group representing private philanthropy and the profit sector, including pharmaceutical houses, insurance companies, and biomedical products producers.

Well-respected and energetic people chaired each of the two groups: the PAG by Drs Giulio Barbero and Robert Cooke and the OAG by Dr. J. Palmer Saunders. These chair people, in turn, selected chairs for the ten working groups related to the topics already identified. For the PAG, the Working Groups and their respective chair people were as follows:

1   Basic Sciences—Drs. John Mangos and Richard Talamo;

2   Clinical Science—Drs. Carolyn Denning and Carl Doershuk;

3) Support Services and Therapeutic Interventions—Audrey
   McCollum and Dr. Katherine Nuckolls;

4 Education and Manpower—Drs. Alexander Spock and Will
   Waring; and

5 Consumers/Delivery Systems—Doris Tulcin and Dr.
   Edmund Pellegrino.

For the OAG, they were as follows:

1 The National Institutes of Health—Dr. Robert Gordon,
   Special Assistant to the Director, NIH;

2 Non-NIH Federal Agencies—Dr. Vince Hutchins, Office of
   Maternal and Child Health Services;

3 Private health foundations and organizations—Dr. Alex
   Maish of the CFF Board and Dr. Arthur Salisbury, Vice
   President for Medical Services of the National Foundation;

4 Professional medical societies and organizations—Dr.
   Charles Lobeck (CFF); and

5 Philanthropic and profit making enterprises—Mr. Robert
   McCreery (CFF).

The working groups were asked to provide information on what was required to fill in the needs or gaps that were identified, such as new knowledge, people, facilities, laws, attitudes, and finances. Then they assessed these suggestions in terms of priorities based on the likelihood of success, practicality, and potential impact on the field, as well as on other less well defined criteria. I served as Principal Investigator on the contract which was approved by the NIH in September of 1976, but not funded until February of 1977. As it was a one year agreement, it was necessary for us to do much of the planning before funding was assured so that the study could be completed in a timely fashion. With the help of numerous lay volunteers, individuals in the scientific and health related disciplines, staff, and a consulting firm, we were able to develop an extensive volume of relevant material which eventually was published and presented to the Congress in the spring of 1978. As promised, I continued to work on the contract even after I resumed my relationship with the University of Tennessee in July of 1977.

During the course of contract negotiations, it was apparent that the NIH would support only those efforts which fell within the mission of the NIH, i.e., research, research training, and technology transfer. The CFF saw a critical need to prepare a related, but separate, report to address the physical, psychological and ethical management of patients, the training of health professionals, consumer education and information, economics and finance, and health care environments. The NIH report entitled "Cystic Fibrosis: State of the Art and Directions for Future Research Efforts" appeared in April of 1978 and was followed by additional publications. One, in 1979, was titled "Cystic Fibrosis: A Disease in Search of Ideas" in

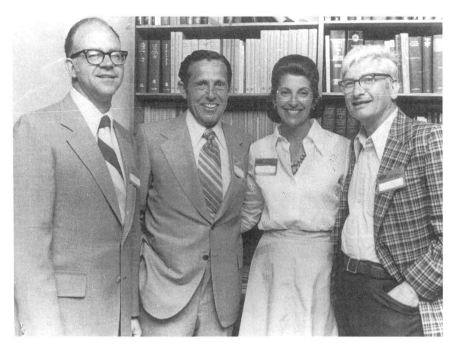

Figure 18.1. *At the Israel Conference in 1976, from left, Dr. Carl Doershuk, chairman of the Medical Council, Dr. Milton Graub, past President, Doris Tulcin, President, and Dr. Amoz Chernoff, Medical Director of the Foundation. Courtesy of Dr. Amoz Chernoff.*

two volumes. The Foundation's own report appeared in April 1978 and was titled "Cystic Fibrosis: A Plea for a Future." This report, too, was followed in December 1978 by an additional pamphlet, the1978 CF Survey Summary, and by the CFF "Five Year Strategic Plan 1979-1983."

All these documents were well received and, as time has gone by, have proven to be of invaluable help to the CF community as a whole. Furthermore, the vast majority of the predictions and opportunities cited in the reports have been achieved. Never the less, even 25 years after the report, there remain many gaps in our understanding of CF and a continued need to pursue the answers with dedication and modern biomedical technology.

As I was completing my time with the Foundation, I had the opportunity on May 15, 1977 to summarize my impressions as both an "outsider and insider" and make some recommendations to the Board of Trustees. Many of my conclusions were drawn from the information and recommendations gathered for the NIH project which we were still in the process of carrying out. While there had been success in care and quality of life issues and the development of some exciting clinical and basic research activities, I chose to focus on the need for careful reappraisal of our programs, directions, and goals so the Foundation would be prepared to deal with the needs of the future. The Foundation's medical budget at that time was approximately $2.1 million. About $1.0 million (roughly 50% of the programmatic effort) helped support a series of over 120 Centers. Some $700,000, or 1/3 of the medical budget, was for grants to support basic research efforts and clinical and research fellowships, while educational and training programs received $370,000. No funds were allocated to clinical research.

One could foresee the coming need for carefully controlled clinical trials that would require a research environment that did not exist at the majority of Centers. Meanwhile, other agencies also assisted the care effort (Maternal and Child Health, Crippled Children's' Services, Medicare, and others) and the NIH expenditures were in excess of $2 billion per year for overall basic research. Since the budgets of these agencies vastly exceeded those of the Foundation, it seemed strategically important to devise a program that would best complement the others and position the Foundation to work closely with them. One could anticipate the need for at least a few Centers with clinical research expertise, need for increasing peer review of the clinical Centers, continuation of the basic research program but emphasizing "seed" money and young investigators, and the initiation of a new program of one or more Basic and Clinical Research Centers with long term, stable funding so as to develop the critical mass of researchers needed. Continuation of the training and education programs was also vital. The above constituted one plan the Foundation might consider and implement. In any event, the time was right for renewed planning and goal setting.

My brief formal relationship with the CFF proved to be of immense value to me, personally, as I not only learned about a disease with which I had previously only been superficially acquainted but also because of the many wonderful and dedicated clinicians, health care workers, and private individuals with whom I had an opportunity to interact and with whom I became friendly. One particularly useful experience was the opportunity to attend the 1976 Conference in Israel. (Figure 18.1) Additionally, the close contact with the various governmental bodies undoubtedly influenced my decision to accept the position of Director of the Division of Blood Disease and Resources at the National Heart, Lung, and Blood Institute at the NIH in 1978, a post I occupied until my retirement in 1988. Following retirement, I immersed myself in gardening, focusing on growing and exhibiting that magnificent flower, the dahlia. Thus, my journey from "Sixty-Five Roses" to dahlias was complete.

19

A Patient's Perspective, Philosophy, and Experience

Bruce L. Baskin

It has been said that the only two things guaranteed in life are taxes and death. I would suggest that life has three guarantees, taxes, death, and life obstacles. Life obstacles face everyone and can occur in many fashions. Failed relationships, job disenchantment, drugs, health problems, and difficulty with children are just a few of these life obstacles. While we all have and/or will be faced with life obstacles, it is how we face and deal with these obstacles which define us throughout our lives. My life obstacle began within the first nine months of my life and began in 1959.

I was born on February 3, 1959 in Cleveland, Ohio. As the second child and first son born to Shirley and Allan Baskin the pregnancy and birth went as scheduled and all seemed well. However, despite a voracious appetite as an infant, I was not gaining weight in the same manner as a typical baby. The local pediatrician could not identify the cause of the weight loss but was astute enough to recommend a visit to Babies and Children's Hospital in Cleveland. The pediatrician had thought about the possibility of cystic fibrosis (CF) being the cause of the poor weight gain and knew of Dr. LeRoy Matthews at the Hospital who was doing research on the disease and had started a successful program of care. A sweat test was performed immediately and confirmed that the diagnosis was CF.

In 1959, the only readily available published data informed readers that CF was a genetic disease which affected both the lungs and the pancreas, and the average child did not live to see their second birthday. Dr. Matthews and his staff were among the few groups in the entire country both intensively treating and researching CF. For parents with children diagnosed with CF in 2001-2002, it should be encouraging for them to recognize the abundance of funds flowing to CF research, and the excellent research and care Centers throughout the United States. We now have an average life expectancy to the thirties and forties, and most importantly the opportunity for a cure for CF within the next decade. This type of optimism could not exist in 1959, and thus this life obstacle appeared much more challenging in 1959 than now.

It became clear during my infant years that the disease had affected my pancreas more than my lungs. Doctor visits were every four to six weeks like clockwork and the discipline to take my medications was drilled into my parents and myself at a very early age. I recall one visit with my mother to see Dr. Matthews and my mother proceeded to tell the doctor how difficult it was to get me to take my medicines. Dr. Matthews, universally recognized as a pioneer in CF work, looked at me from his desk and pronounced, "If you do not take your medicine you will be dead within five years." From that moment in time, I began to mature and grow up faster that most five year olds.

During my elementary school years my parents were faced with and confronted a life obstacle which set the stage for the degrees of success that I have had in my life. They had the dilemma of raising their son either as a disabled child with CF or as a normal child who would live with CF. They chose the latter course and throughout my formative elementary years I was treated both at home and at school as a normal child whose boundaries were unlimited and whose restrictions were few. With the exception of my teachers, none of my friends were aware of my disease nor did I ever have discussions about CF. My treatments were done in the privacy of my home. As a youngster growing up I did not want to feel different than any of my friends and I never wanted to be treated any differently than anyone else. However, I did know that CF was my major, serious life obstacle. Both in school and in sports I read the extra pages on assignments, ran the extra mile, practiced constantly so as to never have CF as an excuse, and always strived to achieve more and more in my life.

Baseball played a large role in my life as I joined leagues at earlier ages than usually permitted and received all-star recognition at all levels. Once again, in living with CF I was acknowledging to myself that I was really different than others and that gave me a drive to succeed that was very intense. Throughout my junior high years I began to realize the true severity of CF. I was hospitalized in seventh grade for two weeks for a lung infection and it was there that I realized how lucky I was. I was 14 years old and hospitalized for the first time since I was a baby. During the hospitalizations I met many children with CF who were not as fortunate. While CF is a disease that kills children, knowing that fact and witnessing that truth are two different situations. Some kids that I met were very young and had spent much of their lives in the hospital. One important observation was that, by and large, these kids accepted their illness, lived fully despite the disease, and spent little time feeling sorry for themselves. CF, like many genetic diseases, presents itself early in a child's life and therefore, most of us don't know what it is like to live without CF. Therefore, like a blind person who has never had sight, it is difficult to feel sorry about missing something you never experienced in the first place.

At one point in my teens, I asked my doctor, Dr. Thomas Boat, a straightforward direct question, "Dr. Boat, realistically, how long will I live?" Without hesitation or reservation Dr. Boat said, "I do not know, but neither do I know how long I will live. I could ride my bicycle home today and get hit by a car, you just never know." The truth in his statement lies in the fact that we do not know. Having CF may not enable me to live into my sixties or beyond, but life without CF provides no guarantee either. Every day the obituary section of the newspaper is filled with people who had no idea last week, last month, or last year that they would not be here today. Worrying about an unknown tomorrow takes away from positive energy that can be used today.

Throughout junior high and high school, I not only played basketball and baseball competitively but I also worked at various jobs after school and on weekends. As CF is a disease which never leaves you it is important, in addition to your treatments, to keep as active as possible. The more time spent constructively is less time spent worrying about the effects of CF on your body. In high school I played varsity sports, was editor of the high school newspaper, and vice president of my high school fraternity. Throughout high school I was very fortunate healthwise, as I never had a hospital stay throughout my three years of high school. It should be noted that throughout my elementary, junior high and high school years I had the absolute fortune of being a patient at the CF Center at what became Rainbow Babies and Children's Hospital/ University Hospitals of Cleveland. Throughout my 40 years, I have only had four doctors in my life, Drs. Matthews, Boat, Doershuk, and most recently, Michael Infeld. These individuals all have the same qualities, they are brilliant clinicians, dedicated to the control and ultimate cure of CF, and exhibit a compassion towards their patients that may be equaled but not surpassed in medicine. Any success that I may have achieved in my life has to be shared with my parents, my wife, my children, and my doctors.

After high school I attended John Carroll University in Cleveland, where I graduated in four years with a degree in Political Science with an emphasis towards Law School. During my senior year I applied for a full time position at a steel company feeling that I would work and attend law school; however, the steel company was looking for an individual who had a high grade point average and was a business school graduate. In addition, they were interviewing at many colleges and there was only one position available.

I immediately went to the recruitment office and asked that I be allowed to interview despite the fact that I was not a business major but I had the credentials. Numerous interviews later, I was offered the job and I accepted it. During my meeting to accept the position at the company I felt compelled to tell the supervisor that I had a disease called CF and that if that presented a problem for him that I would understand. Much to my amazement, the supervisor told me that not only would it not be a problem but that one other employee (non-CF) recently had surgery and had a metal plate in his head. At that time I realized an important lesson that applies to persons with CF or any other illness or life obstacle. That is, despite our own obstacles, we are not alone and that all people have strengths and weaknesses. The best path to a positive life is to realize and accept those weaknesses, while at the same time, consistently accentuate those strengths.

During my junior year in college I met and eventually married my wife, Beth. We have been married for 16 years and for all the success and good fortune I have been blessed with throughout my life, none surpasses the life we have and will continue to have together. Dealing with CF can be very difficult at times and it takes a special person with compassion and patience to help you get through the tough spots. Not a day goes by that my wife's talents aren't appreciated with amazement. We now have twin sons, Brett and Bradley, who recently turned 10 years old. I truly believe that the smiles of children uplift all people and our two boys put a smile on our faces each and every day. The bottom line is that family is all-important in the ability to successfully overcome one's life obstacles. Many CF families are faced with more than one CF child; however, my older sister, Carin, and younger brother Andy were not born with CF. The support of my parents, siblings, relatives, and especially my wife and children have been essential in dealing with CF.

After a year of attending law school and working full time, I left work to continue, and eventually graduate from, Cleveland Marshall College of Law. During this time United Way of Cleveland asked if I would participate in their campaign film to promote the Cystic Fibrosis Foundation and the local United Way. This would mean that my life with CF would be publicized to over one million people via television and corporate campaigns. Up to that time, not even some of my closer friends knew that I had CF and I had always, since childhood, kept my health issues confined to my family and myself. After discussions with my family I decided to participate in the film and devote the next nine months to United Way giving speeches and assisting in the campaign. My real concern was that I wanted to be an inspiration to others but I did not want people to perceive me as disabled. Once again, to my amazement, people reacted positively to my story and I met and came into contact with so many good people that I will never forget. The opportunity to be a part of helping other people through United Way and their programs was tremendously uplifting. Once again, recognition that life obstacles effect all of us helps each of us get through the rough spots a little easier.

During the United Way campaign I came into contact with many tremendous individuals involved with the campaign of their company. Immediately following the campaign, I was offered a position in the Trust Department at Society Bank. I had met both the President and the Chairman of the bank throughout the stint at United Way and was determined to take advantage of the opportunity. Through my subsequent 7 years at the bank, I was promoted 4 times and eventually headed up my department.

In 1990, a search recruiter approached me from New Jersey to interview for a local position with the regional investment firm of Manning & Napier Advisors. The opportunity to work for a major regional investment firm and not have to move to New York City presented me with a tremendous opportunity and I accepted the position. However, despite current discrimination laws, I felt, once again, an obligation to let my new employer know about my CF before accepting the position. Despite current laws, if my employer had been uncomfortable about my disease, I would have understood and not accepted the position. The managing director, Ed George, one of the most honest and direct people one could ever meet, appreciated my candor, and was looking forward to working with me. Ed and I would become close friends and partners over the years and through our experiences we've both learned that nothing is guaranteed forever and that you should enjoy your life and attempt to take as little for granted as possible. In 1995, I had the privilege of being named a partner at Manning & Napier, a firm comprised of not just great minds but great people. In June of 2001, celebrated my 11th anniversary with Manning & Napier Advisors and subsequently was named Senior Vice President.

Throughout this chapter I've described some of the accomplishments in my life that I speak of with great pride in spite of my struggles with CF. As a private person who has always attempted to accentuate the positive I've often felt that talking or sharing about the struggles with CF were a form of complaining, and no one, including myself, enjoys hearing people complain. However, for the purposes of this chapter, it must be recognized that, from the perspective of the CF individual, life is a daily struggle. It is one that begins early in life and affects many parts of the body as a person gets older. In the elementary years, I was fortunate in that the disease had more complications from the pancreas than the lungs. My lung function was basically normal, but I did need to take the pancreatic enzymes at every meal to aid digestion and gain weight. Taking pills seems like an easy task, but for a child to have to take pills in front of his or her friends at every meal can become a real nuisance. Given the alternative of stomachaches and poor or no weight gain, there is no choice. Despite the thick mucus in the lungs of CF patients, the real killer is not the mucus but the Pseudomonas bacteria that begins to infiltrate the lungs for reasons still not clear. Past and present antibiotics are available to attempt to control the bacteria, but currently the bug is tenacious and cannot be completely obliterated in the lungs of a CF patient. Eventually, over a short or potentially a longer period of time, this bug will continue to erode lung function. Once again, I was fortunate insofar as the Pseudomonas bacteria did not appear on my cultures until I was about 13 years old, and at the time I was pretty naive about its long term implications. As medications to fight the Pseudomonas get better and better, and more expensive I might add, the ability to battle the bug becomes enhanced. In my view, with the exception of a magic bullet in the form of genetic alteration, the key to CF research lies in the obliteration or blocking of the Pseudomonas bacteria.

As individuals with CF live longer lives, different physical complications occur as a result of aging and CF. Diabetes and arthritis are two of the most prevalent adult type issues that I have had to deal with throughout my life. The control of blood sugar through insulin injections is, in my mind, an issue that deals with discipline, and as an individual who has taken medications since childhood, the regulation of blood sugar is a nuisance, but an easily regulated problem. Arthritis affects tens of millions of people and can range from a minor nuisance to debilitation. In terms of CF, it is another obstacle that has to be dealt with in a positive light. Adult CF issues like diabetes and arthritis should be perceived in two lights. One, both of these conditions are just one more issue that has to be dealt with, and Two, some twenty, thirty, and forty years ago these conditions hardly even existed for CF people, because few lived long enough to have to confront these conditions for very long.

The bottom line is that CF can be analyzed like a football game, whereby the ball is on the opponent's one yard line and the offensive team cannot seem to get the ball over the goal line. In fact, sometimes you can be penalized and your ball is brought back to the five, ten, or twenty yard line. The key is to continue to line up and attempt to penetrate the goal line, no matter how may downs it may take. One day, the defense will relax, and the line will be penetrated.

Many people could read this chapter and come to the conclusion that, despite living with CF, that I have been blessed throughout my life. Luck is the residue of hard work and individuals with CF have to work harder and harder to overcome an obstacle which gets worse and not better over time. I have been blessed with terrific parents, a beautiful wife, two awesome sons, a great job, and more friends than one could ever wish for. The only thing that is missing for me is that too many children are born with CF and, despite major medical advances, too many children are dying. As an elected Board Member of the National Cystic Fibrosis Foundation for the past four years, I am proud to note that the Foundation is currently raising 170 million dollars per year in the effort to give children a life. For a 42 year old with CF, such as myself, a cure will mean very little to me, but will mean everything to the kids with CF.

20

The International Cystic Fibrosis Association

Early History

Paul A. di Sant'Agnese, M.D.

The year 2000 marked the 35th Anniversary of the founding of the International Cystic Fibrosis [Mucoviscidosis] Association ICF[M]A in Paris, France, in 1965, and a brief history of the early organization, the medical component, and the accomplishments is appropriate.

During the summer of 1960 and in anticipation of my move to the National Institutes of Health as Chief of the Metabolism Branch, I traveled through Europe and made contact with several investigators who were interested in cystic fibrosis. This group included, among others, Professors Guido Fanconi and Ettore Rossi in Switzerland; Professor Andre Hennequet and Dr. P. Feigelson in France; Drs. Archibald Norman and David Lawson in England; Professor G. de Toni in Italy; and Professors H.A. Wejiers, Dicke and Van de Kamer in Holland.

Among the lay community, the initiative for the formation of an international association was taken by the Canadian and US Cystic Fibrosis Foundations, represented by Lyle Blackwell and George Barrie, Jr., respectively. A preliminary steering meeting was held in Paris, in July 1964. The first formal meeting of the international association was held in Paris March 24–26, 1965 under my Chairmanship for the medical and scientific meetings, and of Mr. George Barrie, Jr., Executive Director of the National CF Research Foundation US, for the lay program. Attending were 28 delegates and invited guests representing a total of 14 countries. Also present were representatives of the Office of International Research of the NIH in Paris and of the World Health Organization.

Thus, the ICF[M]A was born: its aims to improve the care of children and adults who have cystic fibrosis, to foster research, and to disseminate information. This international group is patterned on the Cystic Fibrosis Foundations in the US, Canada, and the UK, with a fund raising lay organization parallel to a medical council. Professor Guido Fanconi was appointed as the first Honorary Chairman of the ICF[M]A and George Barrie, as lay President, with myself as Chairman and Prof. Rossi, Vice-Chairman of the Medical/Scientific Council. Officers were elected from different countries to both the lay and medical organizations, with many physicians serving in dual capacity. The ICF[M]A maintained a corporate membership, which included one National Association for each member country.

The first meeting in Paris in 1965 was an important one and established the fight against CF on an international basis. Many of the participants were distinguished pediatricians. Their reputation in the international pediatric community and their interest gave considerable momentum to this organization and to worldwide research and care in cystic fibrosis. At the meeting of the ICF[M]A in Grindelwald, Switzerland, September 1966, it was decided to hold a Congress every three to four years and to publish the proceedings in book form. This plan proved to be astonishingly successful especially if it is considered that there were no significant funds available from the parent organization. There has been keen competition among many countries to host these gatherings which are considered essential, useful, and prestigious.

The first lay President of the ICF[M]A, Mr. Barrie, was succeeded by Mr. Lyle Blackwell of Canada and then by Mr. Robert McCreery of the US. As Chairman of the Medical Council, I was followed by Prof. Ettore Rossi, Switzerland, Dr. Harry Shwachman, of the US, and later by Dr. David Lawson of the UK.

A number of meetings have been sponsored by the ICF[M]A since 1965: the 4th International Congress on CF held in Grindelwald, Switzerland; the 5th in Cambridge, England in 1969; the 6th in Washington, D.C. in 1973; the 7th in Paris, France in 1976, and the 8th in Toronto, Canada in 1980. The ICF[M]A sponsored a previous International CF Conference in Toronto, Canada in 1968 and a meeting in Israel in 1976. Round tables on CF were organized by the ICF[M]A at the 11th International Pediatric Congress, Tokyo, Japan in 1965; the 12th IPC in Mexico City, Mexico in 1968; the 13th IPC in Vienna, Austria in 1971; and the 14th IPC in Buenos Aires, Argentina in 1974.

Now, with a 35 year perspective, it is possible to assess some of the accomplishments of the ICF[M]A. The Association has been successful in stimulating the interchange of ideas on reach and clinical care of patients, in organizing many successful international medical meetings, and developing a medical community which cooperates in many different countries. Back in 1960 and even up to 1965, most physicians interested in cystic fibrosis in various countries did not know each other except through the literature, and there was little awareness of the disease among both the medical and lay public of many nations. The ICF[M]A brought together physicians, paramedical personnel, and lay people and gave them a sense of belonging and a common purpose and dedication. The ICF[M]A was never able to raise significant funds, largely because of the many financial, taxation, and social problems, and the diversity of medical and social services encountered among different member nations. However, the meetings of the ICF[M]A were effective in pointing out what could be accomplished on a national level by a group of people working towards a common goal to increase the public and governments' awareness and support for the fight against CF. Indeed many similar, active and successful, national organizations dedicated to the fight against cystic fibrosis have been estab-

lished in various countries after informal and formal contacts following the foundation of the ICF[M]A.

In conclusion, the ICF[M]A developed into a vital and successful international lay and medical community which has been instrumental in greatly improving the knowledge of CF, the care of patients, and increasing the momentum of
research in this disorder throughout the world. Stimulating the formation of many
national organizations dedicated to the common goal of fighting CF has been one
of its major achievements. It is to be hoped that through the concerted efforts in all
countries and in all continents, CF will be conquered in the near future.

Later Years

Robert D. McCreery, Sr.

When George Barrie was National Director of the National Cystic Fibrosis Foundation (NCFRF), he envisioned a need to bring together physicians and other
interested persons as an International organization collectively focused on Worldwide CF problems. By his efforts, invitations were issued to individuals of various
countries known to be interested in the disease for a July 1964 meeting at the
Grand Hotel, Paris, France to be chaired by George. I was a National Trustee then
and recall some concerns that the meeting would be an unneeded burden on Foundation finances. At the time, I gave a $100 contribution to the newly formed Inter-
national Cystic Fibrosis [Mucoviscidosis] Association and received receipt number
10 from George. The term "Mucoviscidosis" was included in the name to accommodate France and French speaking Switzerland. Later the name was shortened to
The International Cystic Fibrosis [M] Association and later abbreviated to
ICF[M]A.

At the 1964 meeting, it was decided that the Association's purpose would
best be accomplished by limiting membership to one National Association for each
member country. The organization's purpose was defined as "fostering development
of CF associations in countries where they did not exist." Provision was also made
for the election of individuals as associate members, without vote, who would represent their countries until such time as a national association was formed, properly
organized, and accepted by the ICF[M]A to represent their country. The
ICF[M]A was registered as a charity in the State of Delaware after the first formal
meeting at Paris, France in 1965. Representatives of fourteen nations attended.
They then elected George Barrie President. A Scientific/Medical Advisory Council
was created with membership limited to one member nominated from each
National Association to represent their country's professionals at major International Conferences that were expected to be held every three to four years. From the

To obtain a book with details and pictures beyond the scope of this chapter, contact
Mr. McCreery at 3190 Roundwood Road, Cleveland, Ohio 44022

professional group, a member was to be elected Chairman to represent their ICF[M]A interests during the years between major conferences.

The 1966 meeting was held in Berne, Switzerland followed by Toronto in 1967, and Cambridge, England in 1969. During the 1969 meeting, the European professionals organized themselves as "The European Working Group" to hold annual meetings similar to the successful US "CF Club" arrangement. The 1970 Stockholm, Sweden and 1971 Vienna, Austria ICF[M]A meetings provided increased CF interest. George Barrie chose to retire in 1970 and Canada's Lyle Blackwell became ICF[M]A President. Lyle was a former Canadian CF Foundation President and well suited for the position. With Lyle's encouragement, I attended the ICF[M]A 1972 meeting at Hotel Schloss Reinhartshausen, Erbach Reingau, German Federal Republic. About sixty doctors and parents attended from Europe, supplemented by a few US doctors and one from Australia who later arranged an invitation for me to visit CF organizations in Australia and New Zealand. The German meeting provided helpful contacts and the interest of many to attend the planned 1973 Washington D.C. International Congress.

Medical and scientific programs presented at the 1973 Congress generated World wide news coverage bringing CF recognition far beyond earlier awareness. The NIH and US Congress directed expanded interest by adding budgeted funds for CF research and devoted time for special efforts as we visited their Bethesda, Maryland offices. The 1974 Verona, Italy and 1975 Dublin, Ireland meetings increased friendships within and beyond the people of the host Nations, as all involved became more understanding of the International Association's potential contributions.

Frank Deford, sports writer, CF Board member, and later Board Chairman, provided considerable help as Aetna Life Insurance Company hosted the 1975 World Championship of Tennis in Hartford, Connecticut between Australian and American members of the Association of Tennis Professionals. Boston Globe's sport writer, Bud Collins, introduced me to speak on behalf of the Connecticut CF poster child. Later, plaques were awarded to tennis greats Stan Smith and Arthur Ashe, and John Filer, Aetna's President. My acquaintance with both Stan and Arthur increased, as they each devoted time to CF. Stan visited our home when near Cleveland where our laundry equipment cleaned his clothes for the next competition. Later Stan's wife Margie became a National CF Foundation Trustee. Arthur Ashe announced The Association of Tennis Professionals adoption of CF as the ATP charity during a recognition dinner held at the Dallas Fairmont Hotel in September 1975. No one told me a tux was proper dress for speakers and I arrived in Dallas from California shortly before dinner without a tux and found rental shops closed. Someone suggested the hotel had several waiter tuxedos that might be used. The only one available was made from scratchy cloth and was small in the shoulders with oversized pants. None the less, my speech was well received and further cemented my friendship with Arthur Ashe and the ATP executive director, Bob Briner. That relationship later enabled me to arrange for Arthur to take time from the Paris Grand Prix of Tennis at Roland Garros to speak before the 1976 French hosted International CF Conference.

At the 1976 International Cystic Fibrosis [M] Association meeting in Paris, I was elected President for the next four years. The organization had most modest funding. My first efforts were to solicit US friends who graciously responded, joining with Frankie and me, to fund expanded ICF[M]A activities. By using my McCreery Corporation office facilities, administration costs were zero. I wrote member Nation organizations, international friends, and possible new members several news letters each year and distributed CF related information collected from the US Foundation and the NIH.

The 1977 meeting in Dresden behind the "Iron Curtain" was a remembered experience. Frankie originally planned to attend and fortunately decided against the trip. East-West political differences required flying to Frankfort in the West German Federal Republic, then change to a small plane and fly the narrow corridor between the Russian and Western sections to Berlin. Once in Berlin, the challenge was at "Check Point Charlie," crossing into East Berlin and taking a train to Dresden, German Democratic Republic. The challenge was posed by the mass of people, military authority, and travel confusion and was considerable. As I passed through the maze, Dr. Harry Shwachman was observed being retained by police for purchasing East German money at a discount in The German Federal Republic before entering Check Point Charlie. He later commented on the substantial fine levied before being released for travel on to Dresden.

During visits with the Association of Tennis Professionals Executive Director, Bob Briner, we agreed to explore how the ATP and ICF[M]A could profit by joint participation at International tennis matches. Although both France and England were considered for the first effort, the French Grand Prix of Tennis at Roland Garros offered several advantages. By then, I was International CF President and a close friend of Jean Louis Gillerion, President of The Swiss Bank, France, and the French CF Association President. Together we made multiple visits to the French Tennis Association under Roland Garros' leadership. After each trip, I informed Bob of our progress. The combined efforts were successful in 1978 with the first day receipts of the Paris tennis Grand Prix divided equally between The French CF Association and the French Cancer Society. During the next few years, I appeared at the matches as the fund raising expanded. At a later meeting, the French CF Association President, Michael Favier said, "Thank God for Bob McCreery."

I tried to interest Ron Tucker, the United Kingdom CF Trust Director, and the Italian CF organization to participate in events similar to the French success. Italian CF loyalties were divided between a Milan group and those from Rome and areas near the Adriatic Sea north of Venice and I was unable to generate Italian CF interest from the groups for multiple reasons. The Wimbledon tennis matches follow the Grand Prix and seemed a logical fund raising opportunity. Ron promoted the possibility to his trustees and ultimately obtained approval to approach Wimbledon with a plan similar to the French success. The request was rejected by Wimbledon but continued pressure on the English to take advantage of the ATP contacts finally resulted in their holding a Champagne Buffet Party at London's

Gloucester Hotel where Frankie helped greet Arthur Ashe, Stan Smith, Billie Jean King, Jimmy Connors, and other 1978 Wimbledon players.

In London in January 1979, I represented the ICF[M]A at a Mozart Birthday Concert at the Queen Elizabeth Hall with H.R.H. Princess Alexandra and her husband Hon. Angus Ogilvy as Patrons. Angus was ill and did not attend. At dinner following the concert, I was honored to fill his place and join the Princess at a table for two where we enjoyed friendly conversations that she recalled at sub- sequent meetings we attended for the United Kingdom CF Trust.

Dr. Omar Pivetta organized a group of Argentina CF parents after return- ing home from genetics training at Maine's Jackson Laboratories. Omar attended the Washington Conference and the 1979 European Working Group meeting in Noordwijkerhout, Holland where he invited me to visit South America and view their CF needs. After the Holland meeting, I accepted his invitation. Omar arranged for us to meet the CF medical communities in Rio de Janiero, Brazil; Montevideo, Uruguay; Cordoba, Argentina; and his home city of Buenos Aires.

The needs were apparent with the most obvious being organization for coordinated efforts by both lay and professional persons. There were many appeals to acquire pancreatic digestive enzymes that were difficult to obtain and expensive. Omar hoped to organize a South American CF conference if funding could be obtained. After returning home, I visited the Johnson and Johnson Company offices near Philadelphia to explain South American needs for their enzyme prod- uct and the funding required for a South American CF meeting. The appeal gener- ated a $25,000 grant with J&J's interest to be tracked by Charles Wingett, who later established Scandipharm. With this funding, augmented by $5,000 from the American CF Foundation and South American local support, the first South American CF Conference was held in Buenos Aires, Argentina in 1981.

My position as ICF[M]A President provided an opportunity to become a non- voting representative at the Geneva, Switzerland headquarters of the World Health Organization. I soon found that specific responsibilities were divided between Western Nations and Eastern Block Countries with Russians staffing the non-infectious disease division, headed by a scientist from Moscow. During my early visits, the WHO slogan "Health For All By Year 2000" was their motto. In an attempt to achieve the goal, efforts were directed toward communicable diseases, water supply, and food, with little regard to the impact on health by genetic dis- eases. After learning all program planning originated in the Director's office, I requested a meeting with the WHO Director to discuss their position on a genetics program at WHO. Later in 1980, a meeting was arranged with Dr. Ch'en Wen- Chien, Assistant Director General of WHO, and Dr. Anver Kuliev, head of the non-communicable disease group. Following that initial meeting, later discussions defined a need for a WHO genetics program with CF being selected as a model disease for the WHO genetics program, for which I received recognition within and beyond WHO.

In 1981, I accepted the Australian CF Association's invitation to meet with their CF groups in Brisbane, Sidney, Melbourne, and Perth. The visit was extended to include several New Zealand cities, including Wellington, where the American Ambassador hosted a reception honoring my visit.

In 1981, I was pleased to be appointed by the President to a four year membership in the National Allergy and Infectious Disease Council of The NIH. The Council consisted of twelve persons headed by Dr. Richard Krause, who was a friend to CF and became a valued friend of mine.

Berne, Switzerland was the host city for the 1981 European Working Group and ICF[M]A meetings. The Norway voting member to the International had contacts in Arab countries sufficient for the ICF[M]A to fund his travel hoping to bring Arab membership into ICF[M]A. Following his Berne report, the effort was abandoned. Later the extent of CF in Arab countries was better defined with modest progress in Saudi Arabia and care provided to Palestinian CF patients by Dr. Daniel Katznelson in Israel.

The Berne 1981 meeting included a passionate appeal from a well educated Belgium lady, Mimi Versele, with obvious signs of advanced CF problems. Mimi said her great wish was for ICF[M]A to create and support an Adult Cystic Fibrosis Association. The initial response was negative with many believing that emotional issues would defuse ICF[M]A objectives. Mimi's most moving presentation provided the momentum to overcome most objections. Her dream of an Adult CF organization became reality the following year when ICF[M]A recognized her objective and an official organization was created by CF adults from 25 countries attending the 1982 Brussels ICF[M]A meeting. The Queen of Belgium attended their first meeting. During the organizing efforts, Mimi became my friend and she called me her "Cystic Fibrosis Father" after her dream became reality. (Figure 20.1) Unfortunately Mimi died later in 1982, but the organization she envisioned, the International Adult Cystic Fibrosis Association (IACFA) continues to grow and serve a valuable purpose in many countries.

In the spring of 1982, I attended a WHO Geneva meeting when more time was spent on East-West politics than health. Later I confronted the non-infectious disease director, Dr. Anver Kuliev, and said, "Your KBG association is known. Let's rise above political differences and serve cystic fibrosis by arranging a meeting of Russian and Eastern Block CF experts with similar outstanding individuals from Western Nations at an agreed location so we can learn from each other." After considerable discussion, he agreed to approach his superiors about my suggestion. The next day I visited the American Mission's CIA offices and explained my proposal. I was told to proceed but keep them informed. After returning home, there were occasional visits from their Cleveland office asking for information but offering no advice. ICF[M]A participants were chosen with the help of Dr. John Mangos and Ron Tucker. The Vienna, Austria offices of the United Nations were chosen for political neutrality and a productive meeting held in the fall of 1983.

The 1984 International CF Congress at Brighton involved multiple UK meetings organized by Ron Tucker that I attended to provide ICF[M]A input.

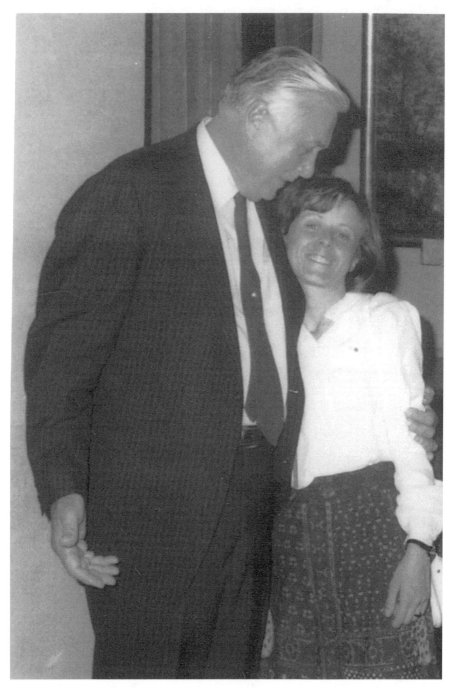

Figure 20.1. *Mimi Versele with ICF[M]A President Robert McCreery in 1981.*
Courtesy of Mr. Robert McCreery.

Fortunately other European CF meetings required being in Europe making it possible to attend most sessions. Related trips included the Irish cities of Cork and Dublin. The French CF Association lead by Jean-Louis Gillerion asked my participation in discussions about their views of ICF[M]A objectives and thoughts on a French scientist being included in the ICF[M]A Medical/Scientific Committee. Those meetings led to Dr. Philip Roussell becoming a valued member.

I first met Dr. Adel Mahmoud when he appeared at NIH on behalf of tropical diseases. He was then Chief of Infectious Disease at University Hospitals of Cleveland and later Chairman of the Department of Medicine. During an evening reception, I introduced him to several NIH and Congressional persons as my friend from Cleveland. Among Adel's interests was schistosomiasis, spread by the waters of Egypt. Questions about American foreign aid programs suggested that a group review problems and potential benefits about funds directed to schistosomiasis control. I was appointed as one of a small group that toured the Egyptian delta areas. My report noted that considerable control could be accomplished by providing free antibiotics to those exposed, coupled with expanded population education. The visit also enabled me to revisit my Cairo home and Egyptian locations that were part of my life when stationed there as an Army officer from 1942 to 1944 before transfer to India Burma China in 1944-1945. I took advantage of being in Egypt to visit the University of Cairo Hospital to explore CF in their country. Dr. Ekram el Salmon attended the Vienna CF meeting as a neutral nation representative. As a Cairo pediatric doctor, she described her CF patient group, noting that the hospital could only provide basic support because of multiple other problem patients brought to her clinic. Frankie and I departed from Egypt to Athens, Greece and a meeting with their CF Association. That very productive meeting was followed by a similar visit in Vienna, Austria and an opportunity to see Vienna in the Christmas season.

The success of the East-West Vienna CF meeting with WHO and Eastern block nations suggested we should extend CF knowledge and opportunity to other areas of the World. Aniver and I were by then friends with common goals. We hoped that other countries could be interested in CF screening of their people and benefits to be gained by detection and treatment. Nicosia, Cyprus was selected as the most neutral meeting location. Our May 1985 meeting included representatives from Egypt, Pakistan, Cyprus, Saudi Arabia, Kuwait, Jordan, USSR, and Japan, with input provided by Greek, UK, Irish, and US doctors.

I had planned for Mrs. Inge Saxon Mills from Rome, Italy to become my successor at the 1986 ICF[M]A Jerusalem Congress; however, because of family health problems, she asked for a one year postponement that resulted in my Presidential responsibilities being extended through 1987.

The second South American CF meeting was held in Bele Horzonte, Brazil in early 1986 in association with a Congress about adult pulmonary problems in the Southern Hemisphere. I selected the ICF[M]A CF participants and arranged funding for their travel with a second grant from Johnson & Johnson through efforts of their representative, Charlie Wingett. Later in 1987, Omar Pivetta's

Argentina group hosted a second CF South American meeting where Inge Saxon Mills was elected ICF[M]A President and my successor. The meeting further emphasized CF needs throughout the Southern Hemisphere countries.

In 1987, I was delighted to accept a three year appointment to the NIH Recombinant DNA Advisory Committee. Each meeting provided depth and insight into gene identification, related problems, and opportunities. It was an exciting group in which to be included as a member.

The 1988 ICF[M]A meeting was held in Budapest during the time that Hungary remained an Iron Curtain country. To travel there, one went to Zurick, Switzerland then squeezed into a canvas slung seat on Hungarian airlines to Budapest. This location enabled Eastern Block persons to participate and profit by interaction with the few that attended from the West. Although Inge Saxon-Mills was then President and had abilities to direct the meeting alone, she asked me to join the effort that she handled with distinction. It was the last ICF[M]A meeting where I had leadership involvement.

After the 1988 Budapest meeting, the continuing US CF Foundation's President Emeritus recognition was my tie to CF until Charlie Wingett, from J&J, asked me to join a new company being formed named Scandipharm, with the intention of focusing on CF pharmaceutical needs. I became a very active Director in the new company with considerable of my efforts directed to opening markets in the US, Europe, and South America. Through a Swiss friend, I learned of the Flutter[R] valve and visited the producer, John Bischofbergher, at their office near Geneva, Switzerland. With my help, Scandipharm later purchased the company and introduced this device that CF patients, by themselves, can use in clearing mucus from their lungs.

I invited talented professional friends to create Scandipharm's Medical/ Scientific Advisory Committee. We then individually or collectively participated in National and International CF meetings that included attendees from Uruguay, Ireland, Brazil, Costa Rica, France, Spain, Denmark, Canada, Sweden, United Kingdom, Belgium, Germany (united as one Country), Switzerland, Italy, Greece, Australia, Turkey, Israel, Mexico, Austria, Saudi Arabia, Venezuela, Japan, India, and perhaps others not listed. Our collective Scandipharm efforts were a major contributor to expanding knowledge of CF to individuals and governments in many countries. My earlier CF roles enabled me to visit friends and contacts that then provided many opportunities for Scandipharm. More importantly the total effort enlarged CF awareness and provided products fairly priced for the daily needs of CF individuals. When Axcan, a Canadian company, acquired Scandipharm in 1999, this ended my CF activities except for the honor of being a US Cystic Fibrosis Foundation Emeritus President.

21

The International Association of Cystic Fibrosis Adults

Barbara L. Palys

The Idea

In 1980, Mimi Versele, a young Belgium woman, accompanied her physician to a conference dedicated to cystic fibrosis (CF). Mimi had CF. She was intensely curious to know more about the disease, and perhaps, more importantly, how to cope with and manage this chronic illness. At the conference, Mimi was impressed by the knowledge shared, the thought provoking exchange of information, and the willingness of the medical participants to share their experiences in treating CF patients. Mimi thought that this type of support venue would be perfect for adults with CF and would help and encourage them to deal with the myriad of problems encountered in battling CF. Her desire was a simple one and she began working towards making her dream come true.

The International Joint Meeting on Pediatric Subspecialties in Berne, Switzerland in 1981 included the annual meeting of the European Working Group for CF, now known as the European Society for Cystic Fibrosis (ESCF). The ESCF is a group of medical professionals from various countries who had joined together and were dedicated to treating CF. A contingent of adults with CF was present at this meeting. This marked the first occasion of a medical/scientific conference open to participants who had the disease—an important milestone in CF history. Maja Smits of the Netherlands, Heidi Karlen and Adrian Sprenger from Switzerland joined Mimi Versele of Belgium. Others joining this group of pioneer adults with CF were Ambrose Kelly of South Africa and, later, Germany (a missionary) and Dr. Petrign Tondury and Dr. Anna Ruedeberg of Switzerland.

It was at this conference that the idea of an association representing adults with CF was born. The initial premise of the group was to focus on the adult patient as a separate and distinct entity apart from the pediatric patient. This was at a time when the median age of survival was hovering in the early teens; however, there were more people with CF surviving into adulthood. Additionally, a support network and forum for education was needed to help these "first survivors into adulthood."

In 1982, the International Association of Cystic Fibrosis Adults (IACFA) was well into its birth pangs. Jean Rudolph Christ of Switzerland, a CF parent, helped the fledging association with incorporation as a recognized non-profit charity and assisted in establishing a bank account. The IACFA came to be befriended by many people like him, willing to offer a helping hand.

Later, the Christ's daughter, Sonia, became treasurer for IACFA and Mrs. Christ (Margarethe) was the bookkeeper for the organization. Thus in 1983, the IACFA was formally born as an association registered in Zurich, Switzerland. Alas, Mimi Versele, the founder, whose idea and energies brought the IACFA into existence was claimed by CF and died. The Belgian CF Association awarded the Versele family a monetary award for Mimi's efforts in the local and international CF community and her family generously donated the value of this award to the fledging IACFA.

The Organization

Early on, two important decisions were made. One was to keep the organizational charter simple to provide opportunity for the organization to grow and expand as needed, and the other was to try to be truly representative of all adults with CF worldwide, with provisions for interaction and participation within the organization. An Executive Committee (EC) was established consisting of 15 positions that included the offices of Chairperson, Vice Chairperson, Secretary, and Treasurer. As only adults with CF could become members of the EC, a realistic guideline of appointing two members per office was instituted, realizing (or recognizing) that compromised health would always be a limiting factor that would affect the association. In addition to the EC, a medical/scientific advisory board was established by invitation of the EC. The EC itself was elected at an annual general meeting of voting members consisting of two representatives from each country. To be a voting member one had to be over the age of eighteen and have CF. It was left to individuals coming from each country to select their two voting representatives. These individuals did not have to represent their home country CF association, thus permitting participation by adults from countries where no organized CF association existed or those disenfranchised by any local organization. An editorial board was later established and appointed by the EC.

The Goals

From the very beginning, the goals of the IACFA were self-evident and set forth in its charter:

> To assist in improving the quality of life by identifying common problems, attempt to define possible solutions, and enhance the exchange of information in the world community of CF adults.

To cooperate, whenever possible, with the larger CF community in defining the new needs arising in the treatment of adults with CF, and raise awareness of the medical profession to the new challenge of treating CF patients who were now adults.

To enable adults with CF to provide unique insights into common problems and potential solutions related to this disorder, which, if recognized internationally, could provide mutual benefit to patients and medical professionals worldwide.

Finally and most importantly, to provide hope for those to come.

It was also recognized that the IACFA would continue to need help to grow and achieve its goals. From the beginning the association had the support of the International Cystic Fibrosis [Mucoviscidosis] Association (ICF[M]A) through its president Robert McCreery (USA). The United Kingdom Cystic Fibrosis Trust and John Edkins, also treasurer for the ICF[M]A, were especially helpful. Peter Kent still serves as an advisor after all these years. The continued support of the Belgian CF Association helped immensely in this formative age. The ICF[M]A, over the years, supported the IACFA with monetary stipends. A wonderful source of endorsement came from the many national associations worldwide by financially supporting their country's adults with CF who were working in the IACFA's Executive Committee. These gifts of financial support helped the IACFA to manage through the formative and difficult first years.

Bringing the Goals to Fruition

As with any organization, it is one matter to have goals and quite another to work towards fulfilling them. To meet the goal of education, sharing experiences, and helping with common problems, a newsletter was established and was simply called the *IACFA Newsletter*.

The first several issues were very much a "home product" typed laboriously on that now extinct instrument called a typewriter. The editor was Heidi Karlen who, by her marvelous personality, was able to coax help for the layout, publishing, and printing. The very first issue is now a collector's copy as only a copy or two remain in existence. The first issue was mailed to approximately 200 readers worldwide. Not only was the *IACFA Newsletter* the first newsletter dedicated to adults with CF, it was also the first—and to date the only—International publication dedicated to CF.

The *IACFA Newsletter* boasts an all-encompassing format ranging from medical and psychosocial articles, to personal experiences, a column entitled 'Sore Spots' where readers wrote of vexing situations, a column called "And the Question Is," National News, Mailbag, and most recently a column on issues related to transplantation, especially lung transplantation. Over the years, debates on emerging issues in CF have been covered in the Newsletter. These included heart/lung transplantation vs. a bilateral lung procedure, living donor transplantation, gene therapy, genetic screening, and cross infection, among others. The newsletter kept pace with changes in the CF community and advocated strongly for adult support and representation within countries, for adult care clinics and practitioners, and adult participation on governing boards of national CF associations. The *IACFA Newsletter* became a quarterly periodical, eventually reaching people in over 69 countries worldwide with a readership in the many thousands.

As it was friendship and sharing at the medical conference that inspired Mimi to create the IACFA, so it is fitting that a conference specifically addressing adult CF issues would be an important venue for the IACFA. The first conference occurred in Brighton, England in 1984. Over 80 adults with CF attended from 14 nations, the farthest from Australia. Ies Fride, who was Chairman of the IACFA for over ten years said in Brighton, "Contacts on an international scale provide a network of information, a wealth of knowledge to be tapped, and broaden the outlook, not only for people with CF but their families, their parents, their friends and the medical profession worldwide." The program for the first conference was very intensive, with sessions on independence, employment, coping with treatments, international contacts, physiotherapy, the relationship between patient and doctor, counseling, relationships with family and friends, sexuality, marriage, and an open forum of questions from participants. These topics represented the important issues adults were struggling with, initially alone, now with help from others. Mimi's dream had indeed come true.

IACFA conferences, held in conjunction with the European CF conferences, have been held biennially with attendance in the hundreds. Additionally, the IACFA has sponsored mini-conferences in numerous countries, including the first ever adult conference in the USA, in Palo Alto, California, in 1995.

Historic Milestones

Although the IACFA had attended an early annual meeting of the ECFS (1981), later discussion within this group of medical professionals focused on whether patients should be permitted to attend the annual European CF Conference. Medical professionals had valid concerns that frank expressions of death and dying would harm CF patients and that the presence of patients might limit this candid but necessary exchange. Also the research presented at these medical conferences had highly technical medical and scientific language that many feared patients would not understand or might misunderstand. While there were other issues, it was these two concerns that dominated the medical discussions.

Finally, at the 1985 conference held in Jerusalem, members of the IACFA and the ESCF engaged in poignant, realistic, and unmitigated discussion. The issue addressed was why patients should be permitted to attend these conferences. It was without doubt the pleas of the IACFA's Chairman and Editor, Ies Fride and John Alaimo that resounded most eloquently. They cited a new era of strong patient advocacy as evidenced by the AIDS movement, the essence of maturity, self-care, and democracy as opposed to alienation, and the ethic of working together. Indeed many adults with CF are medical professionals and researchers. The goals of the IACFA depended on the interchange of ideas at conferences. Quite frankly, the paternalistic era of CF care was coming to an end with the emergence of adult patients who were increasingly able and qualified to represent and advocate for themselves. **It was decided that the European CF Conferences would continue to be open to IACFA participants.** The relationship between the IACFA and the ESCF grew closer over the years and a solid working relationship developed. Without this brave and bold decision from the ESCF, IACFA's struggle would have been much more arduous.

Very much in keeping with the era of the mid-eighties, the IACFA's next historic first happened in Oslo, Norway when the IACFA respectfully asked the ESCF to make their conferences smoke-free. It should be noted that Europe, unlike the USA at this time, had and continues to have a vigorously smoking public. It may seem ironic that medical professionals involved in treating severe lung disease would smoke and even do so around people with CF without taking notice of the effect. We were pleased that this request was honored unanimously and, when announced at the conference, was greeted with clapping and strict adherence.

In 1989, we became aware of the growing concern over cross-infection between patients. About that time there was also the appearance of virulent strain of *Burkholderia cepacia*, a highly resistant bacterium, that spread easily with often severe repercussions for those infected. These issues needed further investigation. Discussion with Dr. Niels Høiby of Denmark, who at the time was a trailblazer on the issue of cross infection and had initiated separate clinics based on bacteria colonization, demonstrated to the IACFA that this was an issue that would have to be addressed in concert with our conferences. **Dr. Anna Ruedeberg and Gerd Doering, both advisors to IACFA, together with the EC drew up a policy of hygiene guidelines designed to restrict cross infection at our conferences. At the same time, conference registration included a request for evidence by bacteriological reports that those attending did neither culture B. cepacia nor the methicillin resistant** *Staphylococcus aureus* **(MRSA).** While it was known and shared that these efforts could not be 100% effective, the IACFA did what it considered morally ethical and responsible to assure an atmosphere of trust at conferences. The IACFA was the first and for a long time the only organization that had such policies. It was only much later that other organizations worldwide adopted the IACFA's policies and hygiene guidelines. Once again, not only did the IACFA introduce a historic first; it also fulfilled the very essence of patient advocacy.

Another historic milestone is that from 1988 to the present, the IACFA has been the first CF patient-based organization to initiate and participate in medical studies. The first such effort, led by Dr. Caesar Romeo of Italy, sought to assess sibling health in CF families as a possible means to better define the then unknown genetic mutation responsible for CF. A subsequent effort focused on parent health assessment and demonstrated that sinusitis was a prevalent symptom in carriers, as confirmed four years later by Dr. Garry Cutting, based on genetic mutations. Other studies included research on the incidence of idiopathic pancreatitis in those with CF and CF carriers, a study on the demographics and epidemiology of those diagnosed late with CF, and a study of patient and family knowledge and perception of gene therapy for CF that was supported by a grant from the US National Institutes of Health. The latter two studies remain ongoing at the time of publication. This series of studies were the first undertaken by an organization composed only of patients with that particular disease, in this case CF. The results were published in peer reviewed journals, such as *The Lancet* and *Pediatric Pulmonology*. The studies were made possible by IACFA's excellent membership database managed for many years by Evelien Alaimo-Grolle, a longtime IACFA advisor and volunteer.

From 1997 to the present, the IACFA assisted with and provided sponsored speakers for parallel conference sessions under the aegis of the World Health Organization (WHO). Additionally, the IACFA participated with and contributed to WHO educational documents including one specific on the care and management of adult patients. **IACFA was the first, and so far only, CF patient organization to work closely with the WHO.**

It has been of especial significance and most gratifying to the membership to observe the personal growth of our Executive Members into positions of responsibility within their homelands. Long time EC members, Mitch Messer and Ami Kolumbus, became presidents of the Western Australian CF Association and the Israeli CF Associations respectively. Recently Mitch and Ami became officers within the ICF[M]A—the first people with CF to hold office in this organization. The IACFA assisted and helped in establishing adult CF organizations in many countries including the USA.

As the Chairperson of IACFA, I was invited to attend and later to become part of the NIH consensus panel on genetic screening for CF. **This participation was the first occasion that IACFA participated in a national effort related to CF.** Later, I became a member of the Massachusetts Genetic Health Program of the Department of Public Health working towards newborn screening for CF. In addition to this Massachusetts activity, the IACFA participated in lobbying for newborn screening in the state of California. As a result of these experiences, I became very interested in and knowledgeable about genetic sciences and have worked on informed consent documents and patient education around genetic issues. In 1998, I chaired a session on ethics in genetic science and biotechnology at a conference on gene therapy in Paris, France. It was largely through this effort that the IACFA was awarded the NIH grant to study gene therapy in the CF community.

Professional Relationships

No man is an island and this holds true for organizations as well. The IACFA prospered and gained members with the help of many special relationships. Primary of these was from the International Cystic Fibrosis [Mucoviscidosis] Association. The first help came with the support of the first president, Robert McCreery, and then with special encouragement from presidents Martin Weibel of Switzerland and

Herman Weggen of the Netherlands. Dr. Robert Williamson, a geneticist then at the Brompton Hospital, was always a ready speaker and effective advisor in the early development of the Association. He was most helpful in educating us on genetic issues and developments. Dr. Dieter Gruenert has served us well as the advisor in the genetic area for the past five years along with advisor Dr. Albert Lowenfels. Dr. Robert C. Stern has been a supportive and knowledgeable behind the scene advisor for many years.

Members of the European Society for Cystic Fibrosis, formerly the European Working Group for CF, have been instrumental in helping the IACFA with medical education and advice. Most importantly, the ESCF opened the doors of their conferences to people with CF. Cystic Fibrosis Research, Inc. (CFRI) of Palo Alto, California, was the first USA based organization to invite the IACFA to hold a conference in the USA. Ann Robinson, past director of CFRI, so enjoyed the IACFA conferences that CFRI went on to organize many other adult and family based conferences. No organization could exist without substantial funding and the Pennsylvania Area Cystic Fibrosis, Inc. (PACFI) and the Cystic Fibrosis Foundation (USA) are generous with their support of IACFA educational efforts.

The Special People of the IACFA

Organizations could not exist or function without the hard work, dedication and cognizance of volunteers. The IACFA has been specially blessed from its conception through the efforts of the founder and first Chairperson, Mimi Versele. Sally Wrigley, who unfortunately died during her first year as president, followed Mimi. The continued growth of the IACFA was assured by the hard work of its third Chairman, Ies Fride of The Netherlands. Ies was there in the beginning, an ardent supporter of Mimi's dream. He continued with leadership in the IACFA during wonderful and stressful periods, managing the growing organization, drawing new volunteers, using well honed diplomatic skills during some intense discussions and policy changes. Ies drew from his love of history and democracy to guide IACFA's development. Filling Ies' big footsteps would not be easy. Ies and I had worked closely together for many years with me as his vice chairperson and we even shared the same birth date. In 1991, I was elected Chairperson of the IACFA, a role I continue to fulfill to this day. I also served for five years as associate editor of the newsletter, becoming editor in 1989, and continue in that role. Not busy enough as Chairperson and editor, I have been IACFA's primary fund-raiser for over ten years.

While Heidi Karlen did a superb job starting the IACFA Newsletter, it was John Alaimo, an American living in Amsterdam, who polished, refined, and made the newsletter into one of professional excellence admired worldwide. The newsletter was actually an Alaimo family affair with husband and wife sharing in the physical work and supporting each other. It should be noted that many of these pioneers in the IACFA personally bought and paid for IACFA equipment, and paid their own travel costs to meetings and conferences. John's experience in the

USA, with its harsh medical insurance situation and disability programs, convinced him that to be considered humanitarian, the USA needs to provide free or low cost health care and support service for people with CF. Moving to The Netherlands with his Dutch wife in order to take benefit from their more realistic and supportive health care measures, John began a diary within the newsletter called "Hospital Corridors." John's earlier volunteer service with Native Americans on reservations honed his focus on those most in need of help. His newsletter years focused heavily on psychosocial articles with a searing, and at times, painful look at the hardship of CF. Eve Alaimo, John's wife managed the IACFA database, a meticulous job needing perseverance and attention to detail with much patience and she continues with this important support activity. Upon John's death, his associate editor, Ann Wren of the UK became editor and I was associate editor.

Perhaps most known for his age – he was and is the oldest IACFA EC member – Ami Kolumbus was also the first EC member to have a family to raise. His experiences brought issues of marriage, sexuality and parenting as a focus of IACFA conferences and articles. At that time, there was little or no focus on these areas within national CF associations or CF clinics. A shared experience with adoption led to articles focusing on this means of becoming parents despite CF. Later, at the IACFA conference in Dublin, Ireland, the IACFA was the first to present a speaker on the then new procedure which provided a means to retrieve viable sperm behind blocked or deformed vas deferens in males with CF. The speaker, Dr. Birgitta Strandvik of Sweden, demonstrated the procedure with vivid color slides. Soon the conference organizers became very much aware that over 65% of the men with CF in the audience had not previously known that they were sterile! The largest assembly of social workers and psychologists were quickly brought together for emergency psychotherapy and support! Ami has always been an example of longevity (currently approaching 60) and positive reinforcement for parenting and fatherhood. Also Ami is the president of the Israeli CF Association and treasurer for the ICF[M]A.

The first person involved with IACFA from both sides of the fence—medical and lay—was Dr. Paul Quinton, the noted biochemist/physiologist who solved the basic defect inherent in CF with elaboration on chloride ion channeling. Paul, nearly as old as Ami, had sat in at a few of the very first IACFA meetings in the early 1980s. Later, Paul was asked and agreed to become a scientific advisor for the IACFA. Over the years, he helped our writers and editors understand the often-complex science associated with CF. Having CF himself, Paul was an excellent example of what people with CF can—and have—achieved. Paul's insight to living and managing with CF was shared at numerous IACFA conferences. His laid-back Texas charm made him very approachable and a favorite speaker. Later we were pleased to have Beatrix Redemann, MD join the EC and share her experiences as a medical doctor, patient, and parent.

The complex planning and detail work that goes into organizing a conference can never be appreciated until tried. Longtime Secretary for the IACFA, Elizabeth (Lisa) Hoyer of Austria, somehow managed to balance the chore of conference organizing and secretarial work. Years of conference organizing experience permitted Lisa to write a "how to organize a conference successfully" guide that still serves the IACFA well. People with CF have special considerations to travel and participate at a conference. Concerns range from oxygen and nebulizer supplies, daily physiotherapy and physiotherapists, a high calorie and generous food supply, clean (fungus and mold free) bathrooms, available emergency care, wheelchair and oxygen canister accessibility, and finally a program that permits time for health care needs and especially for relaxation time. When Dublin was suggested as a conference venue, to accommodate the financial hardship many people with CF endure, dormitory rooms at Trinity College were offered. Lisa traveled to Dublin to inspect the premises and declined the offer after viewing the shared and moldy bathrooms (cross infection), stairs, and lack of refrigeration for Pulmozyme® and insulin supplies. Over the years, Lisa would travel to many of IACFA's venue sites and local organizers shuddered with nervous anticipation of her visits. Lisa retired a few years ago, but not completely (like so many IACFA volunteers), and remains an auditor for the organization.

One of the most difficult tasks for the IACFA is recruiting medical professionals to volunteer for our Advisory Council. One of the first volunteers present when the IACFA was just a concept was Dr. Anna Ruedeberg of Switzerland. Over the years, Anna has helped the organization in so many different ways. At conferences, she is always available should someone become ill. For the newsletter, she proofed articles for medical accuracy, the hygiene guidelines, and patient information questionnaire. She provided oversight of conference registration (for accurate testing to detect *B. cepacia*) and many other medical details for our conferences fell to Anna. She transcended the role of doctor and became a friend to all, a wise counselor, an adept moderator, and a wonderful woman. The IACFA was not the only organization to reap the benefits of Anna's energy. When visiting or dining at the Ruedeberg household, one found the phone was always ringing for Anna and it wasn't uncommon to have her dash out somewhere because she was needed. How she managed all her volunteer efforts, her CF patients, her spina bifida patients and clinic, and her family remains a mystery.

Evelien Alaimo-Grolle has been mentioned previously, however she deserves more. When her husband John volunteered for IACFA participation, it was Eve who financially covered his travel costs, bought the computer needed for the newsletter, and was the sole support of the family. With her social work background, Eve often led workshops or moderated sessions at conferences. The EC quickly realized that Eve's acerbic jokes and comments put a touch of reality on issues being discussed. After John died, Eve continued with IACFA activities. Her management of the newsletter database permitted many of the studies the IACFA has carried out. As with Anna and all of our treasured advisors, Eve was a trusted friend to many. Often organizing EC meetings in Amsterdam, she would open her home to those who couldn't afford the cost of a hotel room. Most importantly, it is Eve who gave a Dutch home to Cream, a Burmese cat from the USA, that then became the IACFA mascot because of its international background!

Conclusion

The hardest part of volunteering for an organization like the IACFA is in dealing with the loss of friends and colleagues to CF. Over the years, there have been too many losses. Death, dying, and grief are issues touched upon at every conference. The reality of the loss of loved ones makes it all the harder for us to cope. Sally Wrigley, Ann Wren, Christophe Comte, Agnes Le Bar, Ies Fride, and Janeth Sperry contributed so much to the IACFA, often working when seriously ill. Each person lived life fully and shared so much with the world through the IACFA.

John, my husband of 20 years and an MIT graduate in physics and astronomy, has been a pillar of support, including financial. He has written the summaries of the European and USA CF Conferences for the newsletter for years, along with extensive behind the scenes support. The IACFA and I cannot praise him enough for the supportive person he has always been.

Has IACFA accomplished its goals? We inspired and helped start adult organizations around the world, the *IACFA Newsletter* is widely read and the most respected lay journal in the CF community, and our international conferences give so much to participants. We did not run from difficult decisions surrounding cross infection. Our advocacy for adults created adult clinics and transitioning programs worldwide. With the help of IACFA's Secretary, Francesco Antognini from Lugano, Switzerland, we have ventured into cyberspace with our own web site. Everything accomplished was unselfishly done by those who came first for those yet to come. In giving, our association has received so much in return.

There will be new goals, especially in third world countries. More advocacy for those with CF to make life a little easier and better. We will continue to make our contributions in the field of research. We will focus on CF geriatric care and hold workshops for grandparents with CF. The IACFA is the future.

How Well Have We Done?

Center Directors Remember

22

Center Directors Remember: Seattle

Jack M. Docter, M.D.

I first heard of cystic fibrosis (CF) in 1938, when, as a second year medical student at Columbia University, I was privileged to hear Dr. Dorothy Andersen present her description of this new disease. She had published a classic paper, "Fibrocystic Disease of the Pancreas and its Relation to Celiac Disease," which described a new syndrome of abnormal bowel movements, malnutrition, and pulmonary disease with scarring (fibrosis). It was my further privilege to hear her discuss this disease many times during the next two years, and it made a lasting impression. I graduated from medical school in 1941 and returned to Seattle for a two year internship at Harborview Hospital.

When war began, I was assigned to Carlyle Barracks in Pennsylvania, but before going there I had sustained a back injury while playing handball. X-rays revealed previously undetected, but significant, problems. These included a congenital problem called spina bifida occulta, other vertebral anomalies, and a herniated disk. I was decommissioned and relieved of my Army assignment and the orthopedic recommendation was for surgery. The superintendent of Harborview then asked me to stay on as Chief Medical resident as twelve of his twenty four house officers were going into the service. He further offered the surgery (disk decompression and spinal fusion) without hospital charges and I accepted the offer.

The Chief Surgery Resident and I alternated night call every other night with the help of the remaining house officers from June 1941 to June 1942. We also did all post mortem examinations of which there were many. As Harborview was a county hospital, the patient population was largely indigent senior citizens. This experience led me to go into Pediatrics and not have to deal any more with senility (my apparent condition at this time). Then surgery, recuperation, and complete recovery took until the summer of 1943.

I became a pediatric resident at Children's Memorial Hospital in Chicago and again was exposed to CF in 1944 and 1945. I spent many hours assisting my colleagues in passing tubes through the nose and into the duodenum (first part of the small intestine) to collect pancreatic secretions for analysis. This was the only known method of diagnosis at that time. I well remember the technique in vogue for getting the tube into the duodenum with a piano wire in the lumen of the tube and direct passage under fluoroscopy. Then the metal tip was guided through the pylorus by a magnet, again with fluoroscopy. The other very time consuming method was to feed the tube into the stomach and wait, for as long as it took, to pass by normal peristaltic action into the duodenum. CF was still considered rare and diagnosed only if the full-blown clinical picture was clear. In the 1950s, the sweat electrolyte defect was discovered and the sweat test established. Subsequently, as a private practitioner, I helped to stuff many a child into a plastic bag to make enough sweat for a sufficient sweat sample.

In January 1947, I took my first airplane ride to return to Seattle, three stops in all, and started in the private practice of pediatrics, sharing office space with an obstetrician. Then in April, I was invited to join two pediatricians as they returned from the service. We were associated for thirteen years, during which time I had joined the staff of Children's Orthopedic Hospital (COH) and been assigned to supervise a ward. COH was a charity hospital with no physicians employed and no resident staff at the hospital. There were about fifty beds and the attending staff had permission to bring private patients there for hospitalization. They were obligated to care for the "house" patients and to run clinics for $5 per clinic. Most refused the stipend. There was no laboratory, and no pathologist or radiologist on staff but the latter came by weekly to read films.

During my years in pediatric practice, I had a few patients with what some still called "fibrocystic disease of the pancreas," and showed enough interest in these patients that my colleagues were overjoyed and began to refer their patients with chronic cough, diarrhea, growth failure, and debilitation to me. There were, in time, enough of these children diagnosed with CF that the families decided to organize to give one another support. They asked me to be their medical advisor. The more I read and the more I observed, I realized that CF was not rare, but was a common, chronic pediatric problem. Diagnosis was made relatively often in my practice, those of my associates, and in various clinics at COH. The clinic began in 1958 and was scheduled once a week on my afternoon off. Gradually, potential CF patients from other clinics were seen and as many as fifteen patients were scheduled each week. Over the next four years, we saw well over one hundred. Soon we were seeing referrals from Alaska, Idaho, Montana, Oregon, and all over the state of Washington, who had, or were suspected of having, the disease.

During these years, other changes were being made at our hospital and a full time pathologist and radiologist were hired. Meanwhile, the all woman board of directors undertook a successful campaign for a new hospital with 125 beds. A medical staff was part of the program, as was employment of a fulltime Medical Director, the volunteer Chief of Staff having persuaded the women that the position had grown beyond the scope of a part time volunteer private practitioner. The new hospital was near the University of Washington campus. I was asked to fill the post of Medical Director. While this required giving up my 13 year private practice, it allowed me to continue the CF program and clinic, a post not sought by others at that time, when the prognosis was so discouraging.

In 1961, Dr. Kenneth Landauer, Medical Director of the National Cystic Fibrosis Research Foundation in New York (the name was later shortened by dropping "research"), called to ask for a site visit of our facility and program. He was also interested in a day of fishing on the Olympic Peninsula. I recruited Dave Shurtleff, a birth defects specialist and fisherman extraordinaire. We met Dr. Landauer's plane rather later than expected and drove to Lake Quinault on the Olympic Peninsula, where reservations had been made. Unable to raise staff at that late hour, we entered unoccupied ground floor rooms by way of an open window, slept for what was left of the night, and took off early with our native American guide. My mental picture of Ken is that of a bare-chested, enthusiastic fisherman, rod in one hand and beer bottle in the other in the bow of the Evinrude-driven boat having the time of his life on the lake.

The following week our CF clinic was invited to join the national organization. Our clinic became a Regional Care, Teaching, and Research Center of the NCFRF with an annual grant of $20,000. Because it was already functioning and serving the needs of the community as a clinic, we decided to use the grant money to study and research the heart and lung complications of the disease, the complications that were killing these patients. To carry on the work, Dr. Stanley Stamm gave up his flourishing pediatric practice to don the white coat of clinical investigator and he served with me in the clinic as well as carrying on the research activities of the new laboratory.

Soon thereafter, I joined the Center Committee of the NCFRF. This position gave me a better understanding of the operation and activity nationwide in the field. Fortunately, my employers were aware of the importance of the CF program and encouraged my participation as a member of the Center Committee of the National organization, then headquartered in New York City. I remember visiting many of the Centers around the country and learning from the experience each time. At a visit to the Children's Hospital in Pittsburgh, I was asked to address their Grand Rounds on the topic of meconium ileus, the complication that some CF newborns present with in the first day or so of life. I had recently seen a newborn from Alaska with a meconium filled peritoneal area as shown by abdominal x-ray. In my presentation, I made the statement that nearly all meconium ileus patients had CF. Their pediatric radiologist leapt to his feet to challenge the statement, adding that I did not know what I was talking about.

I also recall visits to Will Waring in New Orleans, Warren Warwick in Minneapolis, Alex Spock in Durham, and Nancy Huang in Philadelphia. The next best thing to visiting the Centers was having other committee members visit Seattle.

One of the more memorable of my assignments occurred in July of 1971 when I was asked to address the Appropriations Committee sub-committee on Labor, Health, Education and Welfare of the US Senate. I, of course, assumed that I had been chosen by the NCFRF because of my charm and stage presence, but it soon became apparent that the real reason was that the committee was chaired by Senator Warren Magnuson of the State of Washington, an acquaintance, and a good friend of COH. I concluded my remarks with a request for funding of the National Institute for Arthritis and Metabolic Diseases, which at that time included CF in its program, in the amount of $153,000,000. I have no record of the response to this request, but do recall that, in an unrelated request at about the same time, the COH received a $500,000 grant from that committee for a renovation and remodeling project.

These memories cover a 24 year period, 10 of which I was on the Center Committee and for 3 of those, I served as Chairman of the Committee. As Dr. Stamm had returned full time to Pediatric Cardiology and my own personal retirement loomed, I became more and more concerned about the future of our clinic, Center, and CF program. Happily, a young Fellow in Ambulatory Care started attending the clinic. She was working with Dr. Arnold Smith, an inspirational leader in Infectious Disease, who was interested in the organisms involved in diseases of the lung that affected patients with CF. She also knew that her parents and I had been friends growing up in Seattle in the 1930s and 40s. Whatever the influences, she agreed to take over and carry on the clinic and program. I could not have found a more able successor. As the years pass, I realize increasingly that, by far, my greatest contribution to the NCFRF and the CF cause was the recruitment of Dr. Bonnie Watt Ramsey. Watching her career develop and observing her contributions to the field are two of the great satisfactions of my retirement.

23

Center Directors Remember: New Orleans

William W. Waring, M.D.

In 1947 during my senior year at Harvard Medical School, I was invited to join the Boylston Society. Each of its student members had to present a paper to our fellows and guest faculty. After some thinking, I decided to write a paper on "pancreatic fibrosis" (as CF was called at that time in Boston) because of an on-going conflict between Harvard and Columbia about the nature of the disease. The landmark article on "cystic fibrosis of the pancreas" by Dorothy Andersen, a pathologist at Columbia, had appeared in December 1938,[1] and the disease had become a source of controversy between the New York and Boston schools.

Dr. Andersen thought that the pulmonary manifestations were related to a deficiency of the fat-soluble vitamin A, which in turn was produced by a deficiency of the pancreatic enzyme, lipase. She considered that Vitamin A deficiency in turn produced the observed abnormal changes seen in the bronchial epithelium called "squamous metaplasia", which decreased mucociliary clearance from the tracheo-bronchial tree, resulting in retained mucus secretions, promoting stasis and infection, and leading to progressive bronchiectasis (airway damage), respiratory failure, and death. However, Harvard's Dr. Sidney Farber, a respected pediatric pathologist at Children's Hospital, held that the disease was a systemic one that affected all the mucus-secreting glands of the body. It was Sidney Farber who in 1944 coined the term Mucoviscidosis for the disease—a designation still commonly employed in Europe. We now know, more than fifty years later, that Dr. Farber was closer to the truth than Dr. Andersen.

To prepare my Boylston Society paper for its reading on February 26, 1947, I was able to review in detail the world's literature on CF. My review also included reports of patients who in retrospect had CF but remained undiagnosed in the pre-Andersen era. I tried unsuccessfully to fuse the New York and Boston schools of thought. A quotation to these efforts follows from my unpublished paper:

> It is therefore suggested, with some trepidation, that alteration in the character of glandular secretions throughout the body may be an even earlier sign of vitamin A deficiency than squamous cell metaplasia. Such a theory correlates well the observations of both Farber and Andersen. It retains the integrity of the conception of a systemic disease; it accounts for the satisfactory response of the pul-

monary changes to dietary therapy, and it attempts to explain the familial incidence on an inherited anomaly of vitamin A metabolism. Further theorizing without reasonable experimental studies approaches the disastrous.

I had gotten to know Dr. Harry Shwachman at Children's Hospital where he took care of the CF patients. He graciously consented to come to the presentation of my paper, and afterwards he commented on it kindly. He was forever my friend, and from that time CF was "my" disease—the one that I knew more about than any other.

After graduating from medical school, I began an internship in pediatrics at Children's Hospital, just across the street from the medical school, and thus had some opportunity to get to know Dr. Shwachman. Unfortunately my assignments never allowed me to see CF patients along with him and his associate, Dr. Kon-Taik Khaw. At that time children with CF were coming to Boston from all parts of the world just to see Harry Shwachman. I have always felt that the hospital administration failed to support or even acknowledge his pioneering work. The hospital had other luminaries to tout—Sidney Farber himself, now less interested in "mucoviscidosis," was treating leukemia with strange drugs called Am-Fol A and Met-Fol B. In their discussion of their choices of the eleven most important developments in medicine during the past 1000 years, the editors of the *New England Journal of Medicine*[2] cite "molecular pharmacotherapy" as the eleventh. They noted that, "It is hard to believe that 1999 marked the 50th anniversary of the introduction of methotrexate for the treatment of childhood leukemia by Sidney Farber and his group at Children's Hospital in Boston." In 1947 Dr. Farber had a leukemia ward at Children's Hospital to which I was assigned for a stultifying month. During that month I did essentially nothing but refine my venipuncture skills by starting and restarting IVs on scores of leukemic children with few veins and fewer platelets.

At the end of the year, our intern group was ejected en masse from Children's to make room for former house officers who were returning from war to complete their pediatric training. I was accepted at the Harriet Lane Home, the children's hospital of Johns Hopkins, where I remained for four years. Since none of the faculty there was particularly interested in CF and the non-private part of Harriet Lane was traditionally a housestaff run facility, the way opened for me to see and care directly for patients with CF. In today's era of iontophoresis sweat tests and refined gene typing, it is hard to believe that the major diagnostic test then for suspected CF was semiquantitative analysis of duodenal secretions obtained by duodenal intubation. The first edition of the Harriet Lane Handbook, written entirely by the house staff and published in 1952 during my last year when I was the chief resident, describes on page 41 the technique for "semiquantitative analysis of duodenal juice for activity of pancreatic trypsin." The second edition of 1955 describes the technique of duodenal intubation. It cannot be overstated that everything involved in the procedure was done by the house officer, including fluoroscopy and fluid analysis. I quote from the Handbook, page 43, on duodenal intubation:

Restrain patient securely and pass lubricated tube into stomach through nostril. Under fluoroscopic control, place tip of tube at pylorus. Tube can occasionally be passed directly into duodenum; usually it is necessary to place patient on his right side and wait for gastric activity to carry tube forward. Tube is allowed to drain into an iced container placed below patient, and drainage examined at intervals of about ½ hour. If not in duodenum, tube is advanced half an inch and a small amount of fluid is introduced into stomach. Position of the tube may be checked at intervals with the fluoroscope. Duodenal contents are recognized by an olive green color and an alkaline pH.

Duodenal juice analysis, described on page 41 of the Handbook's first edition, consisted of serial tube dilutions of duodenal secretions (up to 1:3200) to each of which was added 7 1/2% gelatin. Liquefaction of the gelatin after refrigeration overnight indicated tryptic enzyme activity. Liquifaction through dilution 1:400 was considered normal. Liquifaction at 1:50 or less was considered diagnostic of CF or obstruction of the pancreatic duct. Of course, it was not realized at the time that we would be missing perhaps 15% of children with CF who had normal or near normal pancreatic function.

My skills in duodenal intubation have not been called on for at least 48 years due to the brilliant, serendipitous discovery in 1953 of the sweat gland abnormality by Dr. Paul di Sant'Agnese,[3] as a result of a heat wave in New York City. This was followed by the subsequent ingenious application of the pilocarpine iontophoresis sweat test by Drs. Lewis "Pete" Gibson and Robert Cooke, as published in 1959.[4] Both are major landmarks in the history of CF.

After a stint in the Army medical corps during the Korean War and a two-year trial of private pediatric practice, I found myself in January 1958 at Tulane Medical School as a full-time Instructor in the Department of Pediatrics under Dr. Ralph Platou. Pediatric subspecialization was just beginning, and neonatology and cardiology were well established. I decided to specialize in pulmonary diseases of children, which of course included CF. With the help of Dr. Margaret H. D. Smith, the pediatric infectious disease expert in our department, a pediatric chest clinic was set up. Our patients included those with CF among many other lung problems. The clinic met twice weekly with CF patients on one day and all other pulmonary patients on the other.

There were four cramped examining rooms, a room that served as a nurse's station and file room, and a waiting area (literally, because the waits could be for hours) just outside with rock-hard plastic benches. By a special arrangement with the medical school, we were allowed to keep our own records in the clinic. Down the hall was the pulmonary function laboratory with adult and child sized Wright peak flow meters and a fine Warren Collins 9 liter bell spirometer, a wall-mounted barometer that would have pleased Torricelli. There was a booklet of charts that allowed us to convert gas volumes from ATPS (ambient temperature and pressure saturated with water vapor) to BTPS (body temperature and pressure saturated

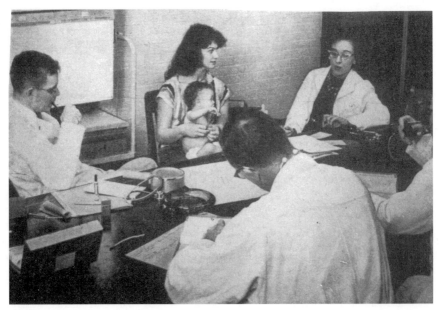

Figure 23.1. *A state of the art CF Clinic conference in the Tulane University pediatric library in 1963. Dr. William Waring, on the left, discreetly smoking a pipe. William R, with CF, in his mother's lap in the middle, and Dr. Bettina Hilman, on the right, with unidentified residents/fellows opposite, one of whom also seems to be smoking. On the table are the usual Wright peak flow meter, stethoscope (not yet a double one), pen to mark x-rays, small card file, tobacco pouch, pipe lighter, used pipe cleaner, and ashtray with ashes. Missing are the Huber lung model and William R's chest x-rays which had been on the view boxes behind. Courtesy of Dr. William Waring.*

with water vapor), an arcane practice that added an element of spurious precision to our testing. With the help of charts of predicted values based on subject height from the excellent text of pulmonary function data by Polgar and Promadhat,[5] we were able to chart the inevitable decline in pulmonary function of our CF population.

For serious prolonged discussions with parents, especially when patients were seen for the first time, we used the departmental library a few doors away from the waiting room. The parents and child were present while the resident or fellow presented the history and physical findings (Figure 23.1). X-rays were viewed and commented on, and these, together with a Huber lung model, were used to show parents what parts of the lungs had been affected. An explanation was made to the parents of the nature of the disease and the severity of its manifestations in this child. The meeting concluded with a specific therapeutic plan and an optimistic (if even faintly possible) prognosis. The process was prolonged and, if there were more than one new patient, the clinic would drag badly. I never learned to speed up such interactions with parents.

As long as the clinic was at the medical school, its operation was low-key. Someone gave me a plastic white pith helmet suitable for safari with the word "CHIEF" written on the front. From time to time I used to wear this while working in the clinic, and I don't recall any questions or expressions of surprise from any of the patients or their parents. It must have been viewed as a part of my uniform. When we moved to the formal atmosphere of the hospital, the pith helmet had to go. I gave it to a fellow, Dr. Jamshed Kanga, who now runs the CF Center in Lexington, Kentucky, where I doubt that he wears it.

Becoming a Center

In 1962, the Foundation in the persons of Drs. Kenneth Landauer and LeRoy Matthews wrote to indicate that the Foundation was interested in establishing a CF Center at Tulane University. I jumped at the chance, if such a Center could represent the two medical schools in New Orleans. Ken Landauer and LeRoy Matthews made a trip to New Orleans, and we had a fine dinner in the Vieux Carré. The upshot was that our Center received its first grant from the Foundation in 1963 and that Dr. Bettina Hilman, not yet in Shreveport, represented Louisiana State University and regularly attended the clinic at Tulane. The grant was for six or seven thousand dollars, as I recall, and it allowed me, for the first time, to have a secretary. In the formation of any kind of Center in the days of manual typewriters and carbon paper, the most important person after the director was (and perhaps still is) the director's secretary.

Shortly after the CF grant award, Bettina and I visited Dr. Gunyon Harrison in Houston to study his care of CF children. These were the days of mist tents, a form of therapy that had been developed and championed by Dr. Matthews and colleagues in Cleveland. Gunyon had had a huge amount of experience with mechanical ventilation for poliomyelitis, had researched nebulizer and compressor equipment, and had developed helpful teaching aids for patients and their parents. In addition, we learned from the skilled respiratory and physical therapists at the Texas Institute for Rehabilitation and Research.

Later, Bettina and I with the assistance of the LSU medical artist, Don Alvarado, developed some excellent teaching aids for chest physical therapy, based on bronchopulmonary anatomy, of which we were very proud. These showed patient positions, areas of the chest to percuss (clap), and for each a superimposed lung model to show which segment of which lobe was being drained. As I recall, sets of these charts were distributed by the CF Foundation to Centers requesting them.

In 1966, Bettina and her husband moved to New York where she worked with Carolyn Denning, the CF Center Director at Babies' Hospital. When she returned two years later to Louisiana to establish her own CF Center at Louisiana State University/Shreveport, she continued to come to New Orleans to see patients and for cooperative research project planning. The association of our two Centers has remained a close one. Her devotion to her patients literally has no equal. For this and for her accomplishments both as a pulmonologist and allergist/immunologist she has received numerous awards and honors, including the creation of Hilman House in Shreveport, a refuge for CF patients and their parents from out of the city or state.

A chronic problem at this time was where to hospitalize CF patients. Tulane Medical School had no hospital of its own. Charity Hospital, across the street, was our inpatient and outpatient teaching institution but accepted only indigent or emergency patients. A solution of sorts was to admit children to the service of one of the Tulane part-time pediatric faculty in a local private hospital. We then served as consultants and essentially managed the inpatient care. The disadvantages of this arrangement are obvious, traveling repeatedly between school and an across town "foreign" institution, and then dealing with strange personnel unused to the sorts of respiratory and physical therapy required by CF patients. Fortunately in 1976 this problem was 0solved by the completion and opening of the Tulane University Hospital across the street from the medical school and connected to it by a bridge. Travel time from my office to the bedside of a patient then became a matter of three or four minutes.

The arrival of the new hospital also spelled the end of the informal clinic and its private charting system, but this was necessary for good care. We now had several examining rooms in the pediatric clinic on the 5th floor, a clinic coordinator, a conference room with 8 x 8 x-ray view boxes on which to set up serial PA and lateral x-rays of our patients. A new lab with modern testing equipment, including a plethysmograph, was established in the hospital respiratory therapy department. The best part was the inpatient facility on the 6th floor with private and semiprivate rooms and a nursing staff highly skilled in all aspects of CF care.

A few years after establishment of the Foundation sponsored CF Center at Tulane, an opportunity arose in 1968 to compete for a training grant from the National Center for Chronic Disease Control (a now-defunct branch of the federal government). Dr. John Herndon, Medical-Scientific Director of the CF Foundation at the time, was probably responsible for this federal action. He wisely sold the CF Center idea as one that would work well for all lung diseases in children, essentially an interdisciplinary approach to care, but with additional teaching and research ramifications. Tulane was successful in the competition and became one of four such federally funded pediatric pulmonary disease training centers in the United States. Others were in Philadelphia (Dr. Giulio Barbero at the University of Pennsylvania, Dr. Douglas Holsclaw at Hahnemann Medical College and Dr. Nancy Huang at Temple University); Los Angeles (Dr. Dan Wiseman at the University of Southern California); and Washington, D.C. (Dr. Frederick Burke at Georgetown University). The mission of these Centers was, as noted above, an interdisciplinary one by which pediatric pulmonary fellows would be trained along with pediatric pulmonary nurses, social workers, and nutritionists. Sponsorship of the pediatric pulmonary centers has passed from the Center for Chronic Disease Control (defunct), to the Regional Medical Centers (defunct), and finally to the Maternal and Child Health branch of the Public Health Service. The PPC program now comprises seven centers. In addition to the Louisiana PPC at Tulane and

LSU/Shreveport, current others are University of Alabama at Birmingham, University of Florida at Gainesville, University of New Mexico at Albuquerque, University of Washington at Seattle, University of Wisconsin at Madison, and Mount Sinai Medical Center, New York City.

The PPC concept grew out of the CF Center program established by the Cystic Fibrosis Foundation. This new grant broadened the scope of our CF and Pulmonary Center. Now, in addition to pediatric pulmonary fellows we had master's degree-bound social work and nursing students with those disciplines represented also on our faculty. Curricula for each discipline had to be developed and became an important part of applications for PPC grant renewal. Some PPC teaching sessions were discipline-specific, whereas others were attended by all students, regardless of discipline. In addition to the annual meetings of the CF Club and pediatric research societies, we now had an annual PPC meeting attended by all disciplines of all PPCs. Fortunately, the complicated planning for these interdisciplinary meetings has been rotated among the several PPCs.

Several years ago I turned over the direction of the Section of Pulmonary Diseases to Dr. Robert Beckerman, who has greatly enlarged and improved the Section's teaching and research activities. Dr. Scott Davis, a former pediatric fellow at Tulane, now competently heads the CF Clinic and the PPC, and Dr. Michael Kiernan, also a former fellow, is in charge of the pulmonary laboratory. These individuals are far better equipped than I to recount the recent history of the CF Center, the PPC, and associated activities.

Clinical Research

Clinical research came naturally as a result of questions that arose from patient observations. I became interested in both the digital clubbing and the barrel chest deformity that occurred in so many of our CF children. At that time Tulane Medical School required of each graduating senior a thesis based on research, usually performed during the summer months. With the help of two students, Stephen Golladay and Stephen Acker, anthropometric studies were made of chest diameters (maximal depth and maximal width measured at the nipple level in standing, quietly breathing subjects) of CF patients and controls. The problem with chest measurements is that both the size and the shape of the chest change with age/stature. Chest width grows faster than chest depth with the result that the chest becomes larger but also flatter with age. An elaborate graph was ultimately produced by us and printed for distribution by the Mead Johnson Company for both boys and girls. With the graph, one could plot chest depth and width as a function of height and calculate the statistical deviations from expected values—for depth, and width, and depth/width ratio. Dr. Warren Warwick of Minneapolis was particularly helpful in sending us elegant, custom-constructed chest calipers that allowed one to read off values directly without having to measure the distance between caliper tips.

It turned out that the critical dimension is the chest *depth* whose disproportionate increase, as obstructive pulmonary disease worsens, changes the shape of the chest from oval toward round. The egregious increase in chest depth after initiation of anabolic steroid therapy led Dr. Judith Harris and me to abandon a study of a steroid drug in CF. We feared that the steroid was making the pulmonary disease worse, but I now believe that, by promoting chest growth, the steroid was only prematurely revealing the deformation that would have shown up eventually without the steroid.

To study "clubbing" (a spoon shaped change of the nails that is most closely related to advancing pulmonary disease), students Robert Wiebe and RobertWilkinson, made measurements on plaster casts of the left index finger of normal, asthmatic, and CF patients of all ages. We found that the most reliable measure was a ratio of finger depths (one at the base of the nail and the other at the terminal [the last] interphalangeal joint.) The former was called the Distal Phalangeal Depth (DPD) and the latter the Inter Phalangeal Depth (IDP). Unlike chest measurements, the DPD/IPD ratio of the index finger remains unchanged throughout life in normal individuals of both sexes and all ethnic backgrounds. The normal ratio is about 0.86, and when the ratio exceeds 1.0, the ratio is about 2 ½ standard deviations above the mean. We found that clubbing is a variable process and that improvement of the disease is associated with reductions of DPD/IPD.[6] Dr. Richard Lemen, while at Tulane, showed that lobar resection for bronchiectasis in patients with IgG deficiency was followed by the reduction and subsequent disappearance of clubbing, just as Dr. Robert Mellins in New York had demonstrated after surgical correction of cyanotic heart disease. The collection and measurement of finger casts remained a standard procedure, like the measurement of chest depths, for every patient on every visit. However, when the clinic was moved from the Medical School to the hospital, the administration discovered that this was an "unbilled procedure" and this practice was brought to a halt. I have kept hundreds of casts from CF patients and hope that, perhaps with this technique as a monitor, we may ultimately elucidate the cause of finger clubbing.

I have alluded to the clinical pediatric pulmonary function laboratory, the first of its kind in Louisiana. It also had a research component with a Van Slyke machine, a Scholander gas analyzer, a gas chromatograph, and a Medtronic pH meter that required several milliliters of blood to give a more or less accurate reading. There was also a wonderful mechanical Monroe calculating machine with at least 10,000 moving parts, the ultimate calculator before electronics took over all such operations. Help in setting up the lab, its operation, and its projects came from neonatologist Dr. Mildred Stahlman at Vanderbilt University, (who had been a co-intern with me at Children's Hospital in Boston), and physiologists Dr. Herman Rahn and Leon Farhi at Buffalo, all of whom I visited at one time or another.

Of interest to me also was chest auscultation. René Laënnec, the inventor and namer of the stethoscope, became a sort of hero for me, because of his extraordinary ability to make observations in the living patient and relate those to morbid anatomy at autopsy. I thought I had invented the differential stethoscope—that is, a stethoscope with two chest pieces, one for each ear. However, I discovered that the instrument had been created in England in the 19th century by Somerville Scott Alison, who described its advantages and application with great accuracy. I consider it a powerful tool for simultaneous observations of breath sound intensity, pitch, and timing in any two areas of the lung. It is the perfect instrument for evaluating possible foreign body aspiration. I tried to teach the fellows how to auscultate methodically by pulmonary bronchopulmonary segment. With the help of the 3M company a Littman differential stethoscope was for a while marketed that had an off-on button on each chest piece. These allowed the auscultator to turn on or off the sound coming from either chest piece without having to lift the chest piece from the patient's chest. The next step was to record and analyze differential breath sounds. With the help of bioengineers Tom Wooten and Mike Wegmann, fellow Humberto Hidalgo, and medical students William Anderson, John Conley, and John Schreiber several publications dealt with breath sound analysis in children.[7,8,9]

In 1967 Bettina Hilman, Hal Brunt (a medical student), and I were first to report a chest radiologic sign that is almost specific for CF—mucoid impaction of the bronchi—finger-like branching or grape cluster opacifications in one or both lungs, produced by the accumulation of radiodense mucopus in bronchiectatic bronchi.[10] This sign is now less and less frequently seen, probably because of the greater emphasis on prophylaxis and on more effective therapy for pulmonary complications of CF.

With regard to therapy, for an insight into why patients with CF are living so much longer, those familiar with CF therapy in the year 2000 may be interested in the "state of the therapeutic art" in 1947, as laid out in my Boylston Club paper:

> Farber has stated four lines along which all rational therapy should be directed: 1) correction of the absent or greatly reduced pancreatic enzyme activity, 2) correction of the malabsorption of vitamin A, 3) correction of the negative nitrogen balance resulting from the fecal nitrogen loss, and 4) control of the upper respiratory infection and obstruction. The administration of pancreatin in the form of enteric coated granules in large doses is helpful, according to most authors, but at least two authors report no beneficial effect. Vitamin A may be given orally in the form of some A concentrate such as Oleum Percomorpum in doses at least five times the normal. Extra amounts of vitamin D should also be administered, as should vitamin B in the form of crude liver extract since there are indications that it may be helpful in nitrogen retention and in the improvement of gastro-intestinal hypotonicity. Large amounts of casein hydrolysates aid in nitrogen absorption and are clinically applicable. Prostigmine has been mentioned above as an aid to fat absorption by increasing gastro-intestinal tone. The dietary therapy has been particularly stressed by Andersen and should consist of enough protein to provide 25 per cent of the total calories, very little fat, and a moderate carbohydrate intake. The entire caloric intake should be at least one and one-half times the amount usually given to a normal infant or child the same age. di Sant'Agnese and Andersen

have reported recently on the use of chemotherapy for the chronic pulmonary infections. They conclude that the sulfonamides are useful in the prophylaxis and treatment of intercurrent infections of the respiratory tract, but that they are ineffective after the stage of suppurative bronchitis has been reached. On the other hand, penicillin may be effective after the appearance of respiratory distress and cyanosis, although failure may occur in infections by drug-resistant organisms. The most satisfactory mode of administration of penicillin appears to be by inhalation, aided by intramuscular injections. They view inhalation as a special case of topical treatment, and suggest that intramuscular penicillin should be used when bacteremia or involvement of the parenchyma of the lung is suspected. Preventive medicine should be practiced in all cases with an eye to decreasing the exposure of the patient to upper respiratory infections. Finally, as may be judged, treatment must be begun as soon as the diagnosis is made, and the diagnosis can never be made too early. Irreparable pulmonary damage may result from a few months' delay.

My most pleasant memories are those associated with the annual meetings of the Cystic Fibrosis Club, which usually attached itself to the meetings of the American Pediatric Society and the Society for Pediatric Research. It really was a "club" in that everyone knew everyone, and there was a spirited feeling of working together with much give and take—all in the name of conquering a miserable disease. The incorporation of the CF Club meetings into a broader and more powerful annual North American CF Conference sponsored by the Foundation—one that included basic scientists and all the clinical specialties—was a necessary one, but intimacy and camaraderie suffered.

The CF Club atmosphere was recreated in 1981 by Dr. Warren Warwick who assembled many, if not most, of those who used to attend the CF Club meetings for his 1000 Years of Cystic Fibrosis meeting.[11] The "1000 Years" was derived from an estimate that the 40 invited researchers together had a total of more than 1000 years of clinical and investigative experience with CF. A review of this colloquium would be most helpful to those interested in the history of CF.

I feel that my greatest contribution is having helped train a number of pediatric pulmonary fellows through the years, many of whom now run their own pulmonary and CF programs. Many of them have been introduced to the differential stethoscope and continue to use it routinely. All of them know how to examine a child's fingers for possible clubbing, having been taught to practice the adage that "examination of the lungs begins at the fingertips."

My work with CF patients and their parents through the years has been both an enriching and a trying experience. The continuity of association through the years that CF care involves tends to forge deep ties with patients and their families. The problem is how to keep that association within reasonable professional bounds. I have learned from patients and their parents to marvel at the strength of the human spirit, at the depth of the suffering and the acceptance of it without whining, at the sacrifices, and at the quiet heroism. In contrast, it seems to me that most of the complaining about illness and life in general has come from my largely healthy patients who in fact don't have much to complain about. As the prognosis for patients with CF continues to improve through the years, the great weight of the imminence of life's end has lifted. The associations are less stressful and the death watches less frequent. What was purely a pediatric disease at the time of our Center's founding now is passing from pediatricians to adult pulmonary caretakers.

References

1. Andersen DH. "Cystic fibrosis of the pancreas and its relation to celiac diseases." *Amer J Dis Child* 1938;56:344-399.
2. Editorial: "Looking back on the millennium in medicine." *New Engl J Med* 2000;342:42-49.
3. di Sant'Agnese PA, et al. "Abnormal electrolyte composition of sweat in cystic fibrosis of the pancreas. Clinical significance and relationship to the disease." *Pediatrics* 1953;12:549-563.
4. Gibson LE and Cooke RE. "A test for concentration of electrolytes in sweat in cystic fibrosis of the pancreas utilizing pilocarpine by iontophoresis." *Pediatrics* 1959;23:545-549.
5. Polgar G and Promadhat V. *Pulmonary function testing in children: Techniques and standards.* Saunders Philadelphia, 1971.
6. Waring WW, Wilkinson RW, Wiebe RA, Faul BC, and Hilman BC. "Quantitation of digital clubbing in children. Measurements of casts of the index fingers." *Amer Rev Resp Dis* 1971;104:166-174.
7. Wooten FT, Waring WW, Wegmann MJ, Anderson WF, and Conley JD. "Methods for respiratory sound analysis." *Med. Inst.* 1978;12: 254-257.
8. Schreiber JR, Anderson WF, Wegmann MJ, and Waring WW. "Frequency analysis of breath sounds by phonopneumography." *Med. Instr.* 1981;15:331-334.
9. Hidalgo HA, Wegmann MJ, and Waring WW. "Frequency spectra of normal breath sounds in childhood." *Chest* 1991;100:999-1002.
10. Waring WW, Brunt HC, and Hilman BC. "Mucoid impaction of the bronchi in cystic fibrosis." *Pediatrics* 1967;39:166-175.
11. *1,000 Years of Cystic Fibrosis, Collected Papers.* Warren J. Warwick (Ed.), University of Minnesota, May 7-9, 1981.

24

Center Directors Remember: Madison

Charles C. Lobeck, M.D.

I first heard of cystic fibrosis (CF) in 1949 when I was a medical student at the University of Rochester School of Medicine and Dentistry. My first memory is of Dr. George H. Whipple doing an autopsy on an infant with the disease. He described what was then termed "fibrocystic disease of the pancreas" as being uniformly fatal before the age of 5 years and emphasized the pathological features of a scarred cystic pancreas and sticky mucus in the lungs. I remembered the scene at the autopsy table but soon forgot all but the salient features of CF. Later, in residency, as I saw more patients with the disease, I puzzled as to how meconium ileus, chronic lung disease, and pancreatic fibrosis could be connected. Because the disease was familial, and followed the rules for autosomal recessive transmission, we thought it must be an inborn error of metabolism caused by a single basic genetic defect, like those described by Sir Archibald Garrod many years earlier. Like many of those inborn errors, it was unremitting once it appeared, and we thought it to be uniformly fatal at an early age. The care of children with the disease was a bad chore. Coughing, foul bowel movements, and fatal outcome took its toll on families and we pediatricians. It was difficult for young physicians eager to cure, to get enthusiastic about such an unpleasant chronic disease.

When I moved to the University of Wisconsin in 1958, one crucial event reacquainted me with CF. I was excited by a seminar in the early 1960s by Professor Lowell Hokin, a well-known biochemical pharmacologist. He was studying membrane transport in the secretory tissues of exocrine glands, most notably the very active nasal gland of gulls and other birds resident in salt water. Of significance, this gland allows birds to drink salt water and excrete the excess salt in their nasal secretions. He had studied other exocrine glands and found increased activity of certain membrane phospholipids in these glands after stimulation with acetylcholine. I was very excited because I knew that there was a lesion in membrane transport of salt and water in the exocrine glands in CF. Dr. Paul di Sant'Agnese had discovered that CF patients had salty sweat in 1953 and a clinically easy method of testing CF sweat had been developed. It appeared that the sweat was always salty and thus a good test for the disease, but also meant that the lesion in the sweat gland must be very close to the cause of the disease. I thought that all we needed to solve the problem was to get a group of patients from whom we could obtain skin samples to test the phospholipid activity of sweat glands. I suggested this to Professor Hokin and he said, "Of course, we should easily be able to detect the abnormality in CF. It probably is in the phospholipid metabolism of exocrine glands." We believed we had a good possibility to find the basic enzymatic defect of CF. A series of events really got the CF project going. John Mangos, a bright young physician who was a superb resident, came to work with me. He became a trainee of the Foundation, the National Institutes of Health (NIH), and the Department of Pediatrics of the University of Wisconsin from 1962 until 1966. I was also blessed with an exceptional laboratory technician, Dorothy Huebner. John went on to become a distinguished pediatrician at the University of Florida and has retired as long time Chair of Pediatrics at the University of Texas-San Antonio. Dorothy later got her Ph.D. and left Madison. All of us were eager to get at the disease.

From the very beginning we needed patients. To get them, I made contact with Joan and Leesely (Buzz) Hardy who were CF parents and were prominent in developing a NCFRF Chapter in Milwaukee. This was our first contact with the Foundation. John and I made a conscious effort not to be intense participants in Chapter affairs and politics. We thought that we could contribute more by remaining detached because we wanted to be in the position of supporting more peer-review of CF research with our support coming from the NIH, and to develop the patient base for our research from the referrals. The Hardys were leaders and they helped us recruit patients for our studies. We found that a relationship with the NCFRF was becoming important in the development of our research and a broad base for patient care. In the early 1960s, we developed a CF Center with support from the NCFRF. We slowly began to be drawn into Foundation affairs. We both participated in the CF Club meetings at the time of the pediatric research meetings, and busily pursued our careers. That seemed enough at the time. We lived the life of the ups and downs of CF care and research, the controversies over ciliary dyskinesia and other research questions, the controversies over patient care, to mist or not to mist, various antibiotics, pseudomonas, the frustrations of grieving CF families, and our own often fruitless research.

The Milwaukee Children's Hospital, which became the Children's Hospital of Wisconsin, had a beginning CF program under the leadership of Dr. W. Ted Bruns. Ted had been a faculty member in Madison and our relationship was cordial from the beginning. Even though there was a potential for intense competition between the University of Wisconsin Children's Hospital in Madison and the Children's Hospital of Wisconsin in Milwaukee, we did not let it stand between the CF Centers. As they developed, the two Centers developed a tight CF research and care relationship. The two institutions now compete for all forms of complex childcare in Wisconsin but the CF care and research relationship is still warm and both CF Centers have thrived. During this period, of active participation in the 1960s, Milwaukee was the center of Wisconsin parent interest in the NCFRF and I had little to do with the development of other CF Chapters or with the national affairs of the NCFRF.

Unfortunately, the project with Prof. Hokin failed. We were not able to show differences between the skin biopsies of control subjects and CF patients, but we were hooked on the search for the cause of CF. The CF Center was booming and we began to study sweat in order to make a more secure diagnosis. We discovered that men, women, and infants had much different sweat composition and published a paper on the subject in 1962. By that time, we were taking care of many CF patients.

We reviewed the literature on CF and were very disappointed in the quality of ongoing research. Much of what was known about treatment was based on anecdotal or biased clinical observation. The parents and their physician colleagues, who had formed the Foundation, were clamoring for advancement in CF research but, in our opinion, the general level of the science was poor. Other than pulmonary physiotherapy, crude pancreatic enzyme preparations, dietary adjustment and antibiotics, there was little to offer the CF patients. They were put in mist tents usually fogged with water that uncomfortably soaked the patient, reducing the visibility of patient, parent and caretakers. It was a torture chamber. I know, I tried one for a few hours.

The national experts, though dedicated clinicians and often brilliant observers, could be dogmatic about their clinical results that did not result from well controlled outcome studies. The Foundation was not as aware at the time, as they are now, of the importance of disciplined well controlled observations. Nationally, sophisticated pediatric researchers in other areas often derided the state of the art in CF care and research. This perception had a profound influence on my next actions.

Because of my feeling that the scientific effort had little support from the NIH and that Foundation support was weak, I became more active on the national scene. I was asked to contribute a chapter on CF to the second edition of *The Metabolic Basis of Inherited Disease*. This was a very prestigious book edited by Stanbury, Wyngaarden, and Fredrickson and led me to look hard at the literature. I wasn't satisfied that anyone was hot on the trail of the cause or even understood the common lesion of the many organ systems. Looking back, I probably was viewed as a curmudgeon by other investigators. Probably because of this critical attitude, I was asked to be on the General Medicine "A" Study Section of NIH and for four years reviewed the applications for CF research grants to the NIH. It was not a happy experience in that many of the grants were poor and were rejected. At the NIH, the sophisticated scientists did not respect national CF research efforts. At about that time, I was introduced to Bob McCreery, the President of the NCFRF, and was appointed to the Research Review Committee of the Foundation. As I became more active in Foundation affairs, I met Doris Tulcin, who impressed me as a sophisticated and remarkably well informed parent of a CF child. She wanted to build the level of scientific effort of the Foundation and improve the quality of grant requests to the NIH. She soon became President of the Foundation and made herself known at the NIH. She encouraged me and I became active on the Research Committee and in other CF Foundation affairs.

While I was pursuing this activity, John Mangos was working hard in the laboratory and demonstrated in 1967 that CF secretions inhibited electrolyte transport across cell membranes. It stimulated his interest in micropuncture techniques then used to study kidney physiology. He was supported by the Foundation and the NIH from 1964 to 1966 to study with Professor Karl Ullrich at the University of Berlin and was off on his career of using sophisticated biochemical and physiological microanalysis to study exocrine secretion.

In the 1960s and early 70s, some of our most stimulating times were working with the patients. John, who is a Greek Orthodox priest, was very talented with patients. He was and is a renaissance man. Our technical staff, chiefly Nona McSherry, was also talented at handling the heartbreak of the disease. We met some wonderful, amazingly strong people who by an accident of nature had produced a child with the disease. This difficult family life was later beautifully described by Frank Deford, the sports commentator and CF Board member, in a book about his daughter Alex, a warmly loved child who died of CF. I got calls from all over the State of Wisconsin about patients and CF became my primary clinical activity. Several anecdotes from those days are worth recounting.

In the late 1960s, I received a call from an older woman who had read an article in the Milwaukee Journal about the growing CF Center. The article described the symptoms of the disease and she said to me, "My daughter has that disease." I was not surprised until she said her daughter was in her late 30s and married! I asked to see her and was amazed to find that she indeed had the disease with all of its manifestations and had never been treated. It was becoming clear that not all patients died young and some lived reasonable lives with very limited treatment.

At about this time, men with CF were found to be sterile because of congenital absence of the vas deferens (the duct leading from the testes) and we began to advise our patients and teach physicians that all males were sterile. One of Wisconsin's best pediatricians called me and asked me to calm down a woman who felt wronged by this information. She was in a rage when she arrived at my office. She had married a young man with CF and was pregnant. She vehemently denied sexual relationships with other men and felt that medicine had suggested that she was a loose woman. Indeed it had! Her husband proved to have CF, but in his case, was fertile so the pregnancy had resulted. An occasional fertile male is uncommon but now is not an unknown phenomenon. It always pays to listen.

For me, the culmination of my clinical experience in the CF Center was an emotional meeting I had years later when I was Dean of the University of Missouri School of Medicine. This was a reunion with our old Wisconsin patients and their parents. We cried together and I was truly emotionally moved but I was still angry that we had failed to make more strides in the discovery of a cause and providing better treatment.

During this time, I was participating in the development of the Cystic Fibrosis Foundation, first as an observer of its management and mismanagement and as a participant in its medical and scientific affairs. My Foundation career ended in 1984 as a member of the Executive Committee and Vice President. It was quite an experience and I stayed on because of my enthusiasm for finding an answer to the disease and frustration with the efforts that were being made. I also felt that the Foundation could become a major force in a sophisticated research effort but was still falling short of that goal. Growing pain is an understatement to describe the development of the Foundation at that time. Moves from New York to Atlanta to Washington were symptomatic of the rapid change and agitation in the leadership. Changes of Executive Directors were frequent and thorny. The Directors of CF Centers could also be an unruly lot. Many were vying for more status and financial support and at the same time trying their best to take care of large numbers of patients. The parents at the grass roots were understandably influenced by their own physicians and were impatient with the lack of progress and sometimes supported one CF Center or another on emotional grounds. The characters were many. I could name a few but fortunately have forgotten most. I developed a strong distaste for "fundamentalist" positions taken by professionals and lay people who tried to advance their position without concern for the mission of the organization and its values. In my career as a medical school administrator, I retained this critical view of large egos and I still have it today.

Despite this critical view there were many who were taking a national and world view of CF. The great leaders and clinical observers of the past like Paul di Sant'Agnese, LeRoy Matthews and Harry Shwachman trained and gave way to a group of new faces like Lynn Taussig, Philip Farrell, Richard Talamo, and Thomas Boat. As they appeared on the scene, the general level of disciplined research rose.

The move to Washington by the CF Foundation was very important, since it brought the Foundation closer to the NIH. The reputation of CF research grew and Doris Tulcin and Bob Dresing, a CF parent from Cleveland, became important leaders. They cultivated the NIH Staff and Directors and promoted disciplined research. Bob Beall, a promising young NIH staffer, came on board as Medical Director of the Foundation and the interest of the biomedical science community grew. There were efforts to cultivate congressional leaders to intelligently promote NIH appropriation for CF at the same time suggesting that CF research should be advanced. This was the goal that we had all hoped for. The rest is recent history. I was pleased when Phillip Farrell went from Wisconsin to the NIH for further training and became a friend of Bob Beall. He returned to the University with an active interest in CF, became the Center Director, and eventually become Chair of the Department of Pediatrics and then Dean of the Medical School at Wisconsin. He continues his sophisticated studies of clinical CF. Through the CF Foundation, Dr. Norman Fost, of the University of Wisconsin, and his ethicist colleagues became interested in the numerous ethical problems of neonatal screening for CF. After I left for Missouri, Elaine Mischler, an expert clinician, Chris Green from Case Western Reserve University in Cleveland, and many others led the CF Center to its high level of expertise today with over 250 patients and 70 adults in Madison and thriving satellites in Marshfield and Green Bay, Wisconsin.

The drive to improve the quality of research into CF has been realized. Since the 1980s some of the best disease oriented research in the US has been in CF. The affected genes and their products have been identified. Study of newborn screening for the disease has been done by the group in Wisconsin with results that suggest some benefit to growth from early detection. Elegant physiological studies by Dr. Paul Quinton have revealed the real lesion in the sweat gland to be impermeability of the reabsorptive surfaces to chloride ion.

I had always hoped we would someday get to this point, but I must admit to my disappointment that these advances have not led to better treatment programs. As I review the current state of treatment, I see attempts to change the course of the disease that are not unlike those of my days. The new knowledge of the cystic fibrosis transmembrane conductance regulator (CFTR) gene(s) has not quickly borne fruit. Tragically, therapeutic regimens are much the same today as they were in the 1960s, even though better drugs are used and results are improved. The improvement in life span and quality of life of patients has been due to refinements of antibiotics and nutrition and in some cases surgery, but not due to the results of the knowledge we have of the fundamental defect. I thought, years ago, that when we reached this stage there would be a quick solution to the problem and enormous strides in treatment. That is not the case. Hopefully this situation will change in my lifetime.

I have learned that successful treatment of genetic metabolic diseases like CF depends upon understanding the pathophysiological events. We can then break the cycle of abnormality with external agents. I have also learned that we cannot divorce our research from the immediacy of patient care. While we wait for gene therapy, which will be here sooner or later, we must work hard to learn more about the fundamental steps of exocrine gland secretion and reabsorption and how they go wrong in CF. Then we can break the chain and develop successful palliative treatment.

25

Center Directors Remember: Philadelphia

Nancy N. Huang, M.D. and Lourdes R. Laraya-Cuasay, M.D.

My collaborator for this memoir of our combined experiences in cystic fibrosis (CF) over the years from 1950, Dr. Laraya-Cuasay, was an outstanding trainee who then joined me as a faculty member at the Saint Christopher's Hospital for Children (St Chris). Later on, she expanded and improved CF care in the state of New Jersey.

I entered the United States in 1947 from my native China. Thanks to Dr. Waldo Nelson, Professor and Chairman of the Department of Pediatrics at Temple University School of Medicine and Director of St Chris Hospital, I was appointed a research assistant at St Chris in 1950, and then Instructor in Pediatrics and a faculty member at these two institutions. The research involved patients with CF and before long I had a growing CF clinic population. After so many early career moves, it was my good fortune to remain at St Chris until my retirement in 1979.

I was born in 1914 in China to a well known civil engineer father and a housewife mother who both believed in educating their sons and daughters equally. Therefore, I went through high school, college, and medical college like my counterparts in the western world and in 1936 entered the Peking Union Medical College, a world renowned institution sponsored by the US Rockefeller Foundation. Our medical curriculum was designed like that of Johns Hopkins Medical College with the clinical and basic science departments headed by highly reputable professors from foreign countries and by our own graduates with further advanced training in the US or the United Kingdom. Dr. Robert Lim, Professor and Chairman of Physiology was trained in Great Britain and Dr. Hsien Wu, Professor and Chairman of Biochemistry, was the Wu in the Folin-Wu laboratory method for assay of blood sugar levels. Drs. Isadore Snapper and Irvine McQuare, who taught medicine and pediatrics respectively in my student years, were both very effective in their respective fields. I was closer to Dr. Snapper because I had my internship and residency in medicine and I participated in a research project on calcium metabolism in patients with osteomalacia that was published in the *Journal of Clinical Investigation*. After Japanese forces shut down the Peking Union Medical College in 1942, I served as a pediatric resident in the Shanghai Public Hospital for Children for two years and then became chief pediatrician in a private general hospital and assistant professor at Tung-Deh Medical School in Shanghai.

When the Communist Liberation Army occupied Shanghai in 1947, I left China for two years of graduate training at Cincinnati Children's Hospital under Drs. Ashley Weech and Katherine Dodd, a most productive, fruitful, and enjoyable experience. Dr. Sydney Farber visited from Boston and gave a series of lectures on CF, which were comprehensive and educational. He suggested that CF was a generalized disease of exocrine glands with inspissation of mucus from mucus secreting glands that had led to the term "mucoviscidosis."

In 1950 at St Chris, I was under the guidance of Dr. Robert High. We worked as a team to see pulmonary disease patients, mostly with tuberculosis and acute infections of the respiratory tract and we soon had a contract to do a clinical trial of oral penicillin in patients with respiratory illnesses. I also began to have CF patients referred, along with others having various chronic illnesses, like rheumatoid arthritis with pulmonary involvement. However, CF was the most frequently referred disease so I developed great interest in them, especially as I saw them improve with oral penicillin. That fall, I had my first experience with a CF patient, a 3 month old boy, who had been discharged from St Chris the day before. After duodenal intubation had been performed and the diagnosis of CF established, he required hospital care for six weeks of intensive therapy for his pulmonary infection and malnutrition. He was again febrile and barely at his birth weight, with frequent paroxysmal cough, rapid breathing, and a distended abdomen. His mother and I were worried about readmission but instead tried a course of penicillin therapy for the penicillin sensitive *Staphylococcus aureus* that had been found on his respiratory tract culture. We were both pleased when he responded well and was much better at his follow up visit. Penicillin was the first significant antibiotic and his mother's beaming smile encouraged me to further pursue its use for CF patients. In a matter of six months, four patients were enrolled in my clinic and all responded to oral penicillin, which gave me confidence and encouragement in the care of these patients. As a result, my colleagues at St Chris began to refer their CF patients to my clinic for follow up care and slowly all patients suspected of having CF also came to my clinic.

In 1955, Dr. Nelson appointed me Instructor in Pediatrics at Temple University School of Medicine and assistant attending physician at St Chris. This was a great step forward in my professional life because the faculty appointment allowed me to independently apply for grant support and to organize my teaching, care, and research activities. Since my responsibilities were not clearly delineated, I could continue to pursue my major interest of care and research around patients with respiratory illnesses, especially those with CF. In 1961, we were proud to be recognized as a CF Center, along with a number of other institutions around the country, as a result of a new program initiated by the National Cystic Fibrosis Research Foundation.

Pre Sweat Test Diagnosis and Diagnostic Challenges

In the pre sweat test era of the 1950s, the most dependable laboratory test was duodenal intubation to obtain a good pancreatic juice sample for tryptic enzyme activity. A deficiency of enzyme indicated pancreatic insufficiency, and with the associated symptoms, was consistent with the diagnosis of CF. However, this test was difficult to perform, time consuming, and difficult for the patients. The non-specific tests for pancreatic function were less reliable and included microscopic examination of stool for fat, the gelatin film test for enzyme activity using unexposed x-ray film, trypsin enzyme test, nitrogen assay, and quantitative fat. So the first step in diagnosis was to at least suspect it in an infant or a young child. This "suspicion" was based purely on clinical manifestations including poor weight gain, early onset of cough, recurrent pneumonia, foul and bulky stools, irritability, evidence of malnutrition, delayed developmental milestones, and increased front to back diameter of the chest.

We had a major challenge when we encountered our first patient suspected of having CF but *without having the symptoms of pancreatic insufficiency*. Since she had typical pulmonary involvement and sputum that grew *Staphylococcus aureus coagulase positive*, she was treated as one with CF. When she died later, postmortem examination of the lungs revealed characteristic changes associated with CF but the pancreatic involvement was minimal and not clinically manifested. We thus learned that the pancreatic insufficiency may or may not be a component of CF. Another family presented with three of their four children diagnosed as having CF at another hospital. They were fairly mild cases and our insistence on repeating the duodenal intubation in all three of them resulted in our determination that one of the three children was actually normal. This child, who was most unhappy with the duodenal intubation at the beginning, was very happy at the end. It was very rewarding to undiagnose CF in this case.

The elevation of sweat electrolyte concentration in CF patients first reported by Dr. di Sant'Agnese in 1953 was a breakthrough in the diagnosis of CF. In the early days, thermal stimulation was used to collect sweat, which was hazardous due to the risk of heat exhaustion, high fever, and even death, especially in infants. Another 2 year old girl was referred by an allergist for wheezing and thick mucus. We were less suspicious of CF because she was, if anything, overnourished rather than appearing underweight that would be due to insufficient pancreatic enzymes. However, several sweat tests were done and all were positive despite the evidence for normal pancreatic function. We were becoming more aware of the different varieties of CF.

In 1959, Gibson and Cooke reported the use of pilocarpine to induce sweat. CF appeared to be a recessive inherited trait in which each parent had to be an asymptomatic carrier for the disease to show in one of their children, so we thought repeated sweat tests and discriminatory analysis could identify which siblings were an asymptomatic carrier like the parents. The CF patients were termed homozygous for the gene because they must have both CF alleles to have the disease. The parents were termed obligate heterozygotes because they must each have one allele to pass on, but each sibling could have just one CF allele (and be an obligate heterozygote carrier and asymptomatic like the parents), or not have a CF allele from either parent and thus not carry the gene at all. However, there was sufficient variation in the sweat test results among the siblings to make the discriminatory analysis technique unsuccessful and we could not accurately identify which siblings were carriers until the gene was identified in 1989.

Several other methods of sweat testing led to some controversy. The sweat test was standardized by the joint efforts of several centers forming a national committee to pool the results from four centers that led the investigators to conclude that a sweat chloride concentration of 60 mEq/L or greater was diagnostic of CF.[1] Repeat positive sweat tests along with one or two other manifestations typical of CF and/or a positive family history established the diagnosis. Standardization has greatly simplified the interpretation of the test provided that sufficient sweat was collected and the gauze or filter paper used to absorb the sweat was accurately weighed and carefully handled. The details in doing the test are very important so we designated Dr. Cecilia Hsu, a medical graduate of National Taiwan University, to perform the sweat test exclusively. Her care and thoroughness maintained our accuracy in the diagnosis of CF.

In another case, the sweat tests were repeatedly normal in a 2 year old infant girl who had a typical early course of repeated attacks of pneumonia with sputum positive for both *Staphylococcus aureus* and *Pseudomonas aeruginosa*. The production of sputum in such a young child and the presence of these bacteria were strong pieces of evidence for CF. By five years of age she developed clubbing of the fingers, which was consistent with significant chronic pulmonary disease. Although she had poor weight gain there were no abnormal bowel movements and without a positive sweat test, a specific diagnosis of CF could not be made. After repeated observations and with the above findings, I told the family that there was no other likely diagnosis except CF and she could be put in our CF program so she could receive free medication. The child had progressive lung disease and died by 9 years of age. Our pathologist, Dr. J.B. Arey, found changes typical of CF in both the lungs and the pancreas confirming the suspected diagnosis, although the sweat tests had remained normal. The patient's 12 year old brother also had chronic lung disease and while he did have elevated sweat chloride levels compatible with CF, in his case the pancreatic function was normal. These two atypical cases occurred in the same family. Thus, we became more aware of the clinical heterogeneity of CF.

From 1950 to 1960, I was most interested in the bacteria present in the CF respiratory tract. Most of the time I served as solo physician, nurse, and secretary. My schedule was to see patients in the morning and perform laboratory studies in the afternoon. This did not change until I received Center funding from the Foundation in 1961. Recognizing the important role of proper identification of respiratory bacteria and their antibiotic sensitivities, in the 1960s I established a separate microbiology laboratory that processed CF patient specimens. I was the director with two microbiology technicians to assist me. The major concentration of our research in this period was to evaluate the efficacy of different antibiotics for CF patients, develop a system to evaluate the therapeutic response to a treatment course of a new antibiotic, and record any adverse reactions or toxic effects. I frequently attended conferences in the Department of Microbiology at Temple University School of Medicine to keep up with new microbiology procedures and my major source of continuing information was from Dr. Spaulding, the Chairman.

Other doctors who supported my interest in microbiology and virology were Dr. Morton Klein and Dr. Ada Deforest in virology, Dr. Ted Anderson in bacteriology, and Dr. Kenneth Cundy, a fellow in Microbiology supported by the CF Foundation, who became interested in the Pseudomonas organism.

My patient load continued to grow. By the mid 1950s, we already had found penicillinase producing strains of Staphylococcus, meaning they had become resistant to penicillin. Fortunately, we were soon blessed by the availability of methicillin, a bactericidal antibiotic, which could overcome the penicillin resistance of the bacteria and provide effective treatment. It also allowed the penicillin resistant strains to be studied in depth and we performed serum and bronchial assays following intravenous and aerosol administration. In those days we based our judgment on patient's response to therapy with chemotherapeutic agents on clinical parameters and chest x-ray changes. Methicillin induced clinical remission and chest x-ray improvement in most patients and even eliminated the Staphylococcus from the respiratory cultures. However, this bacteriological improvement was transient in most patients, and the same type of Staph soon reappeared in the cultures, although all strains isolated after therapy remained responsive to the antibiotic. Adverse hematologic effects occurred so we welcomed the development of nafcillin for intravenous use, as it did not have the side effects of methicillin.

With my early fellows we studied kanamycin, oxacillin, and chloramphenicol, and the staphylococcus carrier rate in CF. About the time (1963) that we observed optic neuritis and impaired vision in several patients on long term treatment of at least several months and wondered if vitamin B deficiency might be involved, Dr. Carolyn Denning reported on four cases. The consensus of CF specialists was that chloramphenicol alone caused the problem when used long term.

With Dr. Ann Sproul, we studied the growth pattern of 50 infants and children with CF. This was the only large study of growth in CF literature at the time and demonstrated retardation of physical growth in both weight and height with the CF medians in only the 3rd to 10th percentiles of children with normal health. Skeletal maturation was delayed in 38% of the children studied. Notably, the growth retardation correlated significantly with the severity of the pulmonary involvement, but not with the degree of pancreatic insufficiency. With therapy, most children had a normal or above normal gain in weight with the greatest gains occurring when therapy was initiated during infancy.[2]

Dr. Carlos Macri from Argentina, a pulmonary fellow from 1966 to 1968, was an effective clinician who studied the effects of chloramphenicol and carbenicillin and participated in a study of survival of CF patients.[3] On his return to Argentina, he organized a CF program that was recognized internationally. Dr. E. Joan Hiller from the United Kingdom continued the studies on carbenicillin, then returned to England to practice allergy and pulmonology. Subsequently, she took charge of a CF and general pediatric clinic and was consultant to the pediatric pulmonary program in Nottingham.

In the 1960s, I collaborated with Dr. Peter Kuo, my husband, in several studies. He was Professor of Medicine at the University of Pennsylvania, a pioneer researcher on the effects of lipids on cardiovascular disease, and a strong proponent that a rice diet can prevent coronary artery disease. We were the first to report on the fatty acid profile in CF and the essential fatty acid deficiency (EFA) resulting from the maldigestion and malabsorption, but did not seem to cause clinical manifestations.[4] We also studied the effect of feeding medium chain triglyceride emulsion (MCT) to CF patients because this emulsion is absorbed as free fatty acids into the circulation without need for prior digestion by the pancreatic lipase. The result of the MCT trial was favorable in that the CF children all showed significantly improved bowel movements and increased weight gain during the period. There was an associated further decrease in essential fatty acids, but they did not show clinical manifestation of EFA deficiency. Most of the children had difficulty drinking the emulsion.

During the 1960s, our CF program expanded rapidly with referrals from outlying community hospitals, all the medical centers in Philadelphia, other hospitals in Pennsylvania including the Lancaster and Wilkes-Barre areas, and New Jersey and Delaware. The Lancaster and Wilkes-Barre areas especially had large numbers of patients, so the Director of the Crippled Children's Program of the State of Pennsylvania authorized satellite clinics of our Center in those two cities. The Wilkes-Barre CF clinic was established at Mercy Hospital in 1966 and was especially successful, with a program designed for diagnosis and evaluation, as well as treatment. The medical staff consisted of one pulmonary fellow, myself, and the nursing coordinator, Ruth Shiffman, assisted by the public health nurse (PHN) from Wilkes-Barre, who did home visits, obtained interval histories, and provided education and care. Other state services included nutrition, physical therapy, and social work using a "team approach" directed to the whole patient and the symptoms.

Upon referral to the program, a home visit was made to assess the situation and a complete history was forwarded to St Chris. Clinic appointments were scheduled once monthly on a Friday and limited to 15 patients. Patient charts were reviewed in the Health Department office prior to clinic and, according to protocol, patients were sent for x-rays, blood work, etc. before being seen by the clinician. Duplicate sweat tests were done on all new patients and the results reviewed by the clinicians to decide which should be repeated. Patients scheduled for follow up appointments had a home visit by the PHN with a progress report sent to St Chris for review prior to clinic. Home visits were made as deemed needed by the PHN between clinic visits for ongoing assessment and instruction and to assist with home parenteral antibiotic therapy. An integral part of the clinic activities was the post clinic conference when each patient's chart was reviewed and evaluated and special needs discussed. Respiratory specimens for cultures were transported to the St Chris CF Microbiology Lab. Patients registered in the Pennsylvania State CF Program received financial aid for most of their medications, chest, x-rays, and labora-tory tests.

The practice of keeping copies of the Wilkes-Barre CF patient records at St Chris served us very well when the Susquehanna River flooded in 1972 and all of the Wilkes-Barre charts were destroyed.

In 1965, I became the fourth president of the "CF Club" and presented my work on the respiratory flora of patients with CF.[5] Later on we presented a paper on survival of patients with CF from 1952 to1967 who were admitted to St Chris in three 5-year periods with progressively increased survival rates due to intensive and continuous improvement in diagnosis and management. In the ensu-ing years, we always submitted one or two abstracts each year keeping the St Chris CF program active in the CF Club.

Further Reflections

Lourdes R. Laraya-Cuasay, M.D.

I had a variety of experiences that led up to my becoming a pediatric pulmonary fel-low in Dr. Huang's program in July 1969 through June 1971. Born on Pearl Harbor Day just three years after Dorothy Andersen described CF, I graduated from the University of Santo Tomas School of Medicine in Manila in 1963, and trained in pediatrics. I entered the United States in 1966 and had further training in pediat-rics at Children's Hospital in Louisville, Kentucky where I met Dr. Walter T. Hughes, then Chief of the Department of Pediatrics at Louisville General Hospi-tal. I was most impressed by the need for chest physicians as I rotated through the Pediatric Chest Clinic that Dr. Hughes supervised and as I cared for pulmonary patients with tuberculosis, histoplasmosis, those associated with multisystem disor-ders, and CF. Being unfamiliar with CF disease, I remember struggling to include CF in my differential diagnosis of failure to thrive or malnutrition, as I was more familiar with infectious or parasitic disease as the usual etiology for these problems. In 1967, I was a second year pediatric resident at the Tulane Division of the Charity Hospital of New Orleans, while my husband continued surgical residency. At the Chest Clinic, directed by Dr. William Waring, I continued to nurture the idea of a pediatric pulmonary fellowship, which at that time was a budding subspecialty. I observed Dr. Waring's great compassion for children with CF, was fascinated by this disease that was looking for a cure, and thought that this was a mission for me. I watched Dr. Waring's technician make casts of clubbing of the fingers (an indirect reflection of the lung disease) and compare the measurements serially to document objectively whether improvement or progression was occurring. Measurement of chest diameter using obstetrical calipers was part of the physical examination. Bronchoscopy was in its infancy then and our adult pulmonology and thoracic sur-gical colleagues were most open to the pediatric application of this technique. Pos-tural drainage was emphasized. Dr. Margaret H. D. Smith was also a great influence in solidifying my desire to take care of children with lung problems. Dur-ing an elective with her, I was involved in fieldwork comparing various methods of tuberculin testing. My rotation at the Contagious Disease Pavilion impressed me with the residual pulmonary problems that occur from complicated pneumonia and the ventilatory complications, including breathlessness and distress, following post bacterial meningitis, interested me. I wanted to better understand the respiratory system and search for effective means of therapy.

My husband transferred to Hahnemann Medical College in 1968 and I accepted a fellowship in Child Growth and Development at the Children's Hospital of Philadelphia (CHOP). At CHOP, I met Dr. George Polgar in the Pediatric Pulmonary Division. He was working on his book on pediatric pulmonary function testing in children, which was co-edited by Dr. Varuni Promadhat. Later, Dr. Polgar was to be my mentor in pulmonary physiology while Dr. Promadhat was my first companion when we attended the CF Club Meeting in Atlantic City, New Jersey in 1968. Dr. Edward Sewell directed the pediatric pulmonary division at CHOP. His expertise was in pulmonary tuberculosis and he acknowledged the great mentorship of Dr. Edith Lincoln to him. He followed some patients with CF. Inspired by the novelty of the pulmonary subspecialty and the examples of Dr. Hughes, Dr. Waring, and Dr. Smith, I decided to become a pediatric pulmonologist.

CF intrigued me as a disease looking for a cure and it was a disease that involved end of life issues. I wanted to share in my patient's lives from beginning to end. I had observed how many Americans disdained the words "dying" or "death." In those days, the word "cemetery" was a taboo to many individuals I met, including those in the health care profession. In my experience coming from the Philippines, both culturally and spiritually death was considered a continuation of life. When the end of a journey was inevitable, then it was also the physician's function to prepare the patient to die in peace.

Pulmonary Fellowship

Dr. Subharee Tongudai (now Dr. Suwanjutha) and I were pulmonary fellows from 1969-1971. Together we worked in the clinics and did clinical research on various antipseudomonal antibiotics, endobronchial lavage, and other clinical subjects. She returned to Thailand to practice pediatric pulmonology and critical care at the Ramathibodi Hospital in Bangkok and recently was co-author with Dr. Huang describing Asians with CF. The main population of our pulmonary clinic consisted of patients with CF from infancy to adulthood. By that time, I was the mother of four children under 5 years of age, did not drive, and Dr. Huang was magnanimous in relieving me from weekends on duty during my fellowship. Instead, she alternated weekend coverage with Dr. Tongudai. I rode in to the hospital frequently with her and she educated me in Chinese cooking, while we also planned more research studies.

Dr. Huang was a great educator and was often referred to as the "queen of Saint Christopher's Hospital for Children" No one said, "No" to her. Before the age of beepers, Dr. Huang's name was constantly paged as she received international and national phone consultations and her name was synonymous with CF in Phila-delphia. All our patient's parents respected her and were awed by her wisdom. However, the patients would hide from her and try to choose us trainees to check them if they had lost weight. Dr. Huang was not known to coax anyone; patients just were admitted when she said so. As fellows, we were the buffers or negotiators for a patient's cause if it was indicated. Dr. Huang was a most compassionate and loving physician in her own way. She did not express her feelings openly but every-one knew that. She received the golden heart award at St Chris in the early 1970s and was always very available to her patients.

During the pulmonary fellowship, we had pulmonary clinics three days each week, one day when we held pre and post clinic conferences, and one day for research studies, journal club, and pulmonary physiology conference. We also had daily pulmonary rounds that could last an entire half day, since we averaged 30 CF inpatients and at least 8 to 10 non-CF admissions and 6 to 8 consults. After or before these rounds, we made rounds on the clinical research floor as needed. We prepared for noon teaching conferences for residents and participated in multi-spe-cialty meetings and conferences. Any manuscript writing was done at home after hours. One pulmonary fellow attended the Wilkes-Barre clinic with Dr. Huang every other Friday while the other fellow was alone to cover every activity that occurred in the interval. After I joined the faculty and became an attending physi-cian, it helped tremendously for us to have two doctors available at St Chris when it was a "Wilkes-Barre Day." The attending physicians rotated monthly for inpatient service but continued their usual outpatient clinic practice. Besides being an attend-ing for the pulmonary service, I also was an inpatient service attending four months each year. It was a most difficult time when more than one CF patient was in the terminal stage and one wished the ability to be in two places at once, or that a day could last 36 hours for everything to be accomplished.

The atmosphere at St Chris was conducive to openness and friendliness with "open door" consultation among the subspecialists. The cafeteria was the place to exchange nonacademic as well as academic information. Dr. Huang was a no-nonsense individual and we did not do much joking around in her presence. Dr. Judy Palmer was an unbelievable human being who was able to maneuver her actions and responses and adapt remarkably well to very different cultures. The psy-chosocial recommendations that she made always took into consideration our cul-tural differences. She made excellent rapport with the adolescents and young adults, and also with young parents. I learned so much from her compassionate and deli-cately balanced approach to human problems and suffering. Much of this teaching came during our long rides to and from Wilkes-Barre. She longed for California and Palo Alto and returned there after I left St Chris.

Dr. Panganiban and Judy were pulmonary fellows together and both were smokers. To conceal this, they devised a mirror system to signal the approach of Dr. Huang whose moccasin clad feet made little sound. But the mirror let them see her approach and they would immediately extinguish their cigarettes. This behavior lasted only a few months because they became non-smoking converts due to the pulmonary knowledge they were acquiring and also from the unfavorable response from the rest of us because we shared offices together at that time. There was a great celebration when their cessation of smoking date was successfully accomplished.

We also used our office as an extension for home intravenous (IV) service before the home care era. We stocked butterfly needles, 20 ml syringes, and normal saline to start IVs for continuing tobramycin doses at home. We did auditory monitoring (no abnormal audiograms were observed) and urinalysis (infrequent and only transiently abnormal results) for those on aminoglycoside antibiotics. These recurring contacts brought us so much closer to our patients. We, as a team, had to create humor out of the seriousness of our daily professional life. Not only was Judy Palmer a distinctive member of our team, she also was the house staff member that Dr. Maria Valdes-Dapena decided to mimic at our St Chris graduation party. Dr. Dapena's outfit included the mini-skirt, the leather clogs, and the Californian style that Judy was known for. This portrayal was the best copycat and the most entertaining performance by an attending that evening.

Several experiences stand out in my memory. When we were recruiting children for the comparative sweat test study, several asymptomatic subjects or siblings were reported to have a normal sweat test at a community hospital, but were later diagnosed as CF when our tests were positive. In one situation, a family had adopted a child who subsequently turned out to have CF. Their second adopted child was included in the study as a control and was found to have repeated positive sweat tests. I had to confirm the diagnosis. On further questioning, the adoptive mother remembered an occasional rectal prolapse when the child was an infant.

During one of our clinics in Wilkes-Barre, I encountered a 25 year old well developed man with surgical scars from a previous appendectomy, gall bladder removal, and intestinal obstruction. He had fainting spells, especially in the summer while working in the laundry area in the basement of a non air conditioned building, a chronic cough, and moderate digital clubbing. An adult pulmonologist, who had trained at Temple University and had rotated through our CF program, had been consulted. He suspected CF and the sweat tests were indeed positive. Another case was of a husky teenage basketball player, who was referred by a nursing student who had rotated through our CF clinic. She observed that he had a productive cough and appeared to have clubbing of the fingers, so she convinced the mother to have him evaluated and his sweat tests were positive. We were encouraged that our educational efforts were effective.

We had gypsies in Philadelphia and a group of them had camped in the park immediately in front of the old St Chris located on Lehigh Avenue. One night they angrily waved lighted torches and shouted threats that they would set the hospital ablaze. We had to urgently summon our Chief of Pediatrics, Dr. Victor Vaughn, who successfully calmed them and was able to discover the cause of their fury. One couple in their group had only two children, a 4 year old boy and an 18 months old girl, and both had recently been diagnosed with fairly severe CF. The mother had received information about CF from tele-med about male sterility, without further explanation or counseling. The anger the group was expressing came from the mother's severe distress because she could not deal, at that time, with the issue of never becoming a grandmother by her own son. We learned to be most careful about when and how the facts of CF involvement are shared with or obtained by families, and to always consider cultural issues. It was our great fortune that Dr. Vaughn had the special talent to negotiate with the gypsies and quell their rage that night. This family stayed with us for another five years until they moved to California.

The Philadelphia Pediatric Pulmonary Disease Cooperative Program

This program played a significant role in my pulmonary training. In 1967, a National Institutes of Health grant became available to fund activities directed towards children's lung diseases. The Philadelphia Pediatric Pulmonary Disease Cooperative Program (PPPDCP) was organized when the four medical schools joined forces to acquire a sizable grant that would finance clinical and research objectives. The purpose was to train specialists in taking care of patients with chronic respiratory disease in infants and children. The collaborators were Dr. Huang of Temple University School of Medicine, Drs. George Polgar and Edward Sewell of the University of Pennsylvania School of Medicine, Dr. Giulio Barbero of Hahnemann Medical College of Philadelphia, and Drs. Herbert Mansmann and Loretta Finnegan of Thomas Jefferson University Medical School. CF was the most important chronic pulmonary disease in this study and had the largest population, with three CF Centers (St Chris, Children's Hospital of Philadelphia [CHOP], and Hahnemann) in the same city. Most adult CF patients were at Hahnemann. Asthma and respiratory allergies (mainly Dr. Mansmann's patients) and neonatal lung disease (Dr. Finnegan) were included but there were not many neonatal patients then.

The grant participants included nutritionists, social workers, physical therapists, and respiratory therapists from the participating institutions. Donna Mueller was the nutritionist from St Chris CF Center. She later earned a Ph.D. in nutrition and was very active in the training and education of nutritionists at the annual National CF Foundation meetings. Jan Tecklin, the physical therapist involved with Dr. Holsclaw in the Hahnemann CF Center, conducted educational seminars on airway clearance methods. The PPPDCP was a gigantic experiment in collaboration. Erlinda M. McCabe administered the program as secretary-treasurer. Meetings of the program were eventful, sometimes turbulent, but generally peaceful. She was amazed at how collegial all the physicians were with each other. All were determined to make the project work. Philadelphia was truly the "city of brotherly love."

Dr. Polgar was the pulmonary physiology lecturer for pulmonary fellows and interested faculty. I recall trekking from St Chris to CHOP every Tuesday or Friday afternoon from September through May for a physiology seminar from 2:00 to 4:00 PM. Those who know Dr. Polgar would know that he would patiently teach us physiology in very physiologic terms, which delighted him. Most of us struggled through these lessons. Despite attentive minds, loud snoring and cessation of respiration were noted from several overly well nourished members of the group. This provided us a preview of what would later be labeled "obstructive sleep apnea." These lectures were conducted for several years until Dr. Polgar moved to Detroit in the 1970s. Dr. Huang stayed at St Chris to allow her fellows to take the physiology course. To provide practical aspects, Dr. Maria Delivoria-Papadopoulos allowed us to participate in her animal laboratory studies at the University of Pennsylvania.

The PPPDCP sponsored postgraduate pediatric lung seminars where the research findings of the pulmonary fellows and attendings were presented. It was at these seminars that our endobronchial lavage experience and other results were presented and the education of public health nurses and patients was conducted. This collaborative program was the setting for mutual exchange of results, comparison of epidemiologic data and informal expert consultations that would lead to a clinical paper on a rare disease or complication.

The Microbiology Laboratory

The CF microbiology laboratory performed bacterial colony counts, pseudomonas antibody titers, and so called phage typing of the staphylococcus and pyocine typing of pseudomonas strains. The phage type of the staphylococcus was fairly consistent within each CF carrier but the *Pseudomonas aeruginosa* organism proved to be very complicated. The pyocine typing was more difficult and also varied in the same patient at different times and we soon discontinued this test. Others adopted the Homma system to study the epidemiology of pseudomonas in CF patients. There was no other method then to distinguish the strains of *Pseudomonas aeruginosa* and we never had the facility or a specially trained biochemist to study these bacteria. Under Dr. Huang's direction, our routine lab procedure identified the bacterial agents and their susceptibility to common antibiotic agents, allowing efficacy study of each new antibiotic. We studied the minimal inhibitory concentration and the minimal bactericidal concentration against the staphylococcus and/or pseudomonas and other pathogens and also the serum and bronchial levels of each antibiotic given intravenously and by aerosol routes. We gained knowledge on each antibiotic relative to the changing morphology of the pseudomonas, such as rough to mucoid form in relation to the duration of administration of each agent, the rate of progression of the disease in each patient, and whether the strains were antibiotic sensitive or resistant.

The microbiology laboratory made possible the study of pseudomonas carrier rates in patients with CF, members of their families, and caregivers. This study was prompted by epidemiologic questions raised during the plan to open our ICU and tracheostomy unit where some children with CF who had a tracheostomy would be admitted along with fragile surgical patients. We showed that siblings with CF may have the same or different pyocine types, and that CF caregivers who do not have CF do not acquire pseudomonas from the CF patient. Furthermore, none of the CF patients carried pseudomonas in the nose, a likely source of spreading when an organism like pseudomonas is present there. Repeat pseudomonas cultures from the same CF patient were often of the same pyocine type, but no single specific pyocine type was predominant in our patient population. Antibody titers to the pseudomonas also were determined.

We also found that most antibiotic agents available then were effective against bacterial pathogens of CF patients. The most effective method of antibiotic administration was the combination of intravenous and aerosol routes. The dosages we used were according to the susceptibility pattern of the organism. We also monitored the side effect of each antibiotic but, along with others, we could not determine why the bacterial pathogens were so difficult to eradicate in CF. The prevalence of pseudomonas in the sputum cultures of CF patients increased with age and the incidence of mucoid strains also increased with age. Occasionally, we encountered a CF patient whose predominant bacterial pathogen was *Klebsiella ozanae* or mucoid Klebsiella species, which were equally as persistent as the pseudomonas. In the 1970s, *Pseudomonas cepacia* (now called *Burkholderia cepacia*) slowly emerged as the prominent bacteria in the sputum culture of patients with more advanced disease. We observed and reported how rapidly most patients who grew *P. cepacia* died and how antibiotic resistant these organisms could be.[6]

We studied carbenicillin in 1968 and found the major disadvantage was the very large dose that was required for intravenous administration. While the resulting excessive sodium load and obligatory excretion may also cause low blood potassium, we did not encounter adverse effects and used it frequently. At the pediatric residents' graduation party in 1969, they presented a skit profiling Dr. Huang holding a gigantic syringe labeled "Carbenicillin" that was attached to a long needle ready for administration to someone labeled "CF." This produced a great uproar of laughter. We appreciated the residents, as they were vital to the accomplishing of our research projects.

Then we were fortunate to have ticarcillin become available since it is two to four times more active than carbenicillin and the therapeutic dose is smaller, so it became preferred for the treatment of *Pseudomonas aeruginosa* infection in the mid 1970s. Shortly thereafter, azlocillin, which is 10 times more active than carbenicillin against *Pseudomonas aeruginosa* and piperacillin, which is similar to azlocillin, became more popular than carbenicillin. The aminoglycosides, principally gentamicin, tobramycin, and amikacin also became available in the 1970s. These rapidly acting bactericidal agents are synergistic with the penicillin derivatives and were used effectively in combination in our studies. For our advanced CF patients, we searched for another method of relieving airway obstruction. In the 1950s Dr. Robert Denton, an anesthesiologist from the University of Pennsylvania and stepfather of two CF children, published his studies on continuous nebulization in bronchopulmonary disease.[7] This was preceded by work with large capacity metal nebulizers and the two studies provided the basis for the use of mist tents in CF. Later, he published his work on the lung mucus in CF [8] and his observations on the use of N-acetylcysteine (Mucomyst[R]) as an aerosolized agent used to thin mucus. With

Dr. Polgar, he studied the lung function of adults with CF and the physical properties of their bronchial mucus.

We then developed a procedure called endobronchial lavage (EBL) through a bronchoscope using a solution of the N-acetylcysteine agent and sodium bicarbonate. We had a cooperative otolaryngologist, Dr. Myles Turtz, who had great respect for Dr. Huang's "infallibility" about CF matters. He performed the bronchoscopy, assisted by the chief anesthesiologist, Dr. Bernard Mayer. The thick mucus blocking the larger airways was suctioned away first and then the smaller airways were lavage with the solution using a volume of 20 ml for small infants to 400 ml in the young adult patient. We soon accumulated data from over 100 procedures in this therapeutic trial. Patients were referred from all over the nation, hopeful of more time added to their lives after removal of the thick mucus. Following EBL, aerosols, physical therapy, and postural drainage were performed every 2 hours for the first 8 hours and every 8 hours in the subsequent 24 hours before returning to the usual treatment schedule. Although the patients reported feeling and breathing better and they had lower respiratory rates, they did not improve in pulmonary function. It was a horrendous experience to watch these advanced CF patients vigorously coughing post lavage, even after aggressive airway clearance methods had been administered, in order to clear the volumes of thinned mucus that still needed to be expectorated. However, their subjective improvement and desire to have the procedure repeated encouraged us to perform more EBLs. This therapeutic modality should have been studied prospectively in a double blind controlled study and we planned a systematic study but were unable to carry it out. It was difficult to draw conclusions retrospectively. The main objections to EBL were the invasive nature of the procedure and possible anesthetic side effects. The pulmonary function parameters used to assess improvement or deterioration may not have been the proper ones to support the subjective reports. We compared our lavage experience with Dr. Lucas Kulczycki, then Director of the CF Center in Washington, D.C., and Dr. Jonathan Randolph, the pediatric surgeon, who performed the lavages there. Our experiences were comparable.

To aid mucociliary clearance, chest physiotherapy and postural drainage were used. A father with two sons with CF from our Center decided to connect a mechanical drill to a plumber's plunger and used this as a mechanical percussor. He could adjust this machine to a low, medium or high frequency and for years this family used this equipment until the advent of more quality controlled percussors. The children reported the converted drill to be just as effective as manual chest clapping.

Antibiotic studies for effectiveness and toxicity continued to be the main focus of our research and involved tobramycin by intravenous and/or aerosol routes and other antibiotics. The highest tobramycin serum levels resulted from the combination of aerosol and intravenous therapy. Later fellows had additional projects including the evolution of pulmonary disease in CF from the newborn period, and the adolescent with CF and CF pregnancy by Dr. Palmer, who later worked with Dr. Douglas Holsclaw at Hahnemann and then she moved to the CF program at Stanford Children's Hospital. Dr. Panganiban studied exercise capacity in CF school children. We collaborated on viral and mycoplasma infections in CF with Dr. Ada Deforest. Dr. Helen Keith was interested in genetics and constructed pedigrees in a large number of CF families. We dealt with an enormous amount of data, including the pulmonary function data collected by Luba Baboychuk, during that pre-computer age when we studied the day to day variability of lung function in our patients. Dr. Shirley Braverman was most helpful with her collaboration in the statistical analysis. With Dr. Hiller, we completed a study of total lung capacity compared to radiologic measurement of the chest. Dr. Nasira Yasmin completed the tobramycin aerosol project with us.

On completion of my fellowship in 1971, I was proud to be appointed the Associate Director and attending physician of the CF Center at St Chris, director of the pulmonary function laboratory, supervisor of the sweat test laboratory, and Assistant Professor of Pediatrics at Temple University School of Medicine.

Dr. Daniel Schidlow became a fellow in 1975 and inherited most of the unfinished studies. When I moved in 1977, Dan succeeded me as the attending physician in the Pulmonary Division and then became the Director of the St Chris CF Center when Dr. Huang retired in 1979. He has successfully maintained the national and international place that St Chris occupies in CF history.

New Jersey

I moved to New Jersey in 1977 to start the pediatric pulmonology division at Thomas Jefferson University of Philadelphia located at Our Lady of Lourdes Hospital in Camden. I gradually increased the CF clinic population to 33 patients, most of whom were transfers from the St Chris CF clinic. My first newly diagnosed CF in Camden was an 8 year old who presented with constipation! And I had several patients who were referred because of a falsely positive sweat test. The geographic location of this CF clinic became problematic as it was right across the Benjamin Franklin Bridge from Philadelphia where three CF centers were located. Soon after, when the University of Medicine and Dentistry of New Jersey at Rutgers Medical School in New Brunswick opened a Department of Pediatrics, I was recruited as the pediatric pulmonary director in 1980. New Brunswick is about 60 miles from Philadelphia and was undergoing a massive rebuilding and architectural expansion with the entrance of the Johnson and Johnson Company in this city. The New Jersey turnpike at Exit 9 and the railroad station at the foot of the small hill to the hospital made transportation easy for patients from all parts of New Jersey. Dr. Huang, by then retired from St. Chris, and I started a CF clinic at the university affiliated hospital, Middlesex General Hospital, which was renamed the Robert Wood Johnson University Hospital when Rutgers Medical School was renamed the Robert Wood Johnson Medical School in 1986. By the tenth year, over 80 patients were registered. Dr. Bayard Coggeshall, the pediatrician directing the CF clinic at Morristown Medical Center, transferred his patients to my care when he retired. In addition, with early diagnosis due to meconium ileus or recurrent bronchiolitis, more mild and moderately ill patients were referred, leading to improving patient survival, decreasing morbidity, and increasing patient numbers. Our CF team consisted of a nurse practitioner, nutritionist, social worker, pulmonary function technician, and respiratory therapist. Support in part was through a New Jersey Special Child Health Services Grant from the Department of Health. Meanwhile, the asthma and other non-CF diagnoses patient numbers were increasing, so the program flourished. For a number of reasons, pulmonary problem patients became so frequent that by 1998 there were 22 pediatric pulmonologists practicing in New Jersey. Our CF program is now the largest university based service in the state and is an accredited CF Center by the National Cystic Fibrosis Foundation.

The Cystic Fibrosis Centers

Dr. Barbero was a medical student at the University of Pennsylvania in Philadelphia from 1943 to 1947. His subsequent pediatric residency and gastroenterology and nutrition training were interrupted by two years of Army duty with a MASH unit in Korea. While there, he helped establish a children's hospital in Pusan that is still providing pediatric care. After joining the faculty of the University of Pennsylvania School of Medicine, his gastroenterology interests led him to develop a program of care for CF patients at the Children's Hospital of Philadelphia (CHOP) and he was the leader of CF efforts in the area. He developed a close relationship with Dr. Graub, a pediatrician and parent of two CF children, and became very active in the growing national CF medical program. He was the 5th Chairman of the Medical Advisory Council of the CF Foundation, following Drs. Shwachman, di Sant'Agnese, Patterson, and Matthews. During the period of time Dr. Barbero was at CHOP, Dr. Huang was developing the program at St Chris. When Dr. Barbero moved to Hahnemann Medical College and Hospital of Philadelphia as Professor and Chairman of the Department of Pediatrics in 1967, he added his young CF patients, to the older CF patients there. The Hahnemann program became the third CF Center in the city and had the highest young adult population. He subsequently recruited Dr. Douglas Holsclaw in 1972 to direct the Hahnemann Center. Dr. Holsclaw had worked in Boston with Dr. Harry Shwachman, with whom he published studies on meconium ileus, hemoptysis, and other clinical papers. Dr. Barbero was a most articulate and eloquent speaker, a very dedicated and caring physician, a motivator, and a great humanitarian. Beyond his gastroenterology research activities, he was interested in the psychosomatic aspect of disease and the impact of chronic illness on the etiology of depression. Dr. Barbero left Hahnemann in 1972 to be the Chairman of the Department of Pediatrics at the University of Missouri-Columbia School of Medicine. In 1996, he was honored with the third Joseph Levy award for his contributions to CF, following Drs Francis Collins and Dr. Paul Quinton. Dr. Barbero died in 1997 at the age of 74 years.

Dr. Victor Rivera, a former pediatric GI fellow at Hahnemann in 1972, recalls one occasion when Dr. Barbero, who was always most solicitous, had to drive him home after 11:00 PM as the trains had stopped running. This occurred because Dr. Barbero had completely lost track of time while talking to a family during evening rounds, as he did not wear a watch. He was nicknamed "Brother Barbero" because he preached about end of life issues in CF. Dr. Barbero used slides from art museums to depict CF, such as oysters in still life.

Dr. Maarten Sibinga worked with Dr. Barbero in the CF program at CHOP. Their research interests were in electrolyte abnormalities in CF, in sweat gland and parotid gland physiology,[9] stool enzymes,[10] and in catecholamines with Dr. Lee Braddock. When Dr. Barbero became the Director at Hahnemann, the CF population at CHOP was split with Dr. Barbero's patients following him and Dr. Sibinga's patients followed him to St Chris, where he directed the Pediatric Gastrointestinal Division. Dr. Sibinga recalled the wonderful years at St Chris beginning in the fall of 1965. Work was exciting and research on sweat gland and parotid gland physiology stirred much interest in the CF arena. When funding for fellows in gastroenterology decreased, he extended his clinic hours to his home. He was one of the first to use home hyperalimentation and was available all hours to his patients. So parents would not need to miss work, he scheduled them on weekends and evening hours. With Drs. Huang and Friedman, he studied attitudes toward hospitalization and laments the fact that managed care has changed much of the individualized care that we used to be able to provide.

Dr. Sewell and Dr. Polgar reorganized the pulmonary aspect of the CF clinic at CHOP before Dr. Polgar went on sabbatical in 1972. Dr. Mary Loretta Rosenlund, a gastroenterologist, took over from the late 1960s to the mid 1970s and was later assisted by Dr. Thomas Scanlon from San Francisco, who became the Director in the late 1970s. Dr. Polgar continued his pulmonary clinical role until he moved to Detroit to become Pulmonary Division Chief and CF Center Director.

While Dr. Polgar was busy on sabbatical, Dr. Holsclaw helped provide coverage for the CF clinic at CHOP. He also consulted at the Harrisburg Polyclinic in Hershey until the CF clinic became organized there. The Hahnemann CF Center was fortunate to have Jan Tecklin as the physical therapist who contributed much to adult care by improving airway clearance techniques. Pulmonary fellow, Dr. Christa Habbousche, and nurse, Diana Kracycky, ably assisted Dr. Holsclaw. With his fellows, he presented clinical studies at the CF Club and published reports on hemoptysis and other pulmonary complications and genital abnormalities in CF.[11] He was active in the CF Foundation, especially as Chair of the Professional Education Committee. He worked with a very slim budget but he managed to publish the CF Bibliography despite the lack of computers and retrieval technology then. This effort included reports from all languages, which further increased the difficulty of completion, but it was a useful resource document and a true labor of love. He was well rewarded when he met Anne Topham who was sent by the CF Foundation, then in Atlanta, to help him with his work and by 1976 they were married. The Quarterly Annotated CF references came from his desk too. He lobbied strongly for the Pennsylvania Adult CF program in the late 1970s. He was proud of the success of this work especially as it soon led to similar important programs in other states.

The St Chris CF Center was the largest of the three and was ranked among the top ten in the country. It was not until the Center was funded by the

National CF Foundation in 1961 that Dr. Huang could acquire a secretary and a fellow. The Center stood at the top third in number of patients with the cumulative survival rate of patients at St Chris being better than that of the national combined survival statistics. We were fortunate to have superb professionals and support staff who were very dedicated to the cause. Foremost among these were the pulmonary fellows, and Donna Mueller, nutritionist, nurses Janet Kramer and Paulette Liberi, psychologist, Dr. Esther Cava, and the social workers, and physical and respiratory therapists. Dr. Cava supported the patients, their families, and the CF staff in our day to day coping with CF care and end of life issues. The Philadelphia Chapter of the American Lung Association recommended that Dr. Huang offer a pediatric pulmonary fellowship as she had the largest group of patients with pulmonary diseases other than CF.

The CF service at St Chris was always busy. Often we would have thirty inpatients besides outpatients and research activities. During rounds, we followed Dr. Huang closely as she moved very fast and we could lose her. Several times we ended up in the restroom, as she could be too preoccupied to announce to us where she was headed.

The CF Foundation looked up to Dr. Huang's experience in CF care. Her aggressive management of the blocked airways led to use of endobronchial lavage, direct instillation of gentamicin intratracheally for tracheotomized infants and children, the use of colistin by intravenous, intramuscular, or aerosol routes, and use of various inhaled antibiotics. We had some patients who required removal of a lobe of lung when the disease was localized only to one lobe. Our cardiothoracic surgeon, Dr. Francisco Niquidula was most careful in accepting for lobectomy only those who were expected to have good remaining lung function postoperatively. Fortunately, only a few with liver cirrhosis needed a surgical blood vessel shunt. Our pediatric surgeon, Dr. Samuel Kresson, was meticulous in operating on newborns with meconium ileus.

Due to Dr. Huang's expertise in CF, she was requested to chair the Drug Committee of the National CF Foundation 1969 to1972 by the Medical Scientific Director, Dr. John Herndon. She invited Dr. ChunI. Wang, Director of the CF Center at Children's Hospital in Los Angeles, and others to serve on the committee to write a reference text *Guide to Drug Therapy in Patients with Cystic Fibrosis* for the Center Directors and their staffs. This was very effective and served, with some modifications, for many years.

On November 8, 1973, Dr. Huang was awarded the Annual Service Award by the American Lung Association of Philadelphia for her leadership and devotion to the care of children with lung disease. Among those who attended were Dr. Waldo Nelson, fondly called "the old man," who mentored Dr. Huang, Dr. John Kirkpatrick, chief of radiology at St Chris, nursing faculty, administrators, pulmonary fellows and the rest of the CF team (Figure 25.1).

The three CF Centers in Philadelphia contributed to the basic science, and clinical and behavioral research in CF. We recognized the enemy and targeted

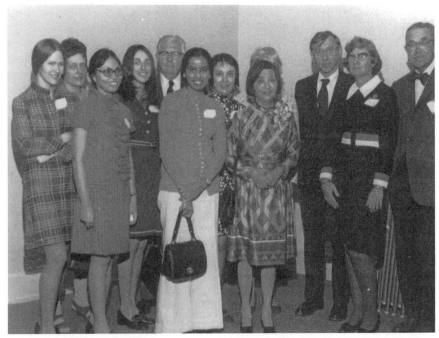

Figure 25.1. *Special guests at Dr. Huang's retirement party in 1979, from the left, front row, Drs. Judy Palmer, Lourdes Laraya-Cuasay, Nasira Yasmin, and Nancy Huang, and Joanne Welsch, R.N. Back row: Susan Saunders, R.N., Sharon Segal, P.T., Charles S. Strickler, Administrator, Adamadia Deforest, Ph.D., Dr. Hope Punnett, geneticist (hidden behind Dr. Huang), Dr. John A. Kirkpatrick, Jr., and Dr. Waldo E. Nelson. Courtesy of Dr. Nancy Huang.*

different goals to aim for improvement in the quality of life of CF patients and their families, and ultimately for a cure. We were committed to hard work and long hours with great compassion towards our patients. We were very available to them and all of us remained very hopeful for increased longevity as we added more to each patient's life and tried to buy added time for them by various therapeutic modalities.

We recognized the clinical heterogeneity of CF and its multisystem effects. We challenged the median survival age that was initially less than a few years, then later improved to teens and beyond. We hated the disease because of the suffering that it gave to the person with CF, the parents and siblings, and all relatives and individuals touched by someone with CF. Together, we were one big CF family that rose to the great challenge of searching for a cure. Inside each of us was the acceptance of the inevitable while ministering to the dying. We were fortunate then to live in an era prior to high technology. Once the decision was made that death was imminent, we held the patient's hands, we called family members who needed to be at the bedside, we gave the patient the permission to let go of life, we paved the way for the last "I love you" and "I forgive you," and we kept a quiet vigil until the journey was over.

Before the hospice era and when the survival age was only up to mid teens, we had one or two deaths, sometimes every two to three months. This was a most difficult time for the hospital staff, parents, and families. Back then we separated the terminal patients and gave them quiet and peace in a separate private room where the families could say their good byes, reminisce however much they wanted, and experience family living as best as was possible without interfering with nursing activities. I recall one time when Dr. Huang was on vacation and we had two simultaneous deaths occurring in different floors. In my exhaustion and deep sense of loss, I instinctively returned to my office by way of Dr. Lawrence Naiman's office and almost immediately fell into his compassionate embrace. Dr. Naiman was the chief of the Hematology-Oncology Division and was well versed in support of staff when a death occurs, as mortality in childhood cancer was very high then. He listened quietly as I expressed my grief and I listened as he shared his losses too. This helped serve as some degree of closure for both of us. Trainees now will never know how it was when CF was such a gloomy disease to deal with and it was especially hard when the patients were so much younger. However, courage and strength of heart came from all those experiences that afterwards drew the CF families closer to us. Many friends that I have now are the parents of those whom I cared for almost thirty years ago. And that gypsy mother who had two children with CF had some uncanny knack of asking at clinic, "Where is so and so," and more often than not she would be correct that the person she asked about would have passed on. This mother would take on a maternal and very supportive role and she would then be comforting us and urging us to keep on working against this monster disease. Such parental support from her and many others kept us at this mission. Many of these children had an inner sense of when they were actually near death. Many planned their own funerals and several that I have cared for asked to return home to prepare themselves and their very important stuff. Their eyes betrayed what they were thinking. And we let them go so they could make their wishes known to their loved ones and be honest with their relatives, if the others were strong enough to handle the information. Oftentimes, just sitting with the family and talking of the good times made the pain more bearable. Mostly supportive care and being just there for them was most important to these families. Yet how did we do it with all the other work we needed to do for those who had more life ahead of them? We managed somehow and without the number of faculty and staff that the present academic world requires.

For myself, participation in Dr. Huang's long term study and learning about CF at St Chris has been most rewarding, with satisfaction and enjoyment. The patients with CF and their parents were a unique group of people and most were highly intelligent and compliant in following our complicated therapeutic regimen. Naturally, there were exceptions who were challenges to us and gave us learning opportunities. Each patient was different and had to be treated individually. It was challenging to manage their disease and deal with their varied personalities. To give good care to all patients and to conduct a good clinical research project required a well planned protocol, patience, perseverance, and long term vigilance.

Although CF remains an incurable disease, the advances in diagnosis and treatment are making great strides and patients live longer. Almost one third are young adults who live a mostly normal adult life. Gene therapy and pharmacologic advances continue to be investigated. We are encouraged with the progress in CF and hope its cure will come in our lifetime.

References

1. Denning C, Huang NN, Laray-Cuasay LR, Shwachman H, Tocci P, Warwick W, and Gibson L. "Cooperative study comparing three methods of performing sweat tests to diagnose cystic fibrosis." *Pediatr.* 1980;66:752.
2. Sproul A and Huang NN. "Growth patterns in children with cystic fibrosis." *J Pediatr.* 1964;65: 664.
3. Huang NN, Macri CN, Girone J, and Sproul A. "Survival of patients with cystic fibrosis." *Am J Dis Child.* 1970;120:289.
4. Kuo PT, Huang NN, and Bassett DR. "The fatty acid composition of serum chylomicra and adipose tissue in children with cystic fibrosis of the pancreas." *J Pediatr.* 1962;60:394.
5. Huang NN. "The flora of respiratory tract of patients with cystic fibrosis of the pancreas." *J Pediatr.* 1961;59:512.
6. Laraya-Cuasay LR, Lipstein M, and Huang NN. "Pseudomonas cepacia in the respiratory flora of patients with cystic fibrosis." *Pediatr Res.*1977;11:502.
7. Denton, R. "The clinical use of continuous nebuiization in bronchopulmonary disease." *Dis Chest.* 1955;28:123.
8. Denton R. "The role of lung mucus in cystic fibrosis." *Ann NY Acad Sci.* 1963;106:751.
9. Sibinga MS. "The sweat abnormality in cystic fibrosis of the pancreas." *Amer J Med Sci.* 1966;252:732.
10. Barbero GJ, Marino JM, Seibel R and Sibinga MS. "Tryptic and chymotryptic activity of stools as a diagnostic tool in the pancreatic insufficiency of cystic fibrosis." 1965;11:787.
11. Holsclaw DS, Perlmutter AD, Jockin H, and Shwachman. "Clin Chem H. Genital abnormalities in male patients with CF." *J Urol.* 1971;106:568.

26

Center Directors Remember: Minnesota

Warren J. Warwick, M.D.

The two clinical giants, Drs. Harry Shwachman and LeRoy Matthews, and research oriented Dr. Paul di Sant'Agnese dominated all aspects of cystic fibrosis (CF) in the 1960s and 70s. The infrastructure of the Foundation was in place before I came on the scene. My role during those two decades was that of a follower of these leaders, usually as an activist promoting one or the others ideas and occasionally as a go between when they were in opposition.

Harry Shwachman, a humble man with great pride in his work, took advantage of the prestige of Harvard Medical School to collect and care for the largest number of patients with CF ever assembled (Figure 26.1). He saw more patients with more CF related problems and knew more about CF than any physician of his day other than Dr. di Sant'Agnese. Where any physician might have seen one or two complications, Harry would have seen 10 or 20. Harry had a strong analytical capability and was able to make judgments that have proven true decades after his retirement and death. Two examples come to mind. First, Harry knew that about two percent of patients with CF will repeatedly have a normal or borderline sweat test. He recommended repeating the tests until there was a positive test and then to stop. Second, Harry said, when patients have bacteria that are resistant to all antibiotics, prescribe erythromycin, leave them on it for a long time, and they will do much better.

LeRoy Matthews, a physically small man, had giant ideas and the powerful personality to make people believe these ideas. He came to CF because a Cleveland group of parents of patients with CF asked him to do something about the way their children were dying. LeRoy always saw directly through a problem to the resolution. He saw that malnourished patients were dying from pulmonary problems and decided that a preventive approach, using all available therapies, could prevent or significantly delay the progressive pulmonary complications. Through the success of his work and the force of his personality this program brought a new generation of young clinicians and researchers into the CF field and, for good or bad, shifted the CF Foundation's focus from Gastroenterology to the development of Pediatric Pulmonology as a new discipline.

Drs. Paul di Sant'Agnese and Giulio Barbero were another effective pair that did not get headlines. Paul was, in my memory, one who would often settle a

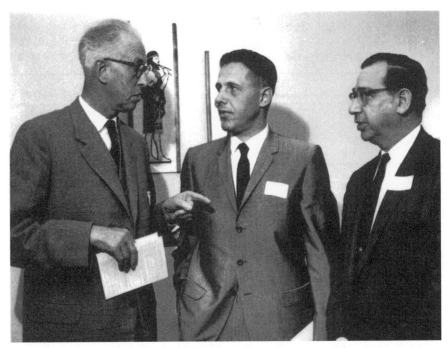

Figure 26.1. *Left ro right, Dr. Guido Fanconi, Switzerland, Dr. Milton Graub, President of the CF Foundation, and Dr. Harry Shwachman, Medical Advisory Council President, 1964. Courtesy of Dr. Milton Graub.*

question in hot debate by quiet, carefully thought out analysis followed by his recommendation. When Paul wanted to do so, he often had the last and the conclusive word. He initiated little but he guided much through his leadership. Giulio also never raised his voice but he was usually the one to start a project on its way and continued to guide the project to a successful end. He was often a counselor to the younger members of the Medical Advisory Council and was equally as effective as Shwachman and Matthews in dealing with the CFF Board and Officers. He could tell you no and make you feel all right.

Early Contacts with CF

While I became a CF physician quite by accident, I have enough clear memories of contacts with CF in the years before I became a CF Center Director to almost believe in fate. As a junior medical student in 1953, I impressed the most brilliant teacher I worked with, Dr. Robert A. Good, by making the diagnosis of CF in an infant named Tony M. I met Tony again in the pediatric outpatient clinic in 1957 when I was a resident at the University of Minnesota hospital. I remember seeing Tony not doing well, my prescription of tetracycline, his distinct improvement, and my feeling of satisfaction.

One of the highlights of my career in the pediatric service of the United States Army, 1957-1959, was making the diagnosis of CF by wrapping a patient in a plastic bag and collecting a test tube full of sweat for analysis. I returned from the Army to work with Dr. Good in the study of transplantation and rabbits. Then in 1961, I jumped at the chance to see patients again. I was to have my own clinic to take care of 16 patients who had CF. I also had a budget of 15 thousand dollars a year, courtesy of Dr. Kenneth Landauer, Medical Director of the NCFRF, who was developing a network of CF Centers for Care, Teaching and Research.

Tony finally and really became my patient when I became Director of the new Minnesota CF Center. As a pre-teenager he had the classic CF syndrome: growth retardation, malnutrition, a potbelly, a barrel chest, clubbed fingers, chronic productive cough, chronic bronchitis, and recurrent pneumonia. Despite the best that I knew to do, Tony got worse and I admitted him to the hospital because there was no treatment that could be done at home. I remember the afternoon when Tony asked me to stay with him that night because he was afraid that he would die. I didn't stay. He died.

The lesson I learned from Tony I have never forgotten. If you claim the privilege of taking care of patients with CF, you have the responsibility and privilege of taking care of them until they die. Since then I try always to be with the patient and the family during the hours when the patient's life ends. I learned much from patients and their families during these hours. The unexpected bonus has been that only once in forty years has a family ever refused my request for a postmortem examination. The families have joined me in trying to find an answer to the question "CF, why?" I believe the lessons I learned from these postmortem examinations played an important role over the years in making survival at the Minnesota CF Center the best in the United States.

The National Medical Advisory Council and Center Program

The critical step made by the Foundation was the hiring of Dr. Kenneth Landauer from the March of Dimes Foundation where he had helped the development of care centers for patients afflicted with polio. His task was to do the same for patients with CF. By 1961, Dr. Landauer established 17 CF Centers funded by the NCFRF, the Medical Advisory Council to the NCFRF, and the CF Center Committee. Thus the direction of the NCFRF was set. All funds raised were to be used to improve treatments and research for a cure for CF. Education of doctors and the medical and the paramedical community was the second priority. Funds were not to be used for patient care except for clinical studies to improve treatments. Harry Shwachman was the leader of the Medical Advisory Council and LeRoy Matthews was head of the Center Committee.

When Ken Landauer set up the CF Center program he had two principals in mind. First, that CF research needed to be done by CF Centers that took care of

318 Cystic Fibrosis In the 20th Century

CF patients and that CFF money could not be used for patient care. Second, the money from the CFF was to be unrestricted to be used by the CF Center Director to develop new research as opportunities developed. That philosophy led to advances in CF research and an increase in the number of researchers associated with the CF Centers.

The few years I spent as a member of the CF Center Committee were the most exciting in my active years with the CFF. LeRoy taught all the members of the Center Committee how to do a good site visit, to look at medical records, the research in progress and planned, how to look for weaknesses to correct, and how to find good projects to encourage. One recommendation that I made in Philadelphia still gives me much pleasure. While visiting the three CF Centers there, I pointed out how they could work together to get one of the Pediatric Pulmonary Centers then being planned. They took my recommendations and were funded. Another aspect of the CF Center Committee is mentioned in the "Then and Now" section.

Concurrently there was rapid development of CF Clinics around the country with many satellites to the CF Centers. Soon the CF Clinics out numbered the Centers by a ratio of 3 or 4 to 1. Then the CFF decided to make all the CF Clinics into CF Centers. The result was a great increase in the funding of the former clinics and an even greater drop in the funds for the original CF Centers that had demonstrated research potential.

This change was good for CF care but disastrous for research in most of the original CF Centers. At the Minnesota Center, this meant being unable to support new ideas brought to my attention by other doctors and researchers who were seeing CF patients in the clinic and hospital wards. None of funds for the Minnesota CF Center have ever been used for support of the Director; all CF Center funds have been directed to clinical or basic research support. For us, and likely at most of the original CF Centers, only those who had developed CF research grants from prior collaboration were able to continue actively with CF research. New research ideas were not explored because we had no exploratory money to test a new idea.

In addition, this meant that graduate student participation in CF research projects almost vanished. Since we also lost funds to supplement the salary of our sweat test technician, we turned the sweat test back to the hospital laboratory until it missed two diagnoses due to laboratory error. Eventually we worked out other means of supporting the sweat test laboratory. But much freedom for seizing new research opportunities never returned. In the past decade under the leadership of Dr. Robert Beall, Ph.D., new research funds have been made available to some of the CF Centers but these funds are dedicated to special goals. Fortunately the funds supporting the CF Centers continues to follow Dr. Landauer's second precept, they continue to be unrestricted.

Early in the Landauer years, I became a member of the CF Center Committee and of the Medical Advisory Council (MAC). I served for several years and helped establish the positions of "Founding Father" for Drs. Harry Shwachman, Paul di Sant'Agnese, and Paul Patterson. I also co-authored a Nutritional Guidebook for CF with Dr. Nancy Huang. My last contribution was to create the Collaborative Study Committee as part of the MAC. Several collaborative studies were started including the first study of Pseudomonas vaccination. The Collaborative Study Committee did not survive my departure from the MAC.

Those were interesting, heady and busy years. I worked closely with Harry Shwachman, LeRoy Matthews, George Polgar, Alexander Spock, Gunyon Harrison, Budge McKey, Nancy Huang, Paul di Sant'Agnese, Paul Patterson, Giulio Barbero, Carolyn Denning, Will Waring, Jack Docter, and Gordon Gibbs.

I have special fond memories of the two great stars:

Harry Shwachman had an absolute memory for everything he had seen and made many astute clinical observations that I wish I could remember today. If he had a weakness, it was in not being able to make the best judgments about experimental studies.

LeRoy Matthews, the greatest genius CF has seen, single handedly established the value of Comprehensive Treatment, laid the ground work for Pediatric Pulmonology, and organized and led the CF Centers as well as planning and directing excellent research. He made only two mistakes. He allowed his "Comprehensive Treatment" plan to be equated to "mist tent therapy" so when the mist tent was discredited many also felt that Comprehensive Care Program was discredited. And he tried too hard to control his diabetes and suffered hypoglycemic brain injury, and cardiovascular complications.

All the rest of us, whatever our contributions, and we made many, stand deep in the shadow of these two giants.

Diagnosis

Concerns about the diagnosis of CF were very prominent in the early years of the CF Centers. In Minnesota, our sweat tests were still done with home made equipment and colorimetric titration by the physicians since the hospital laboratory did not want to take on a test that was not standardized, and which took a lot of time and equipment. The hospital laboratory was more interested in analyzing the duodenal aspiration of pancreatic secretions and that test was our primary diagnostic tool. We hated it because of the time required and the discomfort it caused our patients.

During these early years we did improve the sweat testing technique and published our protocol for the Gibson-Cooke test. However, we still experienced the need for another diagnostic type test when the sweat test was questionable. We wanted one based on anatomical pathology. We obtained biopsies from the labial mucous salivary glands; the collection of the specimens was much faster than the sweat test and almost painless. Larry Meskin did the pathologic studies and Burton Shapiro did biochemical analysis looking for a metabolic defect. After a three-year NIH grant, we found the pathology to be present in almost all patients, specific for CF before age 14 but not specific after age 14. For several additional years, it was useful to help make the diagnosis in difficult to diagnose patients.

Leland Hansen, the research scientist for the CF Center, worked with me to develop a chloride electrode sweat test after we saw the report on use of a sodium electrode for the analysis of sodium on the surface of the skin of CF patients. We started our work in a hot Minnesota summer and found good success, but when the colder weather of the autumn came, the test no longer worked. We then developed thermal stimulation of sweating using 1/2 kilogram aluminum cylinders heated to 104 degrees Fahrenheit. The aluminum cylinder was covered with Parafilm™ and held on the forearm for 5 minutes. The test worked well and with a recording tape we demonstrated stable readings for 10 to 15 seconds thus obtaining a permanent record of the standardization of the electrode and the results of each sweat test.

We used the test to screen all students in grade schools in 12 Minnesota cities but found no undiagnosed patients with CF. Never the less, the publicity given to these screening programs helped the Minnesota CF Chapter increase its fund raising in the rural areas. The publicity also attracted Jane Brody to write a medical science article which received national attention and helped start her long career as one of the country's leading medical science writers.

We also used this technique to successfully sweat test newborn and even premature infants and presented a demonstration at the Chicago meeting of the American Medical Association. Mary Buechelle, our sweat test technician, and I received a "best display award" for our presentation advocating the future use of the chloride electrode for screening newborn infants for CF. The high point of the use of the chloride electrode was the screening of almost all children living in the Canadian Province of Prince Edward Island by Dr. Terry Gillespie, who successfully identified all the known CF patients and one that had not been diagnosed. Joanne Koroshec, the lead nurse for the screening project from our CF Center, went to Nova Scotia to supervise the project. She fell in love with and married a medical student and has never returned.

The test was being tried in quite a number of places and advertised by the Orion Company. Harry Shwachman invited Mrs. Buechelle and me to come to Boston to demonstrate the technology. Harry determined that it might be tolerated but in his work, unfortunately, never used a recorder to obtain a permanent record of each test. About the same time, sweat testing with conductivity was becoming popular and the CFF initiated a multi-center study to compare the three tests. The results showed the Gibson-Cooke test to be about 1% better than the chloride electrode and about 3% better than the conductivity sweat tests. Based on that slim difference the CFF decided to recommend only the Gibson-Cooke test for the diagnosis of CF. We continued to use both techniques doing one each on both arms, for a total of 4 sweat tests, for the diagnosis of CF. We required that all four tests must agree and that all positive tests must be repeated on a later date before accepting the results as confirming the clinical diagnosis of CF.

Along the way, Leland Hansen and I worked with the 3M company to develop a patch for the diagnosis of CF. This patch had 4 test strips, one to signal that enough sweat had been absorbed and the other three to change color at specific sweat chlorides, 20, 45, and 60 mmol of chloride. This patch never made it to market.

Later we worked with the Medtronic Company developing the semi quantitative CF Indicator System (CFIS) sweat test. Some of the innovations Hansen and I had developed were incorporated into the CFIS patent, but we never received credit for our contributions. Hansen and I worked another 10 years developing a true quantitative patch as accurate as the Gibson-Cooke test for sweat testing. Work under progress could result in a patch that would be quantitative for newborns.

In the 1960s and 70s, we made interpretation misjudgments of some of the sweat test results. I recall telling some patients with, what I would now call "clinical CF," that they could not have CF because their sweat test results were always less than 60. I should have listened more closely to Harry Shwachman who said over and over that CF is a clinical diagnosis that is confirmed by a positive sweat test. I have lived with Harry's counsel ever since.

Because of our large population of patients and many families with multiple children with CF we were active contributors of serum from these patients and family members to researchers trying to find the CF gene. Almost all (96%) of these volunteers have now been genotyped revealing that the reliability of gene typing for the diagnosis of CF remains significantly less than that for the standard sweat test. This provides proof that Harry Shwachman was right in stating that CF is a clinical diagnosis that needs laboratory confirmation. Now we can use a number of laboratory techniques besides the sweat test.

From Mucoviscidosis and Cystic Fibrosis of the Pancreas to Cystic Fibrosis

In the early days of CF, the major focus was on CF as a pancreatic disease with incidental, often fatal, lung infections as complications. During this period the mortality rate of CF was high and ranged from 15% to 25% per year. Diagnosis was made by proof of pancreatic insufficiency and treatment was focused on controlling the frequent stools, improving nutrition, and treating the pulmonary infections when they became obvious. In 1957, LeRoy Matthews decided to institute Comprehensive Treatment for his CF patients, i.e., he prescribed all available pulmonary therapies, along with all the other treatments then used, starting as soon as the diagnosis of CF was made. He then continued the program, especially the pulmonary treatments, on a continuing basis at home even though the patients were otherwise deemed "well." The result was a marked decrease in the annual mortality rate to about 2% per year.

In various reports and publications, he and Dr. Carl Doershuk, who had joined him, showed, through this "comprehensive treatment program," that long-term survival was to be expected and that survival to adulthood was only a matter of long-term application of this approach. The emphasis on CF as a pulmonary disease with a potential for good health and long term survival met with disbelief and doubt, followed by accusations of, if not intellectual fraud, at least poor record keeping. Fortunately, the CFF had approved a grant to Minnesota to set up a United States CF Patient Registry to develop knowledge about CF prognosis (see CF Database below). I believe the doubters wanted the database to prove Matthews and Doershuk wrong. However, an extensive review of their patient charts and the database confirmed their reports. The idea that CF was a lung disease that could be better managed began to grow.

During the American Thoracic Society (ATS) meeting in New Orleans, Will Waring, George Polgar. Mary Ellen Avery and I met at the Waring home where I proposed the formation of a Society for Pediatric Lung Diseases. Dr. Avery's feeling was that pediatricians interested in lung disease were too few to make such a society work and that we should instead focus on becoming part of the well functioning ATS, carried this unofficial meeting. Eventually George Polgar carried out part of the goals we discussed at that time with the formation of the journal *Pediatric Pulmonology*, for which he was Editor In Chief for a decade.

Unfortunately the idea that CF is a lung disease has become so strong that the true picture has been almost lost, despite the discovery of the CF gene. In fact, CF is biologically a disease of the cell membrane where the cystic fibrosis trans-membrane conductance regulator (CFTR) protein resides and serves as a chloride channel and a regulator of water transport across the cell membrane. This is the only site where CF gene therapy can work. Since all of the clinical manifestations of CF are acquired and none is unique, clinical CF can, with equal validity, be termed a gastroenterological disease or an endocrine disease.

Thirty years ago, with the foundation of the University of Minnesota's Clinical Research Center, we started a project to understand the propensity patients with CF had for developing diabetes mellitus. This work, led by Dr. Frederick Goetz, failed but the project led to one publication which showed that the clinical worsening we observed in CF patients with diabetes began as early as 5 years before the diagnosis was made. Dr. Antoinette Moran has since taken up the project and now the Minnesota CF Center is the lead center in trying to understand this phenomenon in which we now have more patients with abnormal glucose tolerance tests than we have with abnormal pulmonary function tests.

Once we saw that the deaths due to lung complications could be decreased using the Matthews Comprehensive Therapy approach, Dr. Harvey Sharp, our first gastroenterologist with the Minnesota CF Center and I wondered what would be the cause of death when patients became adults. Liver disease, most likely cirrhosis (the scarring seen frequently in the liver), seemed the most likely disease to kill patients in the future. We started a prospective study of the development of liver disease by obtaining annual liver biopsies. This study was stopped after three years as we saw that the biopsy specimens showed that the liver became healthier as the patient's nutrition improved.

The CFF saw the need to develop better care for patients with CF and other childhood lung diseases. It was active on a number of fronts seeking to train CF Center Directors in this area to evoke an interest in CF and children's lung diseases in pediatricians around the United States. For about 5 years the CFF produced literature and sponsored conferences on Pediatric Lung Disease. The Minnesota CF Center presented one of the larger of these conferences. The result, *Chronic Lung Disease in Children*, was published as a special edition of *Minnesota Medicine* and republished and widely distributed by the Mead Johnson Company as, perhaps, the first book on pediatric lung disease. Another success of the CFF was the incorporation of 10 Pediatric Lung Centers as part of the Cancer, Heart Disease and Stroke program. The Minnesota CF Center was selected to be one of these centers but the Minnesota CHDS supervisory board did not accept the funds because a Pediatric Lung Center did not fit into their plans.

Inspired by George Polgar's book, *Pulmonary Function in Children*, we worked with the Hennepin Country American Lung Association and the school district of Bloomington, Minnesota to do a large study of pulmonary function in children ages 5 through 18 years. At the time, these were the largest numbers of normal and healthy children tested for pulmonary function. These data, published in *Minnesota Medicine*, have not been widely used despite the large data set.

While the subspecialty of Pediatric Pulmonology was still years in the future, I received a 10 year grant from the NIH to train pediatricians in research concerning children's lung disease. My contributions concerned pulmonary function and the lung disease associated with CF, asthma and the immotile cilia syndrome. Joint investigators with me were Dr. Robert A. Good, my mentor in Pediatrics, whose focus was Immunology and Dr. Paul Quie, whose focus was infectious diseases. Altogether we trained one CF Center Director, two Pediatric Pulmonologists, one Medical Director of a tuberculosis hospital in the UK, three academic Immunologists, and three failures who became cardiologists.

During this time Jeffery Budd worked with me to develop an effort-independent pulmonary function test using a mixture of oxygen (21%) and 79% argon to wash the nitrogen out of the patient's lung, followed by having the patient breath room air to wash the argon out of the lungs. We monitored the breath-by-breath changes in oxygen, carbon dioxide, argon, and nitrogen during the washout and wash in of nitrogen and were able to show significantly better identification of early lung disease than we could with standard spirometry. We were successful with testing children as young as 14 months and saw no methodological problems with testing infants.

We recommended that the National Heart Lung and Blood Institute of the NIH create an advisory committee to establish standards for pediatric pulmonary testing and recommended the leaders who might form such a study group.

While this did not happen, we were most satisfied when committees were formed by the American Thoracic and the European Research Societies. They included all the physiologists and physicians we had recommended. Our continuing progress with our tidal volume breathing technique brought both Jeff and me to membership in the *ad hoc* committee of the ATS for setting standards for infant pulmonary function testing and I also participated in the international consensus agreement. This tidal volume breathing test is still under development, failing thus far to catch up with the advances in technology for computers and mass spectrometers. When operational, this test should provide an effort-independent test, very sensitive to developing lung disease at all stages of lung damage for subjects from birth to old age.

Despite the problems patients with CF have with gastrointestinal and endocrine complications, the majority of our patients with CF associated morbidity have pulmonary problems as the major cause. Never the less, the median survival (actuarial) age based on CFF Registry data has reached 39 years and, as of June 2000, we have over 60 patients who have reached the age of 40 years. As a result, we believe that the CF community should begin to think of starting a project to look for the geriatric complications, which will accompany aging in CF patients.

Home Monitoring

The idea of home monitoring for early identification of new complications, or the worsening of present complications, originated when the Minnesota CF Chapter had its offices in one of my laboratories at the University of Minnesota Medical School. The first home monitoring began as an industry-sponsored study of a nutritional supplement. Participants in this study were, as part of the treatment protocol, to do daily measurement of weight and pulmonary function plus recording of symptoms. These reports were sent regularly to the CF Center for collection and analysis. The arrangement with the sponsor was that they would do the analysis in order to reduce the direct costs of the study. Unfortunately, due to changes in management and company priorities the analysis we wanted was never completed. From that experience, we learned to be wary of permitting anyone else to analyze the data from a University research project. Never the less, we were able to rescue enough of the data for a graduate student in hospital administration to complete a Master's Degree thesis on the potential of home monitoring for maintenance care. Stanley Finkelstein and I used this data as the basis for our well published, longer term study demonstrating the value of home monitoring as part of the management of clinical CF disease.

The rigorous effort required for home monitoring has precluded our incorporating the method into our CF care program, except when we have had grant funds to support the concept. However, we did inspire the first home monitoring spirometer and the creation of the first company to market the use of home monitoring pulmonary function for care of asthma and monitoring research. Home monitoring is still ongoing at the University of Minnesota in the Lung Transplant

Program. Recently, in keeping with the philosophy of simplicity in design and effectiveness in detection of changes in lung disease, Leland Hansen and I have recently received a patent on a new concept for measuring and monitoring lung function. This new spirometer measures the time that airflow rates are in excess of three specific airflow rates. Early studies suggest that it can detect changes twice as effectively as the peak expiratory flow or the forced expiratory volume measurements. This greater sensitivity may make early detection of changes in lung function much more efficient. If so, then home monitoring may rise again for CF care.

Airway Clearance

Airway clearance therapy was taught to our nurses and physiatrists by a physical therapist from Belgium. The effectiveness of manual chest physiotherapy was regularly demonstrated by our trained nurses who would take a CF child, referred with untreatable fever, into the treatment room and do manual chest physical therapy while I would do the patient and family history. The patient's temperature wound drop dramatically to normal with just one full treatment and would not return while airway clearance therapy was practiced on a regular basis.

Dr. Justin Wolfson, our Pediatric Radiologist, and I set out to demonstrate how bronchial drainage (BD) worked by making a fluoroscopic motion picture of BD moving mucus out of the airways. Our Belgian Physiotherapist did the BD. No mucus moved during the therapy. We had a good demonstration of mucus vibrating back and forth in the airways but always remaining in the same spot. That is, until the patient coughed. With the cough, the mucus moved dramatically, outward bound. Since then, directed coughing has been part of our practice and teaching of manual airway clearance.

We imported the PEP mask shortly after it was developed, studied it in careful detail and decided that it was not as effective as our BD therapy. We also did a three year study, sponsored by the University of Minnesota Hospital, of intrathoracic percussion as a technology that might reduce the cost of hospital care for patients with CF. That treatment was less expensive but also much less effective and so was dropped as an alternative treatment.

In teaching coughing, we emphasized discovering times for coughing that would not embarrass the patient, i.e., coughing at a time when others are used to hearing someone cough. Examples are the "echo cough" that can be done after another person coughs, and the "telephone cough" that is done, as if to clear the throat, before answering the phone or while waiting for the phone to be answered. More recently, cough teaching has emphasized avoiding coughs that do not stop, and practicing a yawn to total lung capacity then slumping to compress the intrathoracic air followed by coughing.

When Dr. Malcolm King showed that high frequency chest wall oscillation (HFCWO) would move mucus out of the airways of intubated and ventilated dogs, an international race started to develop a vest that would do the same for CF.

Using funds donated by Umberto Marzotto, Leland Hansen and I developed five different versions of a vest that did just that for his daughter, Annalisa Marzotto, who was a patient at the Minnesota CF Center. Eventually this technology was patented by the University and licensed to the American Biosystems Company and sold as the ThAIRapy Vest™. The vest technology has proven to be the most effective way to remove mucus from the lungs of patients with CF and many other lung diseases. The company has since modified the vest, the ABI Vest^R. Leland Hansen and I have recently developed another vest with a changed waveform for which a patent application has been made and a manufacturer found. It may reach the market in 2002 as the third vest. When three HFCWO vests are on the market, we hope to see a reduced cost of this superior airway clearance therapy.

Databases

In the early days of the CF Center program, the CFF's request to Centers for data about the patients cared for were questions such as, "What was the average age of your patients?" "What percent were hospitalized?" "What percent died?" I think most of the Center Directors hated this type of questions because, when I suggested, at the Academic Pediatric Society Meetings in Seattle in 1964, a change in questions so that national statistics could be calculated, I was immediately appointed to do the job for the next year. I developed a one-page questionnaire to be filled out for each patient seen at each Center. The questions included the patient name by the three initials, date of birth, birth complications, date of diagnosis, height, weight, number of hospitalizations, number of days in the hospital, sweat test results, vital capacity, date of death, cause of death, and a few more.

These questions were answered quite well by the smaller Centers, less well by the larger Centers. The complete data were eventually obtained by many letters and telephone calls and were tabulated for a report the next year by my secretary Marjorie Stepek. At the next CF Club meeting we received new directions. The questionnaire had to be simpler and patient and CF Center confidentiality had to be preserved.

Richard Pogue, Ph.D., my computer associate, and I developed a one-page form for each patient which, after the first year of preparation, could be completed simply by inking in just one circle. Each CF Center was given a Center number known only to the CF Center Director, to my secretary, and to my computer associate. Each patient was given a unique patient number, not the social security number. These forms were optically readable and were scanned onto a magnetic tape for computer analysis.

This system worked very well and the CFF funded the database for ten years with about an average cost of $10,000 per year. We were able to do this through the donation of computer time by the University of Minnesota Computer Center and Dick Pogue's *pro bona* services. At the same time Marjorie Stepek was a genius at obtaining work study students to augment her stellar efforts in managing all the data sheets, correcting errors, and communicating with individual Centers.

The program was so well received that all the Canadian CF Centers decided to participate. We analyzed their data separately and reported their data confidentially to the individual Canadian Centers and collectively to the Canadian CF Foundation just as we did for the US CF Centers and the CFF. Some individual CF Centers from Australia, Sweden, and England also sent their data to be analyzed in our database program and several more explored the concept of an International CF Patient Registry.

One of the factors that led to the establishment of this ten year annual grant from the CFF was the desire of some of the early leaders in CF to prove that LeRoy Matthews was a fraud in claiming to have reduced the annual mortality of CF by some ten-fold in his patients. When the Patient Registry data showed that the annual mortality of the Cleveland CF Center was indeed less than 2% per year, they engineered a conference in Philadelphia to show that the statistical studies done in Minnesota were incorrect. A leading life insurance actuary, Cecil Nesbitt from the University of Michigan, was asked to evaluate the questions, the technique of handling the data, and the statistical approach. The conclusion of the conference was that the Minnesota reports were accurate. Cecil did recommend that an alternative statistical analysis had some theoretical advantages and that we should switch to the "force of mortality" analysis. His diplomatic recommendation satisfied everyone with out changing any of the data reports.

I believe that the confidential reports to the CF Center Directors about the survival of their patients was the force that led the CF Centers to accept, however reluctantly, some form of Matthews' Comprehensive Therapy Program for CF. After all, if, when the CF Center Committee made its regular site visit, you could boast if your survival rate was better than the US average and would do so. If the survival rate was less than the US average then you would not, and might wonder how this might affect the CF Center Committee's analysis and recommendations for funding. To improve would suggest having to do something like Comprehensive Therapy.

After ten years of grants funding the United States CF Patient Registry and indirectly supporting the Canadian CF Patient Registry and beginning an International Registry, the CFF decided that the Registry should become the property of the CFF. When the CFF took over the operation they discovered what a bargain the $10,000 grant was. After spending over $100,000 and still not finishing the analysis, they decided to give up the analysis as too expensive. They were shamed into doing the analysis when the Canadian CF Foundation provided the funds and manpower to complete that analysis. The fallout was that the Canadian CF Foundation went its own way and the beginning international CF Registry was abandoned. All the data from the first ten years of the US patient registry, including the magnetic tapes, were transferred to the CFF where they were somehow lost.

One of the many interesting findings reported from the data analysis of the first ten years was that the survival of patients with CF was similar to that of an acquired disease, since the 50% survival from diagnosis was the same regardless of the age of diagnosis.

After about 1970, Jeff Budd worked with me to set up a patient care database for the Minnesota CF Center. That database served as the basis for a CF database program that Stephano Ceri, PhD, of Milan Italy developed and which was presented at two CF meetings in the US. His database was distributed to several dozen CF Centers around the world but never became a standard, in part due to failure of Ceri to maintain and upgrade the program to the needs of its users. The leadership that Minnesota has played in the development of clinical database utilization for CF led to my presenting, in 1983, the keynote address at the Israel CF meeting on the subject of the CF Database. The nature of all databases is that they are never perfect, and they are never finished. That continues to be the state of the CF Patient Care Database at Minnesota.

The Minnesota Center, Chapter, and Midwest Region

The great excitement and enthusiasm that erupted in the Minnesota Chapter of the CFF with the foundation of the Minnesota CF Center started a long close relationship. During these years I attended every meeting of the Chapter and all donations to the Center were passed through the Chapter's books to improve the local and national status. In addition, when funds were scarce I arranged for office space in one of my laboratories for the Chapter Director and secretary, justified by our close association and the local funds that aided our research. The idea of home monitoring came out of this close association. When times became better and a new Director was hired, the Chapter moved off the University Campus. The Minnesota Chapter also funded the publication for local circulation of the *CF Guidebook for Diagnosis and Management of CF* which went through five editions in the 1970s and 80s. The fifth edition appeared for a short time on the Internet.

This close relationship continued. When the Minnesota CF Center had a massive cutback in funds due to the expansion of the number of CF Centers from about 30 to about 120, the Chapter was concerned about the funds for our productive research and training program. As a result, it decided to help the Center raise local funds for research. The CFF leadership however intervened and the funds raised locally for the Center were deducted from the amount allocated by the CFF. These local funds could have maintained our research and training program. I protested unsuccessfully, although I knew of other CF Centers that maintained their programs through direct local support, and thus came to be at odds with the CFF. Coincidentally, I was never again invited to serve on any committee of the CFF and for 15 years the Minnesota CF Center never received any research funding from the CFF.

Encouraged by the CFF, the CF Center Committee, and the Minnesota CF Chapter I made many efforts to set up satellite CF Clinics. The first attempt was in Fargo, ND. Dr. Larry Pray came to the University and worked with me for an entire month learning what I knew about CF at that time. Back in Fargo, he did set up a CF Clinic but promptly left for California never to return. Not another pediatrician in Fargo or Moorhead was interested in directing a CF Clinic and the attempt failed. I had a second failure in Duluth, Minnesota trying to find a pediatrician to run a CF Clinic.

However, I was successful in setting up a very effective CF Clinic in Sioux Falls, South Dakota, directed by an anesthesiologist. That clinic did well until he left the field and for over a year I flew there once a month to run an all day clinic. This preserved the program until another physician became interested and became the Center Director. Another success was in Bismarck, North Dakota where the two hospitals were competing to have the CF Clinic for that state. I site visited and considered the two hospitals presentations. I chose the smaller hospital where an anesthesiologist, Dr. Morgan, and pediatrician, Dr. Margaret Morgan, worked as a husband and wife team. They developed a superb program and, having recently retired, have transferred their work to a combined Pediatric and Adult program at that Center. I also made site visits to the Mayo Clinic and the Medical School in Iowa City, where CF Centers were being established.

The Center was also very active in education. For two decades we ran annual Continuing Medical Education (CME) courses for physicians, nurses, school nurses, etc., on the diagnosis and treatment of CF, and eventually on all childhood lung disease. One of the latter courses was published as a Special Issue of *Minnesota Medicine* (Sept 1969) and was titled "Chronic Lung Diseases In Children and Adolescents" and later republished by the Mead Johnson Company under the same title as, perhaps, the first book on pediatric lung disease. This program gradually disappeared when the CFF funding of CF Centers changed (see above). The climax of these CME courses was held May 7–9, 1981 under the title "1000 Years of Cystic Fibrosis." In this course, we tried to bring together all the CF Center Directors from around the world who had cared for CF patients for over 20 years, since many of them were older and were soon to retire. We estimated that these 40 professors would have combined over 1000 years of experience with CF that needed to be recorded. The charge I gave each was to talk on a subject of their choosing. The result, an unprecedented depth of perspective and knowledge, was published in a limited edition as the *Collected Papers* later that year. It is perhaps of interest that sponsors included many pharmaceutical houses, the International CF [Mucoviscidosis] Association, the National Heart Lung and Blood Institute, and the Fogarty International Center. The United States CF Foundation chose not to be one of the sponsors of this event.

One interesting happening occurred. I chose Dr. Jack Docter, the Director of the Seattle Center and Chairman of the CF Center Committee, to be the opening speaker and Harry Shwachman to be the last speaker. Harry was angry because he felt, as the leading CF doctor in the world, that he should start the program. He was somewhat pacified when I explained that the last speaker had the "Point Of Honor" and that every one would stay to hear him speak. I was delighted to see that did happen. Everyone came, with bags packed, stayed till they had heard what Harry had to say, and most left promptly. Harry was pleased and proud that everyone stayed to hear him give the last presentation.

Perhaps the greatest compliment that can be paid to the organizer of a one time conference is that every year for the past 20 years I have been asked by one or two of the doctors who attended, "When are you going to do another 1000 years program?" I am thinking of doing one on "The 1000 Faces of CF." The speakers would be limited to those who have cared for 1000 or more patients with CF and balanced by the researchers who are trying to understand the nearly 1000 gene mutations that produce the acquired clinical CF disease. Time will tell if this gets done.

Minnesota and the World

For me, and for most of the North American CF physicians, the 1968 International Cystic Fibrosis [Mucoviscidosis] Association meeting in Grindelwald, Switzerland was our first exposure to the world of CF clinicians and researchers outside of North America. I used the trip to visit CF doctors in Oslo, Stockholm, and Copenhagen before and London after the conference. I met Dag Skyberg, Hans Kollberg, Erhard Winge Flensberg, and Archie Norman at their cities and in Grindelwald.

I made one small contribution in Copenhagen where the Gibson/Cooke sweat test was modified by heating the site of pilocarpine iontophoresis with a hair dryer before applying the gauze to collect the sweat. The sweat chloride values obtained were about 10 times the values usually reported. In return I learned from Flensberg of a graphic way to chart the clinical course of CF patients so that the entire history of disease and prescribed cares could be observed in a few moments. I modified this approach back in Minnesota and it provided an early inspiration to develop our computerized patient care database.

At Grindelwald I was most impressed by the quality of the CF caregivers and researchers and determined to learn as much as I could from them. Most of my North American colleagues were impressed with how far the European research was behind our American research and decided to do little with Europe. I encouraged Dag Skyberg and Hans Kollberg in their efforts to establish CF Associations in Norway and Sweden. Hans followed with organizing the First European Working Group meeting in Stockholm. I attended that meeting and each of the next dozen meetings and got to know most of the leaders in European CF research. Perhaps through these contacts, Minnesota became a stopover place for CF researchers from around the world. Almost monthly, during the years when I was an audible advocate of "Comprehensive Care" and the organizer of the International Cystic Fibrosis Registries, we received international travelers interested in CF care and research. I was twice a speaker for the UK Cystic Fibrosis Trust.

Probably because of these contacts I was invited to make a six-week tour of CF Centers in Australia in 1973. I visited all the CF Centers except the one in Perth. One incident, particularly memorable, occurred in Adelaide where Helen Caldecott, a trainee of Harry Shwachman, was prevented from starting a CF Center because the local pediatricians assured her that they, individually, were doing just as well or better than the CF Centers elsewhere in Australia. I asked for the

dates of birth, diagnosis, death, and current age of surviving CF patients and calculated life table survival over one night. The survival rate of the CF patients cared for
by the individual pediatricians was significantly worse than that reported by the
established CF Centers. Armed with this data, Helen was granted the chance to
form the Adelaide CF Center.

Then and Now

It is useful and occasionally amusing to consider the changes concerning CF that
have occurred during 40 years I have worked in the field.

THEN we argued about what to call the disease; cystic fibrosis of the pancreas, diffuse exocrinosis, mucoviscidosis. We knew that CF was a fatal autosomal
genetic disease with no hope for a cure.

NOW we wonder whether CF is one disease, or many diseases, or even if
is a disease, or, if it is a disease, when it becomes a disease. We know of a thousand
mutations all of which alter the cell membrane and all of which are compatible with
a normal life IF the acquired clinical complications are avoided by chance, or by
comprehensive therapy, or eventually by some form of treatment of the cell membrane malfunction.

THEN the patients were infants and children with little expectancy that
they would survive to be teenagers or adults. They were sickly, malnourished,
plagued by chronic coughs, and often pampered and spoiled because they were
about to die. Colleagues would tell us to "Let them die, in the long view it's better
for everyone."

NOW we have patients who are doctors, nurses, teachers, university professors, religious leaders, businessmen and women, founders and owners of companies, lawyers, farmers, and mothers and fathers. We have patients who are planning
their retirement. A miracle not conceivable forty years ago! Now we have the need
to prepare geriatric physicians to care for the acquired old age complications of CF.

THEN we had Billy Graub's and Giulio Barbero's *Guidance, Action and
Projection (GAP) Conferences* to review what was known about CF, to bring clinical
knowledge and questions in association, and to project possible futures for CF care
and research. All of this with the positive goal to interest and recruit basic scientists
to think about and to do research on the problems of CF.

NOW we have consensus conferences to consolidate and agree on the best
of past efforts to ensure that CF care is standardized and with the occasional effect
of intimidating innovative new approaches to therapy.

THEN the CFF and the Center Committee was tolerant and supportive
of differences in thinking and approach. When, as one of the fiercest advocated of
"Comprehensive Care," my commission as Center Committee site visitor to Madison, Wisconsin was to find out why the Center Committee should fund a CF Center that was so out of phase with current recommendations. When I reported that

332 Cystic Fibrosis In the 20th Century

Chuck Lobeck had a valid thesis, that a CF Center should not care for CF patients but rather should act as a teacher for the patient's own physician by monitoring the progress of the patient once a year. Since we would never know if that approach was right or wrong if we did not support the Madison Center, LeRoy Matthews persuaded the Center Committee to increase the funding so that Chuck could study his thesis more effectively. While the Madison Center eventually joined the rest in providing direct care for CF patients, this support helped John Mangos to stay in Madison, to do excellent research, and become a national and international leader in CF care and research.

NOW the Center Committee has a Procrustean approach to deviant CF Centers. When I was Director of the Minnesota CF Center, we had the longest median survival age, with the highest average pulmonary function and the best weight per age or height, with the largest percentage of adult patients, with fewer funds and fewer team members than the Center Committee recommends. Despite these achievements, since we did not have an adult program that met the prescribed format, the CF Center Committee voted to put the Minnesota Center on probation. Perhaps, if LeRoy Matthews had then been in charge of the CF Center Committee, the Committee would have sent more money both to foster the good results and a team to find out what we were doing and how we were doing it. Perhaps then to learn how an integrated continuity program could do so well by following the guidelines Nobel Prize winner Alexis Carrel set forth in his book *Man The Unknown*, "...physicians who know [*a patient with CF*] both in his parts and in his entirety, physically and mentally [*from infancy through adulthood*], are capable of understanding him when he is sick [*and of prescribing to prevent him from becoming sick again*]."

THEN the CF medical community was close knit and those working in the field were most supportive of each other. We knew personally and sometimes quite well all those in CF in the United States. This was fostered by the annual meeting of the CF Club at the Academic Pediatric Societies meeting. This close knit community was most active in promoting new ideas and supporting the investigators. For example, when Alexander Spock needed blood samples to test his cilia dyskinesia theory many of us sent him blinded samples very promptly.

NOW the CF community is a large aggregation of many scientific and clinical communities. Instead of a hundred physicians meeting for a day, we have thousands meeting for several days. We have meetings within the CF meeting for respiratory therapists, endocrinologists, gastroenterologists, pulmonologists, pediatricians, geneticists, internal medicine specialists, cell biologists, and so forth. Now we know only a few of the people at the CF meetings. Giulio Barbero's dreams, of basic scientists working with the CF Centers to solve the CF problem, have come true! While we rejoice in the progress that could only have been made by by-passing the CF Club, the intimacy of the old days, when we knew everyone, has been replaced by many similar intimate groups of researchers working on each of the multitude of problems being discovered as CF-associated. What those of us from the past realize and rejoice in is that we are being passed over so that others will achieve our dreams of finding the cure for CF.

THEN every new idea had a day and all the CF Center Directors had a chance to influence the future. The CF Center Committee awarded CF Centers for innovation by increased funding to explore and develop new ideas. We gave these ideas away in hopes that someday working together we would find an effective treatment, maybe even a cure, for CF.

NOW many new ideas are hidden until each patent has been filed or granted. Perhaps because the CF Centers receive funding based on head counting and properly filled out CF Patient Registry reports, we have a different perception of who we are. CF researchers now protect new ideas developed with funds from non-CFF sources for the newly found goal of financial gain to promote their our own work. We in Minnesota are as bad as the worst with three patents; one on high frequency chest wall oscillation devices to promote airway clearance, one to improve the quantitative pilocarpine iontophoresis test, and one on a new spirometer for home monitoring of pulmonary function.

THEN the CF doctor was often looked at as Dr. Gloom or even Dr. Doom. Patients were expected to be sick and to die prematurely. Diagnosis of CF was a defeat for the family and accepted as a signal for the parents to have no more children. Patients could not eat normal food. Almost inedible low fat diets were prescribed because the pancreatic enzymes were weak. The community was sorry for these dying children and special events, such as Christmas parties with gifts for the children, were regularly practiced. Siblings suffered neglect and marriages often ended in divorce. A normal life, with college, dating, marriage, and a career was unthinkable.

NOW there is an organization of CF Adults. We expect our patients to be normally healthy, to go to college, to date, to marry, even to have a natural family and a successful gainful career. A model of majestic achievement accomplished by dedicated parents, families, and CF team members! But we still have doctors, nurses, school teachers, business leaders, insurance administrators, and even neighbors who do not believe what they see. For example, in May 2000, in a remote Emergency Room in Minnesota, a mother of a child with diagnosed CF was accused of "Munchausen By Proxy" (falsely labeling her child with a condition) because the child had no cough and was "too healthy to have CF." As long as what happened in that ER happens anywhere, we still have much to do and our accomplishments, however great as they are, are not enough.

THEN we fought clinical CF, the many patterns of acquired clinical diseases to which all people are susceptible, in a battle that could never be won.

NOW we have the second front opened and directed by Bob Beall of the CFF, where the risk factor has been identified. So many diverse approaches to treatment are being developed that, in the next decade, one might expect 3 or 4 or a dozen or more treatments that will cure the aberration of function in the cell membrane, which is inherited CF. Fortunate will be the patients diagnosed before they acquire clinical CF for the cure of the cell membrane problem will keep them well. But even those patients who develop clinical CF will be fortunate in that their risks of progression of acquired diseases will be no greater that the risk of progression of these diseases in patients without genetic CF.

THEN our personal heroes were mostly people we knew and were accessible to us. They were colleagues who usually were fighting the unknown "cystic fibrosis of the pancreas" along with us. Included were Fanconi, the collector of syndromes who independently identified the disease pattern; Dorothy Andersen, the wise pathologist who first defined and named the disorder; Sheldon Reed, the clinical geneticist who proved that CF was as autosomal recessive genetic disorder; Harry Shwachman, the gastroenterologist and the best student of the variability of CF who was always at hand when any CF caregiver or researcher needed assistance; LeRoy Matthews, who by teaching us how to care for the pulmonary problems (along with comprehensive care) of CF, laid the foundations for Pediatric Pulmonology; Charles May, who authored the seminal work on pancreatic enzymes; Paul di Sant'Agnese, the consummate scientist who identified the elevated sweat chloride which still is the most reliable anomaly associated with genetic CF; and Lewis "Pete" Gibson, the researcher-pediatrician who showed us how to efficiently diagnosis CF using pilocarpine iontophoresis. These heroes were true flesh and blood people who we knew and could interact and collaborate with.

NOW we have almost too many public heroes as we near the solution to this formerly grim "disease", to get to know. These, our second millennium, heroes, are remote leaders of organizations or teams of researchers with whom only a few CF Center Directors and fewer CF Team members have that same kind of personal knowledge and relationship. Two of the most approachable and effective of today's heroes are Bob Beall, the Scientific Director and President/CEO of the US Cystic Fibrosis Foundation, who is creating the organizational structure that will eventually find the cure for CF, while still attempting to know and appreciate the efforts of all CF Center Directors. The other is Francis Collins, one of the co-discoverers of the CFTR gene and Director of the NIH Human Genome Project, who succeeds in making all CF caregivers and researchers feel like he is a member of their teams.

Most of all, I would like to applaud the unrecognized heroes of CF, the hundreds of CF Center Directors around the world and all their associates at their Centers. It is they who have struggled over the years to create hope when there was no hope, to fight death when death was seen as the only outcome for patients with the diagnosis of CF. It was they who fought for funds to care for patients with CF and to do research on their disease, who cared for CF patients when others recoiled from them, and who never gave up caring. Like the "doughboys" of WWII they are among the noblest of all. Those of us able to contribute to this book are dedicating our memories to all of these silent and unrecognized and wonderful HEROES. I applaud this book which recognizes the efforts of some of those who have worked during these forty years of the CF Center program. But I especially salute the unrecognized heroes of the past, present, and future who have worked, are working, and will continue to work for the caring of patients and families with CF, without hope of recognition or appreciation. They have worked with only the hope of an eventual cure for CF and when that cure comes, they will have their true reward.

27

Center Directors Remember: Cleveland

Carl F. Doershuk, M.D.

> Das Kind stirbt bald Wieder,
> dessen Stirne beim Kussen salsig schmect.[1]
>
> The child will soon die,
> whose brow tastes salty when kissed.

This early German folklore and its literal translation and lament, [2] tells us that even many years in the past there was an awareness of the condition we now know as cystic fibrosis (CF). In 1938, pathologist Dr. Dorothy Andersen expressed the term "cystic fibrosis of the pancreas" to differentiate infants at autopsy who had this pancreatic abnormality in association with characteristic pulmonary changes. This combination of findings clearly separated these infants dying very young from children with a strictly gastrointestinal disorder known as "celiac disease." Cystic fibrosis of the pancreas was later termed mucoviscidosis, chiefly in Europe, and is now accepted simply as CF. Over the latter portion of this century since 1938, there has been an incremental and dramatic improvement in diagnosis, knowledge of the disease, treatment, patient survival, quality of life, basic discoveries, and further basic research. When I entered Western Reserve University School of Medicine in 1952, CF was an almost unknown condition that would later become the major focus of my professional and volunteer life.

After graduation in 1956 and military service in the Navy, I returned to Cleveland in 1959 for pediatric specialty training at then City Hospital (now MetroHealth Medical Center). Dr. Frederick Robbins, who shared the Nobel Prize for his pioneering work at Harvard University with the poliovirus, was the Director. The faculty was excellent and included many who later headed their own departments. Dr. Robbins offered a bit of advice, known as "a pearl of wisdom" to his trainees. He advised having in writing, or at least in mind, a five year list of planned achievements and to review and extend the list annually in order to achieve personal goals and assess personal progress, advice that has served me well.

During my first year of pediatric specialty training, I participated in the diagnosis of a young child with CF who occasionally had pulmonary bleeding and also wheezing. The answer at that time to my question about her future survival was something on the order of, "Not very good." She will be referred to later, as we frequently met again. After being diagnosed, she was referred to a relatively new CF program at Babies and Children's Hospital (B&C Hospital). While I was away in service, Dr. LeRoy Matthews, a young faculty member at B&C Hospital, had been recommended as the one to start a comprehensive treatment program in 1957 for patients with CF. By 1960, he was reporting fairly impressive results. This program was a new development as CF had not been mentioned in medical school, had been covered only briefly in pediatric text books, and there were no CF patients admitted during my two month student rotation just a few years earlier. The faculty at B&C Hospital, headed by the Department Director, Dr. William Wallace, known for developing the flame photometer while at Harvard University, also included many faculty who went on to head their own departments. My training rotation returned me there for six months starting in July 1960 where I had first-hand exposure to the CF program, an experience that provided the major turning point in my medical career.

My interests in pediatrics were in asthma, pulmonary disease, pulmonary function, and care of chronic illness. The CF program was using aerosol inhalations from a nebulizer and compressor (new to me) instead of the hand held devices. Use of these devices was difficult for children because they had to coordinate their hand and breathing together and this was difficult to do effectively. There was also a treatment called postural drainage to help clear secretions from the lungs. Along with others, I had some initial reservation about how effective this treatment to the outside of the chest could be for a disease process deep in the airways. That concern was resolved most favorably as far as I was concerned, as described below. In any event, I could see an easy transition of the aerosol treatments to the care of asthma and other pulmonary conditions. Of further appeal, a state of the art pulmonary function laboratory had been set up and was busy doing clinical studies on CF patients.

There were quite a few CF patients around and it was evident to us in training that the comprehensive treatment program was improving the quality of life and survival for the patients, who, for the most part, were toddlers and young children. It was impressive that the nurses and various laboratory technicians involved were enthusiastic about the program and the clinical improvement they observed in the patients. By report, there had been no deaths in the first year of the program and only 2 deaths by 1960 among the patients entered on treatment, a significant decrease in mortality compared to that experienced prior to beginning the program. The improvements in survival and patient well being were a welcome change from previous local experience and national reports.

Consideration of subspecialty training in a combined asthma and immunology program after residency would again take me and my wife away from Ohio. Drawing on our experience together at Oberlin College and in Cleveland, versus the time away in service, staying in Cleveland with the CF program looked very good, especially since we had strong local family ties. This further specialty training was strongly related to my clinical interests. Like most residents, I had no significant research experience.

Dr. Matthews approached me about a two year fellowship and after some discussion I applied for a US Public Health Service pulmonary training position. The research portion was to design and build a total body plethysmograph (body box) for pulmonary testing of infants and young children, a method that was fairly new even for adults. When I returned to City Hospital for the remainder of my resident training, I learned of the offer and honor of being chief resident in Dr. Robbins' program. The faculty at the hospital was excellent and a further year with Dr. Robbins was very appealing. However, when the award of the training position as a Public Health Service fellow in pediatric pulmonary disease came through, I was eager to move on to the CF program, learn more about pulmonary diseases, and begin care of CF patients.

Fellowship

My two year fellowship began in July 1961 which was the beginning of the fourth year of the treatment program. There was a great deal to learn about pulmonary disease and especially about CF. The active participants in the program were Dr. Matthews, Dr. Sam Spector, an outstanding clinician and teacher, Joseph Potter, Ph.D., completing medical school and supervising the mucus research laboratory, and Joy Lemm, the chief technician. On the clinical side, Mrs. Lee Johnson performed the pulmonary function tests and collected the sweat test samples for chemistry laboratory analysis.

Research was new for me and took a lot more effort than the clinical work. While LeRoy, Dr. Spector and Joe pursued mucus biochemistry and other basic laboratory research projects, my assignment was to facilitate clinical research. The first task was to review what was written and known about total body plethsmography, which had been described for adults a few years earlier. My first project was to establish an infant-toddler plethysmograph (body box) test so that pulmonary function information in infants with CF could be obtained, for the first time, at early ages and hopefully early in life before CF lung symptoms became significant. The results of these tests would provide early detection and subsequent progression of the lung disease. The advantage of the plethysmograph test for infants was that multiple measurements of lung volume and airways resistance could be obtained in a few minutes without need for their cooperation. The second project would be to design and construct an older child-adult size plethysmograph.

There was no prototype for the infant box, so we had to design and fabricate the box and system, while trying to anticipate all potential problems. Older subjects and adults sit in an erect position and can cooperate with breathing instructions. The major technical problem to overcome was that infants and young children could not cooperate, would have to be in a supine (flat on the back) position, and would require some sedation. We used chloral hydrate for the sedation and it is of interest to me to note that pulmonary researchers using infant techniques developed in the past few years again use chloral hydrate for sedation and in about the same way we did back then. A mask would be held in position over the nose and mouth without air leakage and without disturbing the baseline breathing of the subject and the box had to be absolutely airtight at the time of each test measurement. Ultimately, we copied the small sized respirator used for child-aged polio patients in need of respiratory support that I had become familiar with as the senior resident on the polio ward at City Hospital. The unit had a bed-like frame that could be wheeled out for placement of the patient and then closed again. We planned to fabricate the box out of clear plastic, have the subject totally inside the unit when closed, and use a rubber oval opening on the side of the box for airtight entry of my hand and arm to position the mask. The plethysmograph technique was so sensitive to pressure changes that any air leak interfered with the testing. Conversely, even the small amount of body heat from the subject would increase the pressure in the box and invalidate measurements, so a fan for air circulation and a vent to be closed at the time of a measurement were required.

We were fortunate that Dr. Jerome Kleinerman, Chief of Pathology at nearby St. Luke's Hospital and internationally known as a pioneer in lung function studies in small animals, had a laboratory to fabricate the systems needed for his work. Dr. Kleinerman's design experience and his technician, who was skilled in metal working, plastic fabricating, and the various connections needed, were crucial to construction of the box. The advantage of the plethysmograph method was that many measurements could be made in just a few minutes, whereas with the standard helium dilution technique just one measurement required at least 3 minutes, and that was when the subject had normal lungs. The time for the helium test (Figure 5.1) was extended by many uncomfortable minutes when the subject had obstructed airways that develop in CF. In the patients with airways obstruction and over inflation of the lungs, a single helium test could take 5 to 7 minutes or even longer, and two tests were required as a check on reproducibility, a stressful and tiring test for many patients. Both they and we looked forward to the day when the state of the art plethysmograph testing was established.

My own 4 and 6 year old children were a great help by lying on the frame within the infant box so we could check the position of the side openings, the venting device, appropriate sensitivity of the pressure transducers, fan noise, and air leaks. With this preparation, the first small infant sedation and test seemed to go well. The calculation of lung volume was complicated, however, and required entering the cotangent of an angle from the oscilloscope, the pressure changes, and other data into a multi-step series of calculations, increasing the chance for error with each step. Now, with commercialization, these calculations are computer derived and pulmonologists do not have to deal with the computation although it is still good to understand the details. My calculation of the infant's lung volume was in the order of just 50 milliliters, a very small volume compared to the adult range of up to 3 to 4 liters. Consequently, I felt a bit tenuous in reporting such a small number and the other results to Dr. Matthews. However, my initial calculation proved to be correct and the infant testing program was underway.

Some of the young CF children had abnormal lung volume and airway resistance test results but had normal chest x-ray reports. During the time of sedation for the test, we became aware that the patients with abnormal test results coughed during the test even while sedated. Review of their chest x-rays revealed the presence of over inflation of the lungs despite evidence of early bronchitis. This correlation of clinical symptoms, an abnormal pulmonary test, and chest x-ray changes served to heighten our sensitivity to the significance of a clinical history of increasing cough and/or onset of night cough. The result was an intensification of pulmonary therapy for such patients.

The measured lung volumes of our normal subjects differed from the few reports then available. The availability of the oscilloscope enabled us to visualize each test in progress in real time and instantly observe any technical aberration or air leak improving our quality control and accuracy of each measurement. Previous studies of normal infants did not have an oscilloscope, so paper recordings of the pressure and volume changes had to be made after the test was completed, increasing the potential for error.

The main respiratory problem for the CF patient was air trapping behind retained secretions in the airways. Thus there was no need to use the intermittent positive pressure machine that was commonly used for adult asthma aerosol therapy. In CF, the pressure might push secretions deeper into the airways and further aggravate airway blockage and air trapping. Dr. Matthews had presented evidence to the national medical group confirming increased air trapping when positive pressure was used. Their recommendation was to use an inexpensive compressor to create the aerosol and allow the patient to inhale the aerosol normally. This aerosol treatment was more readily accepted by children, easier to use in the home setting, much less expensive, and soon preferred.

A study on older patients using standard pulmonary function tests to evaluate aerosolized Mucomyst[R] (N-acetylcysteine) to thin mucus was ending as I started my fellowship The spirometer data had to be calculated by hand from tracings, each patient had up to eight tests, and there were 30 plus patients in the study. The fellow did the calculations without knowing which therapy was given. There was a large backlog requiring me to quickly learn the calculations and I soon felt I could do them in my sleep. The study was well designed and carried out and some patients improved on the twice-daily nebulizations. However, the parents and patients could not see a clinical difference at home, and there did not appear to be a predictive factor to select patients who would benefit. The product was expensive, could irritate the airways, and smelled like rotten eggs, so neither the patients nor parents complained when it was not recommended very often.

The value of shared experiences between CF doctors became apparent to me early in my training. Dr. Gunyon Harrison from the Houston Center told LeRoy about an antimicrobial, colistin (Colymycin[R]) during one of the many trips they made for the CF Foundation in the early 1960s to enlist Center Directors. The recommended dose, only 0.75 mg per kilogram of body weight, was quite small and the dosage margin appeared to be narrow since there was potential kidney toxicity. After several patients had a course of this treatment, we did not observe improvement. I was nervous when LeRoy asked me to call Dr. Harrison, whom I had not met; however he was very generous with his time. He had increased the dose to 5 mg per kilogram body weight, and then found a beneficial response without toxicity. With this encouragement, we persisted, observed the same benefit, and were able to increase the dose somewhat more. We used this agent for many years for patients whose bacteria were resistant to other antibiotics, before resistance to colistin began to emerge. Years later, others also concluded that this agent was effective, especially by the aerosol route, for CF patients. We got an early start, thanks to Dr. Harrison readily sharing his experience with us. As a result, I always tried to emulate his model of taking phone requests from other Centers and physicians to freely share clinical information and experience during my own career. This is but one example of the many benefits that came from the CF Center network.

On the clinical side, there was much to learn about the many complications that can occur with CF and of the variety of symptoms that an individual patient may present at diagnosis. Poor digestion of fat in the diet was a problem for almost every patient despite a low fat diet and addition of pancreatic enzymes at mealtime. Many families came from a distance for outpatient checkups. They usually had to stop for a meal during the trip and, like most children, the CF child invariably wanted a hamburger. Parents frequently reported they brought along a supply of paper towels from home to pat excess fat from the hamburger. Without this precaution, the child would usually have abdominal cramps and need a bathroom stop well before reaching Cleveland and the appointment.

Then the availability of Cotazym[R] led to considerable improvement in the efficacy of pancreatic enzyme replacement therapy and fewer stool and gastrointestinal problems. Even so, it was still difficult for many patients to tolerate a high fat diet or even the normal fat diet that we preferred in order to help their nutrition. Later, when the more potent, stronger enzymes became available in reasonable sized capsules, it was an important milestone in treatment. The amount of fat in the diet could be increased with good tolerance. It was easier to maintain reasonable nutrition, with fewer bowel symptoms and only with a small increase in the number of capsules required per meal. However, since the amount of enzyme per capsule was now much greater, the total daily dosage easily increased to much higher levels. A number of young patients in the US and abroad were later reported to have a newly recognized injury to the large bowel requiring surgical intervention and even removal of at least a portion of the bowel. The cause or mechanism of injury was unclear but the cases seemed to occur in patients using the higher doses. To my knowledge, after dosage limits were established no additional cases were reported. This complication appeared to be another situation in clinical medicine where too much of a beneficial thing might become harmful. Fortunately, we did not have any patient develop this complication.

Effectiveness of Postural Drainage

Part of my clinical responsibility was to see 8 to10 CF outpatients every Monday AM. In setting up the comprehensive treatment program, Dr. Matthews did not, and we have not, relied on rotating medical students or house staff for the ongoing care of CF outpatients, except in a well supervised training setting. In dealing with this severe and complicated disease he felt it important to have continuity of care and more experienced physicians to provide the care (see Table 5.1). Details about use of antibiotics, enzyme replacement with meals, the use of vitamin supplements, etc. were soon mastered. It was especially rewarding to have time to further educate the families and patients about the disease and the opportunity to practice prevention with the goal of heading off some preventable complication. Specialized support staff did not exist then and considerable time was spent with each newly diagnosed or referred patient and family to educate them in all needed areas in order for them to be successful at home with the treatment program.

My reservations about how effective the postural drainage therapy, with the clapping followed by vibrations to the chest wall, could be were soon answered to my satisfaction. These treatments were hard work for the families at home and took a lot of time when done correctly. So my question was, just how much potential did they really have for being effective in such a serious disease since the secretions to be loosened were deep in the lungs? My reservations were soon overcome based on my repeated clinical experience with some of the younger patients. During the out patient follow up visits, I found that some patients had unexpected physical examination findings of mucus retention (crackles) over the lower lobes, whereas this evidence of active disease was usually noted first over the upper lobes in CF (reason unclear even now). On further questioning the parents, they had been taught only the upper lobe drainage positions because that was the only area of disease evident at diagnosis. So the disease was now showing up in the lower lobe areas where treatments had not been prescribed. When the families were instructed in the remaining positions and used them regularly at home, the lower lung crackles disappeared and the cough improved. This experience went a long way to convincing me that postural drainage treatments, when used with the clapping and vibration components, were effective and important in the long term preventive approach to care of CF patients. From then on, every new family was instructed in all 12 of the drainage positions at diagnosis and encouraged to do all positions at least twice daily. As the patients grew older, vigorous physical activity was encouraged. I came to believe that effective airway clearance therapy, by whatever means and on a daily basis, is vital to keeping the lungs as clear as possible.

Many years later, actual mucus loosening and airways clearance were documented. At our Center, Dr. Michael Konstan used fiberoptic bronchoscopy to demonstrate the effect of various airway clearance techniques. Videotapes during these procedures showed loosening of tenacious secretions from the airway walls and movement of secretions up the airways. In our experience, the Flutter[R] and ABI Vest[R] seem most effective at vibrating the airways and loosening secretions. Long ago, it was demonstrated in adults with bronchiectasis undergoing bronchography, that the major bronchi collapse during the cough maneuver thus trapping secretions behind the blocked airways. With fiberoptic bronchoscopy, collapse of the major bronchi can be seen in even young CF patients. The positive expiratory backpressure generated by the Flutter[R], developed by John Bischofbergher and his group, and other PEP related devices and pursed lip exhalations can help keep the bronchi patent during expiration and allow secretions to move up the airways. Now, the time-honored airway clearance method, postural drainage with clapping and vibration, appears to be less effective than newer techniques, except in infants and children. For older patients, the alternative therapies are important in that they tend to be less time consuming, have better acceptance, and are self administered so the patient can be independent in doing airway clearance treatments.

In the early days, to expand the role of postural drainage and chest physiotherapy for our patients, we recruited Eloise Draper, a physiotherapist trained in the United Kingdom where she had experience in working with respiratory patients. She developed and led several courses in respiratory physical therapy to spread this information to a wider group of physical therapists. One challenge was soon evident. The hospitalized CF patients had treatments four times daily, seven days a week. By tradition, physical therapy department hours were typically 9 to 5, five days a week, it took some effort to gain acceptance of a schedule requiring two shifts a day, seven days a week and the necessary increase in staffing. Although we lured her from her planned retirement, Eloise was a vigorous and spirited professional and a great help to the program for several years.

Value of the Chest X-ray

Chest x-rays taken at regular intervals in follow-up became an another important tool in evaluating the course of the disease. Most of the patients were thriving after the initiation of their home care treatment and their weight came to near normal for their height. Mortality was certainly decreased and survival increased. However, I could not determine why the intensity of recommended treatments and the use of antibiotic therapy differed from patient to patient until LeRoy, Joe Potter, and our radiologist, Dr. Arthur Tucker, had an evening session of chest x-ray scoring. We used the Shwachman-Kulczycki score method, which along with the pulmonary function tests, categorized patients by severity and permitted following the course of the pulmonary involvement. Each patient's chest x-rays differed, since some had been diagnosed before any lung damage was evident, others had a lot of involvement initially but had improved to near normal, while others had advanced changes and had not improved much after treatment had been started. Then it became obvious that the intensity of recommended treatment and antibiotic therapy varied because LeRoy and Joe had a mental picture of the severity of x-ray involvement to guide therapy in addition to knowledge of the patient's current status.

The pulmonary function test results enabled us to monitor and detect change over time, but the serial chest x-rays revealed the extent and localization of irreversible injury that required the most ongoing treatment and would ultimately influence survival. It became apparent to me that the term "early diagnosis" did not simply mean diagnosis at a very young age. To have a true early diagnosis, it was important that the chest x-ray still be in the normal range, or if not, it was best for it to return to near normal within months after initiation of intensive therapy. Only with an early start before irreversible changes occurred could comprehensive treatment have a significant long term impact on such a serious condition.

Regarding the serial chest x-rays, one patient's course was greatly upsetting. She had been diagnosed elsewhere and moved to Cleveland after one year of age, when her chest x-ray was virtually normal, she was normal for height and weight, had no cough, and seemed to thrive for the next several years. Then a cough did develop and her respiratory cultures became positive for *Pseudomonas aeruginosa*, not a good development. While other patients had this organism and were stable for relatively long periods, this young child developed progressively worsening symptoms, rapidly developed heart failure (the first I had encountered or heard of at her age) and died within a year of the onset of the increased respiratory symptoms. I could not understand this rapid downhill course and wondered about what we had overlooked in her treatment. Contact with the previous physician revealed that, even before she was six months of age, this little girl had serious chest x-ray involvement, including an enlarged heart (evidence of heart failure) secondary to the lung involvement, documenting the seriousness of her initial condition. Although the x-ray responded dramatically to treatment, none the less, the critical damage had occurred. For me, this experience further reinforced the importance of diagnosis at an age early enough before irreversible pulmonary damage has time to occur. Also it was important to be aware of the early severity of involvement when parents asked about the prognosis for their child.

A subsequent trainee and later faculty colleague, Dr. Robert Stern, demonstrated the value of the chest x-ray and the benefit of a near normal x-ray at the time of diagnosis using the results of the chest x-ray scoring on the first 95 patients who entered the treatment program 1957–1961 and reported on their survival outcomes.[3] By 1974, these patients had a minimum follow up period of 13 years and were divided into two groups, Group 1, with 45 patients achieved a chest x-ray score of at least 19 points (of 25 points by the Shwachman-Kulczycki method) within the first year of treatment, was termed the "better group," suggesting relatively minimal pulmonary involvement. The remaining 50 patients fell in Group 2 because they had not been able to achieve a chest x-ray score of 19 or more points (indicating initially at least moderate, and for many, severe initial pulmonary involvement) and failed to improve significantly during the first year of treatment.

During the 13 year follow up period to September 1974, 26 of the total 95 patients had died (just two percent per year), but the other striking finding was that all but one of these deaths were in Group 2 patients (25 deaths among these 50 individuals). There was just one death among Group 1 patients. It was stated that, "Even in Group 2, where all of the patients came to diagnosis and treatment after irreversible pulmonary involvement had occurred, the observed survival is better than that presently [1974] reported for unselected large populations of CF patients."

By the end of 1991, all of the 50 Group 2 patients (more advanced initial disease by chest x-ray) had died, except for one survivor, a patient who had successful lung transplantation about that time (and fortunately still survives). Meanwhile, of the 45 Group 1 patients, 23 (50%) remained alive in 1991, including individuals who had an initial abnormal chest x-ray score but were able to improve to near normal during the year treatment was started. Nine years later in 2000, there were still 16 survivors, over 1/3 of the original 45 patients. All remained active except one who retired in 1999 due to disability, as compared to the single survivor (the lung transplant patient) beyond 1991 among the Group 2 patients.

A larger sample further emphasized the benefit of earlier diagnosis. Among the 535 patients treated from 1957 to 1975, there were only 13 deaths in 280 Group1 (mild chest x-ray involvement) patients while there were 106 deaths (at least a seven-fold greater mortality) among the 255 Group 2 patients (irreversible involvement) over the 18 year follow up period. Treatment begun before irreversible damage by chest x-ray resulted in a striking 93 percent survival rate after 18 years of follow up.[4]

Results such as these strongly support the value and importance CF diagnosis before irreversible lung damage (in this case using relatively simple scoring of the chest x-ray at diagnosis and during the first year of treatment). In these patients, the diagnosis was followed by the initiation of the comprehensive treatment program devised by LeRoy Matthews in 1957. Data from the National CFF patient registry indicate that, as recently as 1998, some 40% of CF patients remained undiagnosed until after the first year of life. It would seem intuitive that during a year or more delay in diagnosis, before effective and prophylactic intervention is begun, there would be an increased chance of irreversible lung damage and abnormal nutrition. An efficient and universal newborn screening program could benefit all newly born CF patients.

Joining the Faculty

During the early years and for a number of years after, LeRoy, the fellow, our secretary Ruth Fagan, and I all worked out of an eight by ten foot office, as space in the old B&C Hospital was at a premium. It was fortunate that we were all compatible. The two telephones were considered a lot in those days, there were no beepers of course. We had to use the hospital operator to make even a local phone call, and long distance calls were discouraged. Since the culture, pulmonary function, and/or chest x-ray results were not known for several days after an appointment, we devised a mail system to make treatment recommendations and avoid the inefficiency of the telephone arrangement. Answering machines could have helped, because when an important telephone call was required, often no one was at home.

By my second year of fellowship, the improved survival and increasing referrals caused a rapid increase in the patient population, the research was going well, and I had an offer to join the faculty. LeRoy had won National Institutes of

Health (NIH) research support for the mucus research he and Joe Potter were doing, and his application for a Program Project Grant from the NIH was the first in the nation for CF. The pulmonary function lab was becoming much too small and more equipment was needed. LeRoy was always resourceful in raising capital improvement funds, the lab was expanded and equipment added, and I became a faculty member as an Instructor in Pediatrics at a salary of $8,500, a further improvement on the $2,400 per year as a resident and $6,500 as a fellow. When I asked about a contract or a document to sign, Dr. Matthews assured me that, "nothing was more guaranteed than Dr. Wallace's word." He was absolutely right about Dr. Wallace. Life was a lot more informal with fewer restrictions and legal concerns in those times.

We continued the clinical research development with the plethysmograph study of the CF patients and control subjects. To study the newborn controls we had to move all our equipment to the nursery at MacDonald House, the delivery hospital in the next building, to have enough infants in the first days of life. Fortunately, there was no need to use sedation as the infants were almost uniformly quiet after they had been fed and wrapped snugly in a blanket. The test results seemed correct, but there was always concern about accuracy, such as a calibration error or other defect. Although it was time consuming, to be certain we moved all of the equipment and studied another group of infants getting identical results. The availability of the oscilloscope ensured accuracy.

Jim Johnson, the engineer husband of our technician, Lee, facilitated the design and construction of the large box. This box would serve for children old enough to cooperate, usually over six years of age, and for older subjects. The design and construction was easier, as the entire unit could be made of plywood, and the subjects sat erect and could easily follow breathing instructions. By 1964, with the two systems in operation, data were collected on normal subjects from infants toddlers, children, and adults. Tests on individuals with CF, asthma, other obstructive pulmonary conditions, and other disorders followed. For the CF patients, the ease of this new procedure led to their immediate acceptance. These two plethsmographs were among the first to be used in clinical care, certainly in children and infants. Use of the small box added to understanding of early changes in lung function as did the large box, but of more importance to the patients, plethysmography made it much easier for them and made recruiting of patients and controls easier too. The infant method we established added new information, but it was not easily adaptable for routine use. It was some twenty years later before new approaches for the study of infant and toddler lung function have led to more clinically feasible methods.

The American Association of Respiratory Care was organized in 1955 but respiratory therapists were few. There were fewer than 150 registered respiratory therapists in the country in the early 1960s and their training was essentially adult oriented. We were fortunate that Bernard (Bernie) Kew, one of the national therapy leaders, had developed a training program at nearby St. Alexis Hospital. After

LeRoy gave a talk about CF at the annual Ohio Association meeting in Columbus in 1963, he met with some students and mentioned looking for two people. This was one of the important events of the developing pulmonary program. By 1964, Marvin Lough, a Bernie Kew trainee, became the head of the pulmonary function laboratory (likely the first lab in the country dedicated to children). He also headed the respiratory therapy unit newly created by LeRoy (probably the first respiratory therapy service dedicated to pediatric patients and again the stimulus came from CF patient care needs). The addition of Marv to the staff was one of the best things that ever happened for the CF program and for the hospital. Soon after, Angel Martinez, who had a special way with everyone, especially children, was recruited for a respiratory therapy position. But he soon mastered the complexity of pulmonary function testing and became the mainstay of the pulmonary function lab for many years, producing quality test results and fabricating whatever new piece of equipment was needed for a project. Young patients especially loved him and it was everyone's great loss when he died of cancer at an all too young age.

In 1964, two anesthesiology residents elected to spend six months in the lab to learn about pediatric pulmonary testing, physiology, pathophysiology, and clinical lung problems. They were well prepared in general pulmonary physiology. In return for what they were learning about pediatric diseases, they quizzed Marv as he prepared for the respiratory therapy registry board examination. Although he was more than capable enough to pass the exam, their attention ensured that Marv would become the 162nd Registered Respiratory Therapist in the country. As soon as he gained some pediatric experience he considered himself primarily a pediatric respiratory therapist and lobbied the national American Association of Respiratory Care (AARC) to sanction, for the first time, a Pediatric Section. Once his request was approved, Marv provided the national level leadership necessary to develop a successful program. His recognition of the pediatric training needs and his foresight and leadership in the AARC were recently acknowledged when he was honored and named a Fellow of the National AARC.

Marv also initiated what was probably the first academic-based respiratory therapy program to include a strong emphasis on pediatric respiratory care. He enlisted Bernie Kew, Dr. David Gillespie, Dr. Paul Fumich, along with me and later a few others to start an Associate Degree Program in Respiratory Therapy. With his leadership, a complete curriculum was developed by 1968 for Cuyahoga Community College and later for Lakeland Community College. He led all of the pediatric training which was located only at Rainbow Babies and Children's Hospital. Marv was also the initiator and chief editor of a popular and successful *Pediatric Respiratory Therapy* textbook for students in 1973, with two subsequent editions. Later, he developed an annual three day pediatric course for therapists from around the country until every area had sufficient pediatric experienced personnel to put on their own training courses. Subsequently, he participated in the Philadelphia Pediatric Pulmonary Center annual training course with Dr. Douglas Holsclaw and therapist, Jan Tecklin. Much of this pediatric respiratory therapy activity was a direct outgrowth of the needs created by the national CF Center program and the growing numbers of CF and other pulmonary patients being seen at the CF Centers.

The Blood Gas Test

When I was a medical student, I had a summer job in adult pulmonologist Dr. Scott Inkley's laboratory at University Hospitals of Cleveland. One task was to analyze arterial blood samples for oxygen content from patients undergoing cardiac catheterization. Called the Van Slyke method, this technique was complicated, time consuming, and exacting. It could not measure carbon dioxide in or acidity (pH) of the blood. Also, a large blood sample was required and the equipment was extensive. The days I was assigned to the Van Slyke machine seemed very long. Consequently, in 1964, I was very much interested in a new micro instrument that could not only rapidly measure oxygen tension but also carbon dioxide pressure, which together are known as the "blood gases," and included the important additional value of determining the pH of the blood. Of special import, this testing could be done on very small samples making it feasible for repeated testing in infants and children, in particular, those with CF. Soon after it would aid the management of premature infants, an advance increasingly important in pediatrics as the survival of these challenging premature infants was rapidly increasing due to the expert care provided by neonatologists, Drs. John Kennell and Marshall Klaus. We obtained funds for the first blood gas analyzer in the city and probably the entire state and surrounding region and this technology gradually became widespread. It was another large step forward in patient care and once again the impetus was from the CF program.

Terry Gillespie, the trainee fellow following me, came to us from Halifax, Nova Scotia. Terry was great to work with, had a wonderful sense of humor, and had many amusing stories including automobile and moose encounters in Nova Scotia and from his experiences working across Canada on the railroad. His assignment was to standardize the gas analyzer and develop a method using a thin capillary tube to collect a very small arterialized blood sample since the capillary sample could be entered directly into the machine. Thus we could avoid repeated arterial punctures requiring a needle and syringe and a larger sample. When we began using this blood gas technique in the care and study of the CF patients, the neonatologists soon became aware of it and asking for daytime tests. It was so helpful to them that Marv, the therapist who knew how to do the test, was increasingly called in from home at night. To fill the growing demand from the nursery, the hospital soon agreed to add respiratory therapy positions. This improvement in pulmonary care and the growth of pediatric respiratory therapy positions, also originated from the stimulus of the CF program, as undoubtedly occurred similarly elsewhere all around the country.

Terry was a welcome help in caring for the increasing number of CF and other patients that were being referred to us. LeRoy was ever more active with the National CF Foundation, including serving as Chairman of the first Center Committee of the Medical Advisory Council. He developed the first annual report forms for use by the Centers beginning in 1963 and an interval record form to be used at each outpatient visit to remind the clinicians of the history, physical exam, and treatment information to be recorded. Terry and I split many of the patient care activities as we continued to gain knowledge and share clinical experience. When Terry returned to Halifax, he established an exemplary CF program there.

The two issue edition in Dr. Andersen's memory by the Journal of Pediatrics in 1964 reflected the esteem in which she was held by her colleagues. It provided an excellent opportunity to describe the comprehensive treatment program to the pediatric world in the first issue,[5] followed by evaluation of the first five years of the program in the second.[6] This journal was prominent and easily referenced for others to access. In preparing the manuscripts, my days were spent with morning rounds, a full day in the lab, follow up evening rounds, and a brief supper followed by outlining and writing several nights a week, usually at the Matthews' home. Lee's wife, known affectionately by all as "Rock", always had popcorn to keep us going. These two reports were followed by the evaluation of the prophylactic and therapeutic program in 1965 and several reports by Drs. Warren Warwick and Richard Pogue at the 1969 Cambridge, England International CF meeting and elsewhere using the national patient registry data. The report by Dr. Stern on the survival outcome of the first 95 patients[3] in 1974 added additional evidence of the beneficial effect of the treatment program, especially when initiated early in the course of the disease.

The "Heparin Lock"

Special mention is appropriate regarding the development of the "Heparin Lock" for intravenous therapy. Excellent fellow trainees continued to be attracted to the program and the training grant was of significant help. Drs. Sue Miller and Sue Pittman followed Dr. Gillespie. Both went on to head or support the CF Center in their new areas. Bob Stern, a former resident, returned from the Air Force and was the next CF and pulmonary trainee. The blood gas measurements were a continuing research interest but posed a problem in young children who usually cry during blood drawing and that could alter their true resting values. A possible approach was to place a small intra arterial needle that could be left in place so samples could be drawn without disturbing the child, but the only set up with a small needle had very long tubing. I asked the sales representative for a needle with only a very short length of tubing and, soon after, we had a newly designed small caliber needle and short tubing with a resealing rubber diaphragm at the end. While of some help to the blood gas project, this unit became of much greater importance to the overall care of patients. There had been an increasing need for a better way to provide intravenous antibiotic therapy, especially after the introduction of the semi-synthetic penicillins. Carbenicillin was proving to be effective against Pseudomonas infections. However, large and frequent doses were required and patient activity was limited because fluid had to run constantly to prevent clotting in the tubing between doses. Dr. Stern had devoted significant time to research possible solutions

Center Directors Remember: Cleveland

to this problem and was able to quickly incorporate the new needle and short tubing into his strategy. His ingenuity resulted in a new concept for intravenous (IV) therapy, since the short tube allowed him to add a very small amount of heparin to keep the IV from clotting when not in use. The patient could be freed from the continuous drip of fluid previously essential and could have normal activity between dosages of medicine. With the short tubing, the dose of heparin required was too minimal to be a hazard. He called the method the "heparin lock" (see his Chapter for reference). Thanks to him, his idea revolutionized IV therapy for our patients and allowed them to be ambulatory most of every day. After the method was published in 1972, the use of the heparin lock spread to other CF Centers and ultimately to the care patients of all ages with all sorts of illnesses and conditions.

The Child Life Program

During my residency training at City Hospital under Dr. Frederick Robbins, I had the opportunity to observe the development of a unique program for hospitalized children. It became known as the Child Life Program. For any child requiring hospitalization in the middle 1950s, educational and distraction activities were generally lacking in pediatric units everywhere and hospital stays were generally much longer than those of today. Dr. Robbins had the foresight to hire Emma Plank, a Montessori teacher from Europe, to develop a comprehensive program for these children. With Dr. Robbins support, her ideas and concepts met with growing acceptance. After I joined the faculty at B&C Hospital, I was privileged to observe her concept beginning to spread there. Positive responses from patients, parents, and hospital staff provided increasing acceptance and development. By 1969, with active support from Assistant Director of Pediatric Nursing, Dalia Zemaityte, this initially informal so-called "Play Lady" program grew into the professional Child Life program under the direction of Edward Gratzik at B&C Hosp. It began to spread elsewhere, and became widely known. The requirements for staff and space grew from just one playroom in B&C Hosp, to one activity room on each patient-care Division in the new hospital. Hospital life for our children was forever improved.

Later, in 1977, one of my CF patients, 24 year old Kim Kerr, who had volunteered in the program while completing her college work, subsequently applied to Boston's Wheelock College for additional training and Child Life accreditation. After her return to Cleveland, I was pleased to watch her establish the first hospital-based, Child Life program in northeast Ohio outside of Cleveland.

Pseudomonas cepacia

A bacterial organism named *Pseudomonas cepacia* led to a disaster of major proportions that built up at our Center from the early 1980s. A telephone call from the Hospital for Sick Children in Toronto suggested the possibility of fever and rapid progressive pneumonia leading to death in some adolescent CF patients. This clinical course was unusual and appeared to be caused by a different Pseudomonas organism, called *P. cepacia* (now called *Burkholderia cepacia*). At that time, several of our patients had this organism on respiratory culture, but had not shown an increase in symptoms and did not have an accelerated clinical course. Indeed, our earliest patient to be colonized with this agent still has it and has never required hospitalization or seemed to have progressive symptoms due to it.

About that time, several Centers in nearby states could no longer admit patients after the age of 18 years. Since adult based care was not yet well developed, 18 year old patients from these areas frequently turned to our Center for care. Unfortunately many were culture positive for *P. cepacia*. With the influx of these patients, we had an average inpatient CF census of 12 to 15 patients and soon up to one half of them had *P. cepacia* positive cultures. With the usual two week or longer admission and this degree of exposure, almost every non-colonized but exposed patient became culture positive by the time of the next outpatient culture. Ultimately, 25% (125 out of our then 400 patients) were culture positive.

A number of patients, especially adolescent and young women, developed the fever, elevated white blood cell count (indicating significant infection, but not seen then in the usual CF patient requiring admission), and increasingly severe symptoms leading to unanticipated death much earlier than expected, as we had learned from Toronto. By 1983, up to three new colonized patients were occurring every month. Since there was no precedence for this situation, it was a very difficult decision to separate our colonized patients from the others with the hope of halting the spread. Implementation forced the separation of friends, disrupted inter family relationships, essentially led to the demise of the successful group educational meetings, the closing of the summer camp to colonized patients, and many other less visible interactions. The separation of colonized patients did ensure our completion of transitioning the adult age patients to one of two divisions of the adult medicine section of the hospital, a move appropriate for this age group in any event.

The health threat posed by the spread of the *B. cepacia*, the need for separation of patients, and the associated adult transitioning was very traumatic for the patients, their families, and, equally so, for every staff member. On the positive side, and to our great relief, once the affected patients no longer had contact with the others, the spread of the organism stopped completely. Sadly though, some of the colonized patients died with the rapid and precipitous decline, and while others deteriorated more slowly, it was much sooner than would have been anticipated. Some other Centers had similar experiences. Centers that had few such patients did not have the spread of *B. cepacia* to their other patients and fortunately have not had to endure the heartbreak of such an experience. More recently, others have reported the spread of the more commonly seen *P. aeruginosa* occurring between patients when they have close contact for a week or so, again raising the issue of separation of patients.

There was another casualty from the spread of *B. cepacia*. In 1967, our respiratory therapist Jim Bolek, who later was supervisor of the clinical part of the Pediatric Respiratory Therapy Department, organized what was probably the first ever summer camp for CF children. The Matthew Salem CF Camp was named in honor of a patient who loved camping. For many years, the camping experience was a high point for children not well enough to otherwise be away from their home and their daily treatments for a week. They learned more about CF, interacted with many others, received all of their recommended daily therapy, experienced a wide variety of activities, and enjoyed good fellowship. Sadly, this superb program was severely impacted when the B. *cepacia* patients could no longer attend with the others. For this and potential legal ramifications, the camping program had to be discontinued as part of the CF program.

Intestinal Obstruction

Unfortunately, a number of the newly referred children with CF had severe, advanced, and relatively irreversible pulmonary disease. None the less, there were no deaths in the group during 1961, and only three deaths in 1962. Optimism was high, but everyone recognized the seriousness of the disease. From the early days of the program, we held monthly parent meetings to provide more information about CF. These were heavily attended through out the 1960s, with attendance ranging from 60 to 100 per meeting. At one meeting, all of the equipment and the large plethysmograph were disassembled and moved to the basement amphitheater for a demonstration. This required a major effort to set it up and working again in that setting, but the meeting was heavily attended and it proved to be one of the most popular programs. At another meeting, pediatric surgeon Dr. Robert Izant, always an excellent speaker, drew a large crowd. His graphic color slides of the surgical problems that presented in CF and how he dealt successfully with them resulted in a parent father becoming light headed and passing out, affording opportunity to tease Dr. Izant about the effect of his graphic delivery and beautiful color slides. Bob was one of the first surgeons to specifically train in pediatric surgery, an important development for the care of infants and children. His skill was of great importance to patients, especially in successfully dealing with the problem of meconium ileus. At birth, some CF infants cannot pass the first bowel movement (meconium) due to a failure of the last section of the small bowel (the ileum) to develop. Soon after birth, such an infant usually requires surgical correction. I knew, had read about, and had seen several infants with meconium ileus.

Dr. Izant confirmed my diagnosis in a somewhat similar situation but presenting in an older CF child. While still in my first year of fellowship, I admitted a three year old girl who was irritable and had a history of no bowel movement for two days. Her abdomen was distended and bowel sounds were poor, indicating poor intestinal motility (ileus). However, she had no fever and her abdomen was soft with no signs to suggest, to me at least, an acute abdominal process requiring urgent surgical intervention. None the less, in such a situation, a surgical consult was indicated and I called for one, as I was not comfortable with an etiology, a specific diagnosis, or what further evaluation she might need, let alone a plan of treatment.

When I was checking the abdominal x-rays before calling LeRoy at home (it was late evening), two surgical residents arrived. When they saw the marked increase in bowel contents and marked dilatation, both suggesting to them an obstruction that would indicate surgery, one resident proceeded to telephone for an operating room for emergency surgery. Since I had the advantage of examining the patient (they had not done so yet), I objected to this rush to surgery. They were clearly astonished and obviously wondered where this doc (me) had received his training. So they immediately called Dr. Izant for help while I called Dr. Matthews. Both attendings returned to the hospital immediately and, to my great relief, agreed that this was not an acute surgical abdomen. The residents disappeared. However, just as for me, this was a new complication for Bob and LeRoy. They agreed that stool blockage and lack of intestinal motility were the problems and that repeated enemas seemed safely indicated in this circumstance. But all of us were concerned, so both the attending doctors stayed the night along with me worrying about the outcome. Nothing happened for hours and Dr. Izant, with the surgical responsibility, began to express more concern, while LeRoy still felt pretty confident that surgery was not yet indicated. Later, their opinions reversed as they literally hung over the sides of the crib and discussed possibilities. In retrospect, it was a humorous scene, but not at the time. Finally, after many enemas the child had an enormous bowel movement and the situation was resolved. Since the clinical findings and abdominal x-rays were suggestive of the meconium ileus pattern seen in the newborn, and with no evidence of a similar case in the literature, we termed this condition "meconium ileus equivalent" and published a report. This complication was encountered more frequently as patients became older and better enema treatments were devised to expedite resolution. Ultimately, the term DIOS (distal intestinal obstruction syndrome) better described the problem. However, the profound relief I experienced when the two attending physicians agreed with my initial assessment that this was not an acute surgical abdomen has not been forgotten. Also, not having to undergo abdominal surgery may have contributed a bit to the fact that the little girl who presented with the abdominal problem that night is still alive today.

Other Experiences

Early in my training, I did not inquire much about cigarette smoking by the CF patients, as most were too young to be smoking, so I thought. Also, smoking was very prevalent in those days, and was very common in the waiting rooms and even occurred in the doctor's exam room. Physicians, nurses, and others smoked on the wards and during patient rounds. Our then chief of staff of University Hospitals, Dr. Scott Inkley, and another leading physician, received a great deal of criticism for even attempting to have cigarette machines removed from the hospital! Although I had stopped smoking years before, cigarette smoke was so prevalent that it was not as noticeable as it is today. One early teenage patient, KP, was old enough to have his appointments without the parents being present. At each visit, he immediately would have a terrible paroxysm of very productive cough to the point of getting red in the face and occasionally even blue for a bit. The cough never improved despite any treatment measure I recommended. After he could catch his breath his first question always was, "Doc, when are you going to help me with this cough?" One could only feel very bad about his cough and have a sense of guilt in not being able to help him. Then one day, the mother of a little girl whose appointment usually followed KP's, appeared upset and finally said, "Doctor do you know what KP does at every visit just before you call for him?" Of course I did not have a clue and was stunned to learn that he stubbed out his cigarette in the waiting room just before every visit! Added to his significant CF lung problems, it was no wonder he had such a bad cough and my guilt feeling about being unable to help him abated. Despite the cough and repeated entreaties, he would not give up smoking (during a later admission his nurse told me he was found smoking in his oxygen tent). And the question about smoking was added to my CF history taking from then on.

As new CF patients were diagnosed, each family was encouraged to join the Chapter and support the program as much as possible. Sometime in the 1960s, I admitted an 18 month old newly diagnosed boy. It appeared that either one of his parents would be a good candidate for a Board of Trustees position. It was reasonable to anticipate that the mother would be busy caring for the CF youngster and the others at home, while the father, who was successful in business, would have more time and many contacts. One day while the mother was sitting in a rocking chair with her sleeping child, we were discussing plans for discharge and I asked whether the father might be interested in serving on the Board. Her immediate response was, "*We* would be glad to serve." I was in a bit of panic, as the policy was that only one member of a family at a time could serve as a Board member. The mother was very gracious when I explained my dilemma. Thus, Sarah Dresing's husband, Bob, was the one who became the Chapter Board member and showed his creative and administrative effectiveness. He then went on to the National Board and subsequently served effectively as President of the National CF organization. Sarah chaired many fund raising projects and had many other CF activities locally. At the same time, she was totally supportive of Bob's involvement at the local and national levels.

The number of pediatricians interested in pediatric pulmonary disease and CF were relatively few in the 1960s. There were four major organizations available to us at that time, the American Thoracic Society (ATS), the American College of Chest Physicians, the American Academy of Pediatrics, and the Cystic Fibrosis Foundation. Those of us in leadership positions tried to use our attendance at the meetings of these organizations as a time to coordinate our efforts and activities. The goals were to promote awareness of pediatric pulmonary diseases, the need for research and training of health professionals, and the need for pediatric pulmonary or chest sections in the appropriate organizations. I especially remember discussions with Martha Franz from Dayton and Gordon Young from Columbus in the early and mid-1960s that served to benefit all three of our Ohio Centers. Will Waring, from New Orleans, was very active in the ATS as a Council member and was aware of a new plan to establish special interest groups in that organization, to be called "Scientific Assemblies." He had the foresight to recommend a "Scientific Assembly on Pediatrics" and the leadership accepted his proposal. As a result, since I was in Cleveland and the next annual meeting of the ATS (and the American Lung Association) was to be held in Cleveland in 1969, Will prevailed upon me to accept responsibility for convening the initiation of the Assembly (by laws, etc.) and planning the first meeting to be held in 1970. Of the convening participants, I recall only Henry Levinson, Warren Warwick, and Bettina Hilman but there were a few others who joined our deliberations (Will was busy elsewhere). After we agreed that we would support the Assembly concept, we developed a mission statement and worked out a set of bylaws, including the provision that elected officers should be under forty five years of age. We believed that this was an important concept for the younger members who would follow and it still seems to be in effect. The ATS Council readily accepted our plan and the first meeting in 1970 was successful. The Assembly has grown and proved important and effective ever since. It is gratifying to know that there are now over 1,000 Primary members and some 500 Secondary members (these totals include some 25% from outside the US) with a continuing active and productive leadership. Meanwhile, the other organizations have also provided continuing support and other venues for furthering pediatric pulmonary issues.

From the beginning of my involvement, I felt that there would be two particularly challenging times in the early life of each patient. One was during the first year or so of life when immunity was being established and physical activity was limited. Viral respiratory illnesses and the possibility of the damaging secondary bacterial infection were frequently possible. The second period of challenge, I felt, would be during adolescence, whether its psychosocial onset (and period of rebellion and rejection of the need for regular daily treatments) began early or did not become manifest until mid to late teens. I watched many of these young people do well and maintain normal pulmonary function through childhood. My hope then was that, once full lung growth was achieved and with a normal or near normal chest x-ray, even if the person abandoned their needed daily health care for periods of time, they might still do well.

Unfortunately my expectation was wrong. The transition from more sheltered home life to college or independent living proved to be a third period of challenge. This was especially true for patients who had already developed chronic respiratory colonization of *Pseudomonas aeruginosa*. Even with daily treatment, the tendency for progression was much greater since we were not successful in eliminating the Pseudomonas. With neglect of health care for periods of time, obvious pulmonary deterioration became evident. However, it was gratifying to see that once an individual was able to develop a stable life style of his or her own (after completing college and/or getting stable employment for example), most were able to maintain their health in a steady state for long periods of time.

However, the interim penalty during the transition period was to incur further loss of lung function and, despite our counseling, essentially each individual seemed to have to work through this period for themselves and gradually understand their body and its health needs.

The addition of Bob Stern, Tom Boat, and Bob Wood to what had grown into the Pulmonary Division and Cystic Fibrosis Center by 1959 was especially timely, as LeRoy became Department Chairman in 1970, after the death of Dr. Wallace, and we were all kept busy. For a long time, Ruth Fagan was our only secretary for the whole program. She somehow managed to keep us in line, type and send out all of the correspondence, and deal with the increasing number of abstracts and research grant proposals, while Sid Gest single handedly administered the entire Pediatric Department. Ginny Petrie, our first Division Coordinator, continues her outstanding support of the Division today. We have always consistently been blessed with excellent and dedicated Center Nurses.

Writing and completing the manuscript "State of The Art: Cystic Fibrosis" for editor Dr. John Murray and the journal *The American Review of Respiratory Disease* in 1976 with Bob Wood and Tom, with editorial and bibliography support from librarian, Judy Wood, was a special time for me. And it was a timely achievement for CF, thanks to them.[6]

As each of us trainees came into the program we found the use of aerosol antibiotics to treat the more resistant Pseudomonas organism to be relatively new to us. Each expressed reluctance to accept the concept that the small amount of antibiotic inhaled onto the large surface area of the airways could possibly provide an effective measure against this significant bacterial infection. As the first convert to the effectiveness of antibiotic aerosols, I found it interesting to observe each following trainee express skepticism about its potential effectiveness. Later, when confronted with their own patients with progressive, difficult to control, pulmonary symptoms from the persisting low grade infection, each in turn observed a beneficial effect when they added antibiotic to the aerosol treatments and, just as with each of us, those who followed, also became converts. It was quite some time later before a study performed elsewhere demonstrated positive results and the use of antibiotics by aerosol became more wide spread.

Further, each of us came to the independent conclusion that, despite whatever dietary recommendations were made, the patients grew and gained weight best when we aggressively kept treating any sign of increased pulmonary symptoms. This included using the hospital for the addition of intravenous antibiotics and intensive postural drainage treatments as often and for as long as needed to improve or stabilize pulmonary function. There also was agreement that the use of two intravenous antibiotics together against the bacterial infection, as LeRoy had observed in Boston, and as others were also finding, gave better results than one antibiotic alone.

Dorr Dearborn, Ph.D., M.D., was recruited from the NIH after Don Carlson became Chairman of the Department of Biochemistry at Purdue University and Dorr continued the excellent leadership of the Biochemistry Lab. He and Dr. Margaret Bruce were probably the first to observe and report on high levels of uninhibited elastase activity in CF pulmonary secretions and the elevated elastin degradation products in the urine. Neutrophil elastase products (from the white blood cells that enter the lungs to fight the infection) have subsequently been recognized as a major source of airway damage in CF and have been the target of several treatment measures.

One frequently gains better insight from patients about their view of the disease. In one such instance, this came to me from a two year old boy. One day, standing at the doorway of the exam room with his mother holding his hand, he kept pulling back while repeatedly saying something. Finally it was clear that he was saying, "Not sick, not sick, not sick" over and over. He had been diagnosed at a very young age before any real pulmonary symptoms had developed. So, young as he was that day, he was correct that he was not sick and in fact was free of symptoms. As far as he was concerned, he did not need a doctor at all and wanted to leave right then. This revelation brought the realization that for most CF individuals no matter what problems and symptoms they might be contending with at any given time, more often than not they just factor them into their daily life, usually do not complain, and frequently accomplish more than their peers. Most carry that attitude of "Not sick." It is not readily apparent to the average person and often even to those of us who are care givers, just how much the CF individuals deal with every day and how fatiguing the daily treatment routine and the almost constant low grade lung infection can be. One cannot help but respect and admire each one of them.

Initial education and establishing a positive attitude toward long term survival are important with a chronic disease such as CF. None the less, continued reinforcement is important because the pulmonary involvement differs from patient to patient and some patients show progression of the disease and death at a young age. Misperception about early fatality came up in the case of KS, a girl from another state diagnosed before two years of age. Her treatment was started before significant pulmonary disease had developed, and she was seen regularly in follow up. When KS was 12 years old, her mother seemed concerned and asked, "When will it happen?" At first, it was not apparent what her question related to; perhaps onset of adolescent change, onset of poor weight gain, onset of pulmonary symptoms, or something else. Then it became clear that her family had observed what probably many others have worried about. They had seen a number of early adolescent CF children in their local community who seemed to be reasonably well, fairly quickly have progressive symptoms, and soon after were dying. This progression was difficult for them to understand, very frightening, and could be assumed to be typical of the course of CF in adolescent age patients, such as their daughter. Our experience with patients with normal or near normal chest x-ray scores after one year of treatment on comprehensive treatment as described above, was helpful in providing an answer in context. This girl had an essentially normal chest x-ray at diagnosis, had not experienced any significant clinical or x-ray progression since then, and her pulmonary function test easily remained within the limits of normal. She had come to us only a year or so after those patients who were included in the outcome report of the initial 95 patients [3] and she was included in our later experience.[4] Her course was progressing similar to that of the ones in the "better" (good chest x-ray) group.

Based on these experiences, my response was of the hope that, barring an unforeseen severe complication or untoward event, there was reasonable expectation that she could live long beyond that of her care provider (me). As demonstrated by the patients in the better chest x-ray group, she has continued equally as well. Despite developing diabetes in her mid teens, she is now over 30 years of age, and continues with a near normal pulmonary function test. She only recently stopped full time employment so that she and her husband of some ten years could adopt an infant and she could be a full time mother. She is an excellent example, along with many others who have followed, of the more than 50% of our Center population who are greater than 18 years of age.

Linda, the little girl I met at City Hospital who had the threat of life shortening complications in early childhood, is now married and over 40 years of age. She has persisted despite the initial odds against her. We recently met and she shared these thoughts:

> Living with CF is like a battle, one that must be fought every day without reprieve. Bacteria, our living and oh so powerful enemy, tend to literally set up shop and colonize our lungs. They are indeed "unwanted and uninvited guests." It can be a frightening battle at times, because even though you fight vigilantly you realize, in the dark recesses of your mind, that you still may lose in the end. I am truly grateful for all of the work, research, and hours of effort that our CF doctors, care givers, and researchers have put forth through the years. They have helped make living into adulthood a realistic probability and a more tolerable one as well. Sitting in the wings with whatever weapons at my side, I wait for a cure someday.

This woman's determination as she faces each new day is typical of those with CF. Over time and with increasing pulmonary symptoms, most individuals with CF quietly fight harder and harder despite facing what is still an ultimately losing cause. While giving way to CF does not come easily to them, as their time grows short, their loved ones (family, spouse, and even close friends and care takers) may be reluctant to give the verbal assurance of having made the best fight possible. Many patients at this very late stage almost struggle more for those around them, not wanting to hurt them. Yet they silently have need for permission that will let them go. "Giving up" has been a phrase used unfortunately by others to describe the terminally failing patient. This language may express the hurt felt by family and friends over impending loss, but it is an inaccurate characterization of those who have struggled against the severe chronic condition that is CF. Before an overflow audience at the memorial service of one patient, his closest friend, Tom K., put the final days in perspective. "When someone dies of a prolonged illness, it is easy to fall back on the euphemism that the person has 'lost the battle' or 'given up' to their disease. My friend won his battle with CF just as he successfully lived his life of hope and inspiration to others. Dying is not the larger tragedy, the lifetime of waiting for an early death and trying to spare others pain can be more burdensome."

My national CF Board involvement led to an invitation to serve on the NIH National Heart and Lung Disease Pulmonary Disease Advisory Committee from 1976-80. This opportunity was especially important to me as Dr. Richard Talamo, an outstanding individual and leader, was the other pediatric representative and we worked closely together to support pediatric pulmonary interests in research and training. Subsequently, there was a further opportunity to serve on the Pulmonary SCOR Review Committee from 1980-85. However, I felt most fortunate to return to the CF Foundation for my final national level activity, that being with the Center Committee from 1986 to 1994. This was another rewarding and fulfilling time, especially with the continued learning and sharing opportunity provided by site visits to the personnel of other Centers. The award of the Richard C. Talamo Distinguished Clinician Scientist Award in 1997 was a totally unexpected honor of which I remain most grateful and proud.

After 15 years as Division Chief and 29 years as Director of the CF Center, it was time to retire from the daily care scene. It was especially important to me be able to turn leadership of the LeRoy Matthews Cystic Fibrosis Center to those with whom I had long worked and respected. I was confident that they would not only be able to maintain but would further improve the program. Indeed, with Dr. Michael Konstan, as Center Director (Figure 27.1) and Dr. Michael Infeld, as the Adult Section Director, it has been a real pleasure to observe that the patients and the Center have continued to thrive without interruption. To have so successfully sustained the program, these two caring clinicians and experienced researchers have had the support of others equally dedicated. This includes the other continuing physicians Bob Stern, Dorr Dearborn, Carolyn Kercsmar, John Carl, Tom Ferkol, Laura Milgram, Jim Chmiel, Dan Craven and Division Chief, Pam Davis, and our excellent nurses, Sue Koziol and Karen Vosper. My hope is that each member of the clinical and research parts of the Center program will have continuing satisfaction and great success in their activities.

The years have passed all too quickly and have been filled with too many patient losses to fully make up for the degree of success we have experienced in trying to improve the outcome for all CF patients. It has been a source of great satisfaction to have cared for so many CF adults now in their 30s, 40s, and even 50s, a half century of life experience and beyond. The clinical Center continues to have more than 50% of the patients over 18 years of age. And it has been most rewarding to have shared so many wonderful relationships and to have had the opportunity to participate in what must be recognized as the most successful continuing fight ever achieved against a disease of genetic origin by a voluntary health agency, the National Cystic Fibrosis Foundation.

Being involved with the comprehensive treatment program within a few years of its inception, working with my mentor LeRoy Matthews and the excellent staff we were blessed with over the years, accomplishing the pioneering infant pulmonary function research studies, and my involvement as a volunteer with the CF Foundation, the Medical Advisory Council, and the leaders of those days, made for especially exciting, productive, and satisfying times. Most gratifying was the opportunity to participate as mentor with so many excellent trainees, most of whom have

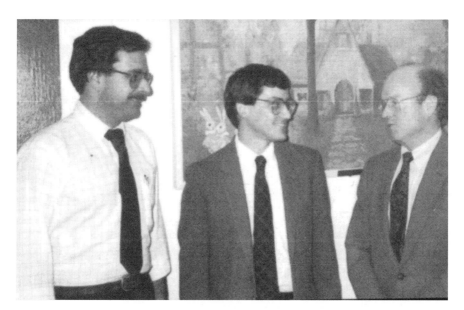

Figure 27.1. *From the left, Dr. Mel Berger, Dr. Michael Konstan, and Dr. Robert Beall. In 1988, Dr. Konstan was the first Harry Shwachman Clinical Investigator awardee from the CF Foundation. Courtesy of Dr. Carl Doershuk.*

continued their CF involvement, many as Center Directors. Ideal patient care cannot improve without the research arm that has always been equally as important to Dr. Matthews' treatment program. Thus, it has been additionally gratifying to be able to observe the many clinical research trials progress as guided by Michael Konstan, at our Center in collaboration with the other Therapeutics Development Network Centers and in conjunction with the Research Development Program Center led by Pam Davis. While CF still poses many challenges, the devoted efforts of the ever growing numbers of talented and caring professionals worldwide will yet lead to victory over this disease.

References

1. Rochholz EL. *Almanac of Children's Songs and Games from Switzerland.* Leipzig, J J Weber, 1857.
2. Taussig LM. "Cystic fibrosis; an overview." In *Cystic Fibrosis*, Taussig LM, ed. 1984, Thieme-Stratton Inc. New York.
3. Stern RC, Boat TF, Doershuk CF, Tucker AS, Primiano FP, Jr., and Matthews LW. "Course of cystic fibrosis in 95 patients." *J Pediatr* 1976;89:406-11.
4. Wood RE, Boat TF, Doershuk CF. "Cystic fibrosis—State of the Art." *Am Rev Resp Dis* 1976;113:833-78.
5. Matthews LW, Doershuk CF, Wise M, Eddy G, Nudelman H, and Spector S. "A therapeutic regimen for patients with cystic fibrosis." *J Pediatr* 1964;65:558-75.
6. Doershuk CF, Matthews LW, Tucker AS, Nudelman H, Eddy G, Wise M. and Spector S. "A 5 year clinical evaluation of a therapeutic program for patients with cystic fibrosis." *J Pediatr* 1964;65:677-93.

28

Center Directors Remember: Nova Scotia

C. Terrence Gillespie, M.D., C.M., F.R.C.P. (C)

While I was born and raised in New Brunswick (N.B.), my subsequent medical training and medical career were centered in Halifax Nova Scotia (N.S.). These two provinces are part of the three Maritime Provinces, the other being Prince Edward Island (P.E.I.). Their population is largely of English, Irish, and Scottish origin with Acadian French speaking minorities. N.S. has a population of about one million people. Except for their connection by the narrow Isthmus of Chignecto, N.B. and N.S. are separated by the 150 mile long Bay of Fundy, famous for its tides. Halifax, the largest city of N.S. and the provincial capital is on the Atlantic coast, and is the home of Dalhousie University and Medical School. Sydney is the second largest city and 275 miles to the northeast while Yarmouth, 220 miles southwest, is the Canadian terminus of the ferry to Portland, Maine, about 200 miles due west across the mouth of the Bay of Fundy.

The late Dr. Joe A. MacDonald of Glace Bay reportedly made the first diagnosis of cystic fibrosis in N.S. in the mid 1940s. This diagnosis signaled some awareness of CF in the province. A second era intensified the awareness of CF and brought the first organized approach to diagnosis and treatment of this serious disease in the province in 1958 when Dr. William Cochrane was recruited to the Halifax Children's Hospital from Toronto. He had the foresight to open a special clinic for CF patients in the fall of that year, just the third CF clinic to be started in Canada. Dr. Alan Ross at the Montreal Children's Hospital opened the first clinic in 1957 and Dr. Douglas Crozier the second at the Hospital for Sick Children in Toronto in 1958, shortly before Dr. Cochrane left Toronto for Halifax.

Dr. Cochrane was the first pediatrician to hold a full time appointment in the Faculty of Medicine and the Department of Pediatrics at the Dalhousie Medical School. Earlier at the Hospital for Sick Children, he had an established record of research in metabolic diseases of children and was highly regarded by the house staff as an innovative and stimulating teacher. Under his tutelage at Dalhousie, the postgraduate training in pediatrics was greatly enhanced, resulting in more physicians seeking further postgraduate pediatric training in Halifax. By 1963, he was appointed Professor and Head of the Department of Pediatrics at the University and Physician in Chief at the Halifax Children's Hospital. When I was completing a two year residency in pediatrics with Dr. Cochrane, he encouraged me to obtain subspecialty training in children's chest diseases and CF with Dr. LeRoy Matthews at Babies and Children's Hospital, Western Reserve University, in Cleveland, Ohio from 1964 to 1966. On my return to Halifax in July 1966, Dr. Cochrane assigned me to direct the CF clinic, marking the beginning of the province's next era of CF history, to 1992.

Dr. Paul Patterson, from Boston, revealed the 1951 "state of the art" of CF in N.S. in a report to the Minister of Health. In keeping with long established tradition, Boston physicians frequently visited Halifax as guest lecturers at Dalhousie University Medical School. At that time, Dr. Patterson was studying pathology at Harvard University and the Children's Hospital in Boston. His purpose was to discuss CF and seek answers to questions arising from observations made at the Boston Children's Hospital by Dr. Harry Shwachman regarding the family backgrounds of patients with "pancreatic fibrosis" (i.e., CF). In the introduction of his report, Dr. Patterson noted "detailed family histories of children with pancreatic fibrosis seen at the Children's Hospital, Boston, Massachusetts, revealed the information that nearly 80% of the children had ancestry in eastern Canada (Quebec and the Maritime Provinces), especially Nova Scotia and Prince Edward Island. A survey of Nova Scotia and Prince Edward Island was planned in order to find some explanation of the etiology of the disease pancreatic fibrosis."

Dr. Patterson conducted the survey in the summer of 1951. In his report he described pancreatic fibrosis as a fatal disease of infancy and childhood characterized by pancreatic insufficiency and chronic pulmonary disease. He stressed that many of the symptoms and complaints these children had were found in many other conditions, such as asthma, whooping cough, tuberculosis, and other defects or infections of the pulmonary system. He added, "For this reason, the disease may not be diagnosed unless the physician is acquainted with this entity, does a duodenal intubation, and examines the aspirated fluid for increased viscosity and the absence or reduction of pancreatic enzymes."

In his survey, Dr. Patterson interviewed physicians from each of the 15 counties of N.S., visited several communities throughout the province and, whenever possible, examined children with CF. He remarked that he found it difficult to determine the incidence of CF because "only two of the general practitioners interviewed had heard of the disease."

On visiting the Children's Hospital in Halifax, then the only children's hospital in eastern Canada, he found charts of CF patients from the period of 1948—1951 and interviewed staff members and some of the families of known patients. He felt that "the disease was being overlooked in the same way as in other children's hospitals in the United States."

This, then, was the state of awareness about CF among physicians when I entered medical school in Halifax in 1952. Throughout the next 5 years of medical school and internship, that state remained unchanged. I can recall only two references to CF, one indirect and one direct, during that entire period. The indirect one happened a day or two after initial enrollment and before classes started. As was the custom at the time, groups of first year students were taken on tours of the various teaching hospitals. When our group toured the old Halifax Children's Hospital, we were shown a plastic tent canopy spread over a metal supporting frame with two or three rows of standard light bulbs attached to the metal frame. The intern conducting the tour told us that this heating apparatus was being tested as a method to produce a sufficient amount of sweat for laboratory analysis in certain babies and small children, but there was no mention specifically of CF. Later I learned that this method was being considered for investigating suspected cases of CF but was abandoned shortly afterward when reports about fatal complications (acute salt loss) accompanying its use appeared.

The second reference to CF was a direct one in a discussion of "Celiac Syndrome" in fourth year in 1955. In the discussion, the attending pediatrician listed 5 possible conditions to be considered in the differential diagnosis of an infant or child with this syndrome, which was characterized by foul smelling, greasy, bulky and floating bowel movements. Several different diseases could cause these abnormal stools. First on the list was celiac disease itself (later called gluten enteropathy) and last was "cystic fibrosis of the pancreas." There was no other mention of CF, either then or during internship through 1957.

Following graduation, I served five years in the armed forces as a Medical Officer with the Royal Canadian Air Force. This period included two years at Goose Bay, Labrador, a year of postgraduate work in cardiopulmonary physiology at the University of Western Ontario in London, a year at the Institute of Aviation Medicine in Toronto, and a final year as Senior Medical Officer at R.C.A.F. Station Summerside, P.E.I. In those years there was only one occasion when I considered CF as a possible diagnosis. That was at Goose Bay, an isolated airbase in Labrador where most of our work was with the dependents of air force personnel. The distraught parents of one infant reported greasy and malodorous bowel movements in their infant son, who was otherwise well. I briefly considered CF but quickly dismissed that possibility because the baby wasn't "sick." Eight years later, I met the family again in Halifax when I knew much more about CF. The child was well but a sweat test was done "just in case." Fortunately the result was well within normal limits.

During the year in Toronto, I began to consider my options after my military service ended in 1962. I was interested in pediatrics and discussed pediatric residency with a Dalhousie classmate who was then doing his pediatric training at the Hospital for Sick Children. It was then that I first heard of Dr. Cochrane, who was highly regarded as a teacher by the resident staff and had recently gone to the Children's Hospital in Halifax. My classmate recommended that I take pediatric training with Dr. Cochrane rather than in Toronto. While posted to Summerside in the following year, I attended the annual Dalhousie Refresher Course in Halifax where I had the opportunity to meet Dr. Cochrane. We discussed the pediatric training in general and the program at the Children's Hospital. Dr. Cochrane felt that, because of the unusual variety of cases, it was one of the best places in North America to start pediatric training. When my military service commitment ended in June 1962, I began two years of basic pediatric residency with him at the Children's Hospital in Halifax. I was unaware that a new era in the CF story in N.S. had been underway since 1958. Little did I realize that in the future CF would become a major part of my professional life.

Recently I reviewed the early years of CF in N.S. in a conversation with Dr. Cochrane who left Halifax in 1967 to become the first Professor of Pediatrics at the new medical school at the University of Calgary, Alberta. Subsequently he became Dean of Medicine and then President of the University of Calgary and currently resides in Calgary.

The Cochrane CF Program: 1958-1966

Shortly after arriving in Halifax in the summer of 1958, Dr. Cochrane diagnosed CF in an 11 year old boy. In searching the medical records at the hospital, he found files on 13 other CF patients living in the province who were the survivors of the 75 known diagnoses from 1950 to 1958. He was able to determine this number during his visits to communities throughout the Maritimes, a part of his teaching role in the Dalhousie Continuing Medical Education program. Challenged by the complex problems of CF, its devastating consequences, and poor survival, he started a special clinic for these patients and their families later that year and started a CF database that I continued to maintain through 1992.

Dr. Cochrane had a pivotal impact on the development of pediatrics throughout the Maritime Provinces. He spearheaded the recruitment of fulltime staff, strengthened the laboratory and investigative facilities at the Children's Hospital, and was active in strengthening the role of the community pediatricians. Dr R.L. Ozere (pediatric infectious disease) joined the fulltime staff in 1961. After Dr. Cochrane's appointment as Professor and Head of the Department of Pediatrics and Physician in Chief at the Children's Hospital in 1963, he recruited Dr. Margaret DeWolfe (immunochemist) in 1964, Dr. K.E. Scott (neonatalogy) in 1965, and Dr. Philip Welch (genetics) in 1967. Increasing numbers of physicians seeking postgraduate training in pediatrics enrolled as residents in Dr. Cochrane's program. With these additional staff members and with the assistance of the community pediatricians, he undertook major revisions in the pediatric undergraduate curriculum. With his major research interests in metabolic and inherited diseases, he secured research and fellowship grants that enabled him to enlist research fellows to develop a growing research capability.

Among others, he obtained a grant from the US Cystic Fibrosis Foundation (CFF) to support his work in CF. In 1964 I had the pleasure of meeting Dr. Kenneth Landauer, Medical Director of the CFF. Dr. LeRoy Matthews introduced us, remarking that I had trained with Dr. Bill Cochrane. Dr. Landauer expressed his pleasure on learning that the CFF grant to Dr. Cochrane had produced a trainee who was now training with Dr. Matthews. He obtained further grant support from the Canadian Cystic Fibrosis Foundation after it was incorporated in 1960. In addition to starting the CF clinic, he actively participated, with Mrs. Freda Vickery, Director of Social Services at the Children's Hospital, in the formation and activities of a Parent's Council and Advisory Committee for CF in the fall of 1958. This group, which provided strong support to the families, later evolved into the Cystic Fibrosis Society of Nova Scotia. Membership in the Council included representatives from across the province with a local executive committee in Halifax to conduct its day to day business. Although a relatively small organization, it was very active and secured the cooperation of service organizations and persons not personally involved with CF. Mr. George Smyth, parent of a child with CF, was principal author of a history of the CF Society of Nova Scotia from 1958 to 1983. He noted that they were "grateful for the contribution of persons not directly involved with the problem, and we are especially indebted to service clubs and similar organizations that seemed to arrive on the scene at a time that we needed a booster shot in terms of finances and morale." The Parent's Council negotiated an agreement with the Halifax Visiting Dispensary (a local voluntary non-profit charitable organization) to obtain drugs for CF at cost. Through fund raising efforts, the Council assured supplies of medications for the children with CF especially when the family was unable to carry the heavy financial burden. This dispensary later became the Metropolitan Dispensary and was able to secure space for its operations in the new Izaak Walton Killam Hospital for Children (IWK Children's Hospital) when it opened in 1970.

Mrs. Vickery and a physiotherapist attended the weekly clinic staffed by Dr. Cochrane and his fellow. Dr Arthur Shears, a specialist in physical medicine, saw each new patient and prescribed postural drainage procedures for those with respiratory problems. In clinic the physiotherapist taught the parents the techniques for doing these treatments at home on a daily basis but patients with serious respiratory problems were admitted to hospital for treatment and parental teaching. Funds were raised to obtain aerosol and mist tent nebulizers and Mrs. Vickery maintained a storage cupboard in her office for these items. The Metropolitan Dispensary dispensed pharmaceutical grade U.S.P. propylene glycol diluted to a 10% solution used in the mist tents along with all the medications (antibiotics, pancreatic enzymes, and water soluble vitamin preparations) used to treat CF. Medications were available at cost and when family resources could not meet these costs, the CF Society provided financial assistance so that all patients received the prescribed medications. Members of the Parent's Council assisted families with newly diagnosed children in setting up and using the inhalation equipment for home use. If the patients lived outside the Halifax area, members of the Parent's Council traveled to the homes to assist the families in setting up for their newly diagnosed child.

In his discussions and correspondence with physicians throughout the province, Dr. Cochrane sought their cooperation in referring patients with CF to the clinic. He stressed that the clinic was formed to gather and record clinical information that would provide impetus for research into the underlying cause of CF and create conditions for improving treatment of affected children. He was careful to assure the referring physicians that the clinic would not "steal" their patients by assuring them that the patients would return to their family physicians for continuing care. This assurance resulted in all known patients in the province being referred to the new clinic and they provided the basis of the CF database for all patients with CF diagnosed in N.S. since July 1958.

In addition to medical education, Dr. Cochrane actively sought to increase public knowledge of CF and helped the members of the CF Society in public fund raising endeavors and educational campaigns. The small CF Society, beset with the terrible emotional, social, and financial burdens of this devastating disease, submitted annual briefs to the provincial Minister of Health seeking financial support but no funds were forthcoming until 1968.

After the Canadian Cystic Fibrosis Foundation (CCFF) was incorporated in 1960, Dr. Cochrane was active in its Medical Advisory Committee. Mrs. Vickery served as a resource person for home care in CF and was called upon to speak to several chapters of the Foundation across the country. The CF Society of NS served the entire province, whereas the CCFF was organized into local "chapters" elsewhere in Canada. While the two bodies cooperated, the CF Society of NS, because of its province wide jurisdiction and with particular ties to both N.B. and P.E.I., remained as a separate organization until the mid 1970s. Then the Society was reorganized and became the nucleus of what became the Metropolitan Chapter of the CCFF. Funds of the former Society, remaining after formation of the new chapter, were incorporated into the Stephen Russell Memorial Fund to provide vocational and educational training for patients with CF. This fund was established in 1973 by the parents of a 26 year old young man with CF who died that year and has been well utilized to support training and education of many young adults with CF.

Confirmation of the diagnosis of CF, as indicated in Dr. Patterson's 1951 report, was difficult and time consuming. It necessitated admission to hospital for duodenal intubation and analysis of duodenal fluid and, apart from the Children's Hospital, few hospitals were able to undertake this procedure. In 1953, Dr. Paul di Sant'Agnese reported that loss of salt in sweat was responsible for the salt depletion so common in CF. That led to studies to measure the salt lost in the sweat and in 1959 Drs. Gibson and Cooke published their report of a procedure called "pilocarpine iontophoresis," to measure the concentration of salt in sweat. Their report of the range for normal values and the range of elevated values observed in CF confirmed Dr. di Sant'Agnese's findings. This diagnostic method subsequently became the "gold standard" of diagnosis. It could be performed in an hour on an outpatient basis so hospitalization was not required to confirm a diagnosis. Dr. Cochrane had been following these developments closely and in early 1959, he obtained a portable kit for sweat testing from Dr. Shwachman in Boston. This portable kit was contained in a fishing tackle box and contained a battery operated ammeter to deliver a small current to the skin, and lead strips to serve as electrodes. This unit remained in use until 1967 when it was replaced by more up to date equipment.

The complete sweat test consists of two parts, collection of the sweat sample followed by laboratory analysis of the sample for its salt (sodium chloride) , usually the chloride, concentration. Dr. Cochrane's fellows collected and weighed the sweat samples and sent them to the laboratory for analysis. While this kit was available at the Children's Hospital, confirmation of diagnosis in other communities in the province remained problematic. To enhance physician awareness of CF and thereby improve the timing and the rate of diagnosis, Dr. Cochrane encouraged the use of the "sweat disk" as a screening test for CF. Although neither as accurate nor as reliable as the pilocarpine iontophoresis method, it was simple and virtually cost free. Small disks of salt free filter paper, approximately 2 inches in diameter, were soaked in a solution of silver chromate that imparted a dark brown color to the disks. As recalled from high school chemistry, when silver and chloride are mixed they precipitate to form a whitish salt, silver chloride. The screening test took advantage of this simple reaction. The child's hand was briefly wrapped in plastic to promote sweating. Then, with the plastic removed, the disk was placed between the child's thumb and forefinger. If high levels of salt were in the sweat, as in CF, a yellowish fingerprint appeared on the brown disk. This raised the possibility of CF and the child could then be sent to the Children's Hospital for the definitive sweat test. While Dr. Cochrane was aware of the limitations of this screening test (there were both false negative and false positive reactions), it promoted much needed awareness of CF among physicians, an improvement over not doing any testing at all. The disks were prepared and shipped to hospitals throughout the province and were widely used.

Dr. Cochrane kept abreast of research and clinical progress in CF and introduced inhalation and mist tent therapy, physical therapy (segmental postural drainage to assist in clearing mucus from the lungs), and antibiotics (given either orally, by injection, and/or in aerosols) to combat infection. The standard dietary approach then in use stressed a low fat, high protein diet with added enzymes to aid digestion of the food. Additional vitamins were also prescribed as part of daily treatment. A fundamental feature of his program was that, after treatment was initiated at the CF clinic or in hospital, the daily care routine was continued at home. Children with obvious respiratory disease or malnutrition were admitted to hospital for immediate treatment that was continued at home after discharge. Others, with less severe findings at diagnosis, had a modified treatment regimen prescribed in the outpatient clinic. After assessment by Dr. Shears, the parents were instructed in the techniques and procedures of segmental postural drainage by the physiotherapist. Even then, throat or sputum culture and antibiotic sensitivity tests were made at each clinic visit and, based on the results, antibiotics were prescribed on a long-term basis. If the cultures showed different sensitivities of the staphylococcal bacteria to the antibiotics in use, changes were recommended. Dr. Cochrane prescribed special aerosolized antibiotics if respiratory symptoms became prominent and he also encouraged parents to keep the children active. For some patients with increased respiratory symptoms, he recommended breathing exercises in addition to segmental postural drainage.

The introduction of this fairly intensive program, the first of its kind in the region, embraced the hospital, the home, and the community. Families were pleased with the knowledge that at long last something was being done for their children with CF. The program resulted in improvements in longevity and well being of the affected children with survival into adolescence being seen in more children than had been the case earlier.

Although we had seminars on CF during pediatric residency, we had relatively little contact with the affected children and families. For the most part, because of the special needs of these children, and the unusual therapy (aerosols, postural drainage, enzymes, tents, etc.) used only in CF, Dr. Cochrane and his fellows looked after the hospitalized children. Apart from writing the routine admission orders, we did not have much of a role in their management. During my two years of residency to 1964, I recall seeing only 5 or 6 hospitalized patients with CF. Unfortunately, all but one of them died. In my last 6 months at the Children's Hospital, I had occasional chances to attend CF clinic but I was still bewildered by the unusual medications, dosages, and treatments.

The necessity for duodenal intubation to obtain secretions for analysis to diagnose CF had all but disappeared with the advent of the sweat test. However the sweat test procedure itself was a matter of concern to me. Usually, Dr. Cochrane's fellow did the tests, but occasionally we residents were called upon to do them; I received two such calls in two years. The procedure involved the use of an analytical balance to weigh the small samples of sweat. I had last used such a delicate instrument some ten years earlier in the first year physiology course and had serious concern about the reliability of my use of the analytical balance. Because others developed similar concerns, I was prompted to establish a better solution to this problem later in my career.

During residency, I developed interests in immunology and hematology. When a two year National Institutes of Health (NIH) fellowship in the combined fields of hematology and immunology was announced at the Children's Hospital and the State University of New York at Buffalo, I arranged to go for interviews. While discussing this with Dr. Cochrane, he showed me a letter from Dr. Matthews at Babies and Children's Hospital, Western Reserve University in Cleveland, Ohio. Dr. Matthews was seeking trainees for a fellowship in children's chest diseases and CF. Dr. Cochrane suggested that I should visit him after the Buffalo interviews. I was not interested and responded with the comment "that isn't my thing Dr. Cochrane." On two subsequent occasions in discussing the fellowship in Buffalo, he again suggested the side trip to see Dr. Matthews. By this third time, the "penny dropped" and I finally realized that he really wanted me to see this Dr. Matthews. Prudently, I complied with his thrice repeated suggestion. In December 1963, I went to Buffalo for interviews and the fellowship was offered. I deferred acceptance until I had a chance to discuss the matter further with Dr. Cochrane and my family. Then came the short flight to Cleveland in the evening. At 8:30 AM the following morning, I met Dr. Matthews at Babies & Children's Hospital (B&C Hospital) and spent that entire day with him. We toured the clinical and laboratory facilities of the hospital, attended Grand Rounds, and met the Professor of Pediatrics and Department Chief, Dr. William Wallace, as well as a number of other staff members. In the afternoon, we made rounds on the fourth floor ward where CF patients were located. I was struck by the normal appearance of several of the dozen or so patients with CF whom we saw. Although hospitalized, they did not resemble what I naively believed all patients with CF looked like (thin, ill looking, and coughing). Some, outwardly at least, appeared quite normal. I couldn't help wondering what were they were doing in hospital. Given my limited background in CF, I was puzzled but I realized something was different in Cleveland. We finished the day about 6:30 PM. and Dr. Matthews then told me his deadline for applying for National Institutes of Health funds for the fellowship was the next day. He needed an answer, and put the question, "Are you interested?" My answer was brief, "Yes I am."

I returned to Halifax to complete the remaining 6 months of my basic training. During that time, I attended CF clinic several times and became closely involved in the care of a gravely ill 4 year old girl who was admitted in the final stages of respiratory failure. She died about 4:30 AM a few days after admission. I had been at her bedside all night and called Dr. Cochrane. He came to the hospital and we had early breakfast together in the hospital cafeteria. I remember him remarking that he didn't understand why we weren't getting the same results as Dr. Matthews in Cleveland. He said, "We're doing everything he's doing but we're not getting those results. I want you to find out why."

Fellowship

With that mandate, my family and I left Halifax in late June 1964 to begin the fellowship in Cleveland. Dr. Carl Doershuk met us. He had completed his fellowship training earlier and had joined the faculty, working with Dr. Matthews. He told me what to expect at CF clinic on the coming Monday morning starting at 8:30 AM. That Monday was my "baptism of fire" in CF as we saw patients steadily finishing about one o'clock in the afternoon.

The two years in Cleveland were filled with a fascinating variety of pulmonary cases and experiences, but much of our work related to CF. The caseload was heavy (we followed about 280 patients regularly every 4 to 6 weeks, and another 40 or so from out of state who were seen less frequently) and we saw patients 6 days a week. There was a very active research program with Dr. Don Carlson (biochemistry), Dr. Bernard Boxerbaum (microbiology), and Dr. Joe Potter (biochemistry/immunology) actively engaged in research projects related to CF. Dr. Matthews had established a pediatric pulmonary function laboratory directed by respiratory therapist, Mr. Marvin Lough, and this was used intensively to monitor the progress of individual patients and in studies to measure the efficacy of various therapeutic interventions.

I was not there very long before I found out why the program in Halifax wasn't getting the results being obtained in Cleveland. The fundamental difference was a matter of degree rather than kind. Dr. Cochrane had been using all of the basic measures that Dr. Matthews had initiated in Cleveland in 1957, but only in some of the patients. Dr. Matthews, on the other hand, had developed the concept of starting full treatment on the day of diagnosis for *every* patient, regardless of the clinical condition, and all were admitted to hospital to begin this treatment. This was not so in Halifax or in other clinics where treatment of the respiratory component of CF was begun only when the respiratory disease was quite evident. Dr. Matthews believed that since we knew that practically all infants and children with CF would develop lung disease sooner or later (usually sooner), it made sense to begin respiratory and nutritional treatment as soon as possible, even if there was no readily apparent respiratory trouble. Since most deaths were due to lung destruction and consequent cardiorespiratory failure, respiratory treatment had a certain primacy. This use of measures (aerosols, postural drainage, mist tents, antibiotics, etc) which hopefully could interrupt the vicious circle of obstruction and infection in the bronchial tubes so characteristic of CF, was logical. Dr. Matthews had a unique and profound grasp of postnatal lung growth and development. In his closing lecture to second year medical students at the end of the Respiratory Section in the spring of 1966, he presented a masterful account of the enormous postnatal growth that takes place in the respiratory system in infancy and early childhood. He taught that the obstruction and infection associated with CF interrupt and distort normal growth and development of the respiratory system, especially in the smallest bronchial tubes. Since mucus in the infected CF airways became stagnant, like poorly flowing water, he emphasized that the best way to prevent this development was to keep the stream (the airways) flowing cleanly. Thus his treatment philosophy and methodology combined both preventive and active interventions, aimed at preserving the capacity for normal growth but at the same time actively treating obstruction and infection. The survival results, better than those attained elsewhere, demonstrated the effectiveness of this intensive and comprehensive therapeutic program. Because it was very unlikely that a so called "mild" case would remain so, he stressed the importance of using the various measures in all patients from the outset.

During my stay in Cleveland, I saw the dramatic results of these measures in many, many children. A particular 10 month old infant with CF, who was referred and admitted on New Year's Day, 1965 is permanently etched in my memory. In her home area she had had surgery at birth for bowel obstruction (the meconium ileus that occurs with CF) and was diagnosed at that time. She had surgery again at 5 months of age. At birth, she weighed 6 pounds and unfortunately still weighed just 6½ pounds at 10 months of age when she arrived at B&C Hospital. In the next year and a half, she had two follow up admissions. The improvement during her first admission was dramatic enough, but was even more so after two subsequent admissions later in the year. I last saw her at 23 months of age when, apart, from the scars of surgery, she was to all intents and purposes a normal child in every respect. My reaction at the time was simple. If this is comprehensive therapy at work, then I'm all for it. Skeptics abounded, but most of those who came to see firsthand what was going on, quickly lost their skepticism. However, one morning while I was working in the pulmonary function lab, Dr. Doershuk came in with two visiting pediatricians from out of state who came to look at the program. When he was called away to see a problem on the ward, one of the visitors asked me, "Do they work like this all the time?" When I assured them that indeed they did, he commented, "Now I understand why they get the results they do. When I get home, I don't intend to work that hard." For me, the challenge on returning to Halifax would be to emulate the comprehensive treatment program, so that we too could achieve similar results.

Table 28.1 Age of Patients

Age (years)	July 1958 Number	%	July 1966 Number	%	July 1974 Number	%
Under 1	1	8%	4	9%	2	3%
1 – 5	7	54%	19	41%	12	16%
5 – 10	5	38%	9	20%	24	31%
10 – 15	--	--	7	15%	21	42%
15 – 21	--	--	7	15%	10	28%
21 – 28	--	--	----	---	7	9%
Total	13		46		76	

On my return to Halifax in 1966, Dr. Cochrane and I both attended CF clinic on July 4. When it was over, his comment to me was brief, "Okay Terry, it's your baby."

The Comprehensive Clinic 1966–1992

It was the best of times to be returning to Halifax. Canada's forthcoming Centennial Year (1967) loomed just beyond in the New Year, and the citizenry eagerly anticipated Expo 67. Locally, construction of a modern new Children's Hospital (the Izaak Walton Killam Hospital for Children or as known locally, "the IWK") made possible by the generous bequests of Izaak Walton Killam (a Nova Scotia born industrialist) and his wife, was already underway. Each Canadian province had a specific Centennial project and for N.S. that project was the erection of the Sir Charles Tupper building to house the Dalhousie University Medical School. Named in honor of Sir Charles Tupper, a physician from N.S., a past President of the Canadian Medical Association (1867–1870), and later Prime Minister of Canada (1896), it was scheduled to open in 1968.

In 1958, Dr. Cochrane was able to identify 13 surviving patients with CF in the province. None were over 10 years of age. By July 1966, he had 46 patients under his care with an increasing age span up to 21 years of age. (Table 28.1). The care of these patients and direction of the clinic were now my responsibility. After another 8 years in 1974, the age range extended to 28 years of age and 37% were over 15 years old.

On my arrival there were two infants in hospital who provided me the opportunity to begin working with the house staff, nurses, physiotherapist, and two new inhalation therapists who had just been employed. The infants had been diagnosed earlier in the year and had been readmitted because of major difficulty with wheezing. With intensified treatment, changed aerosol therapy, and improved mist tent equipment, the response was gratifying and the nurses were quick to notice. Before discharge, the parents were taught continuing home care management and the maintenance of the new equipment. During this period, I had the first of many teaching sessions, particularly with the nurses, which were held on the ward as circumstances permitted.

The next six months were busy with 18 further admissions, 17 for known patients and one for a newly diagnosed and quite ill 13 month old boy. These patients were all treated with intermittent aerosols 4 times daily (more often if necessary), postural drainage, pancreatic enzymes, vitamins, and antibiotics, and nightly mist tent therapy. The antibiotics were given either intravenously (IV) or by intramuscular (IM) injections. At that time, oral antibiotics for resistant "Staph" (staphylococcal bacteria, a major problem in CF patients) had become available, but for inpatients we relied on the IM or IV preparations with preference for the latter. During this time, whenever the opportunity presented, I had informal training sessions for the nurses, including administering aerosol treatments, mixing the pancreatic enzymes in applesauce, and control of the room temperature so that the children could sleep comfortably in the tents. I especially wanted to convey to them my own belief in a much more hopeful future for those with CF than was generally believed. Their knowledge and attitudes had a very important bearing on therapy; their skills, efforts, and concerns in applying the therapy measures were a sine qua non of exemplary treatment. And it was a two way street, as their observations and skills were vitally important to me. Despite carrying an increased workload because of the more intensive treatment employed, the nurses quickly responded to the improvement in the well being of the patients and the parents quickly sensed these more hopeful attitudes, usually without a word being said.

Several of the readmitted patients were seriously ill and required very intensive treatment. In addition to the management of their respiratory problems, nutritional problems were of major concern. The then prevailing attitude that diet in CF should be low in fat had to be countered with a more positive approach that stressed, first, the needs of the child. The children needed, perhaps above all else, to grow. For that to occur, a high protein intake was vital (reflecting the "wisdom of the body" many children with CF made up for the loss of nutrients in their bowel movements by demolishing a steak with surprising ease). It took a considerable period of time to redirect attitudes from the primarily negative one of fat restriction to a positive one of first providing increased protein the child needed for growth, with as few fat restrictions as possible. Water-soluble forms of vitamins A, D, E, and K were ordered for all children to replace the fat soluble forms lost with the excessive fat excreted in the stools. Of particular importance was vitamin K. Lack of this vitamin could result in excessive bruising and bleeding, and at diagnosis or with episodes of infection, laboratory tests were done to detect any problem. In newborn infants who had surgical removal of part of the small bowel because of meconium ileus (intestinal blockage), interference with the normal absorption of vitamin B12 was a potential consequence, so these patients received a 3 day course of intramuscular B12 with 2 weeks of oral folic acid.

For comprehensive treatment program to be transferred to the home, a great deal of time is needed to implement it and to train each family. Given the far reaching and long term chronic aspects of CF, admission to hospital at the time of diagnosis provided the necessary time and opportunity to begin parental education. I felt that a minimum of two weeks was necessary to assess and treat the patient and for the parents to get realistically informed about CF and trained in the techniques and methods of its management at home. Many infants and children, critically ill at diagnosis, required lengthy stays in hospital before they could be managed successfully at home. It was very gratifying to see parents leave the hospital with a child so much better than on admission. The teaching hospital atmosphere provided opportunities to work and consult with my medical confreres and colleagues, junior and senior housestaff, nurses, physiotherapists, respiratory technologists, social workers, and a host of others in meeting the challenges of CF. It did not take long for a remarkable team of individuals to develop, united by the aim of providing exemplary care for the patients.

The problem with sweat testing done by resident physicians referred to earlier, soon became an issue for me to resolve. Before anyone with CF could be treated, a diagnosis had to be made and that required a reliable diagnostic standard. As with any other sensitive diagnostic test, such a procedure is best done by experienced laboratory staff. The Gibson and Cooke sweat test was by this time accepted as the "gold standard." After the first new case of CF was diagnosed that September 1966, there was an increase in the number of requests for sweat tests. Unfortunately, this increased volume had to be performed by the resident staff and resulted in an acute work overload for them. In the meantime, I was trying to have the entire procedure (both collection of the sweat samples and analysis in the lab) done by qualified laboratory technicians. That would provide the best guarantee of reliability and accuracy, and the procedure would be covered by the provincial hospital insurance plan, so that no charges would be levied on a family for the test. By January 1967 this was accomplished to everyone's satisfaction. We then updated the equipment and adopted the modifications of the Gibson-Cooke method, as published by Dr. Warren Warwick and his co-workers in Minneapolis.

As a teaching tool, I formulated clinical guidelines that incorporated the philosophy and methodology of Dr. Matthews. I wanted to emulate his comprehensive treatment program so that we could achieve similar results in survival and improved well being, although our circumstances were very different from those in Cleveland in population, number of pediatricians, and patterns of medical practice. For example, only two of the thirteen pediatricians in N.S. were located outside Halifax, a neonatologist in Sydney at the north end of the province, and a general pediatrician in Yarmouth at the south end. N.B. had only eight pediatricians and P.E.I. just two. My guidelines were:

> Each patient, regardless of clinical condition, to be admitted to hospital at diagnosis.
>
> Initiation of long term inhalation therapy and postural drainage with clapping and vibration.

Antibiotic usage to be specific (whenever possible) and intensive but intermittent.

Full physical activity encouraged in and out of hospital.

Frequent follow up in clinic every 4 to 6 weeks recommended.

Readmission to hospital, especially in infancy and early childhood, to be early and when deemed necessary, to prevent or minimize complications versus delayed or "last resort" admissions.

These guidelines encompassed my understanding of the Cleveland program as adapted to our circumstances. They were not carved in stone and I was prepared to change any of them if there was evidence that this was desirable. But until there was such evidence, I planned to implement and maintain these guidelines and I did so. They remained in effect during my tenure as clinic director to 1992, with the exception of the tent therapy for newly diagnosed patients. This therapy had become controversial, prompted to a considerable degree by flawed studies.

The P.E.I. Mass Screening Project

As their official Centennial project for Canada's Centennial in 1967, the Medical Advisory Council (MAC) of the CCFF proposed to conduct a survey in P.E.I. province to determine the incidence of CF. This information would be valuable scientifically and in medical and public health planning for the future. The proposal was to do sweat tests in a statistically selected sample of children of the Island to obtain a measure of the incidence in the Canadian population. P.E.I., Canada's smallest province with a population of about 130,000, descended mainly by settlers from the British Isles and northwestern France, was ideally suited for this project.

Dr. Cochrane had a medical student, Jim Nugent, on a CCFF sponsored summer research project assessing a newer but untried sweat test (the conductivity method) that was being considered for use in the proposed screening project. Since weighing of the sweat sample was not necessary, it would be simpler and take less time than the standard pilocarpine iontophoresis method. I was aware that Dr. Matthews had found it less accurate than the established method and I was intrigued by the possibility of using another method altogether.

Dr. Warren Warwick, CF Center Director at University Hospitals in Minneapolis, was using a heated gel pack to stimulate sweating and a new chloride specific electrode to analyze the chloride concentration. This method of sweat testing required only 5 minutes of heat stimulation followed by a virtually instantaneous determination of salt concentration using the chloride electrode. With this method a complete screening of the entire childhood population of P.E.I. might be feasible, rather than the small sample by the standard technique. Dr. Warwick sent his technician, Ms. Joanne Koroshec, R.N. to Halifax to conduct preliminary tests in January 1967. Using Dr. Warwick's method in our CF clinic, in Charlottetown, P.E.I., and in St. John's, Newfoundland, the salt concentrations were elevated in the children with CF, but not in their unaffected siblings. Dr. Cochrane's recommendation to the CCFF Medical Advisory Committee to use this technique for the mass screening project was accepted. Mr. William Hardy, past president of the CCFF, obtained the endorsement of the P.E.I. government, and enlisted the services of Mr. Wiley Barrett to act as the on site field director and coordinator. Events moved swiftly and included a meeting of personnel from government departments and various community agencies, pediatricians Dr. J.H. O'Hanley and Dr. Ross Parker, a number of other interested parties, including the Women's Institutes of P.E.I., and Mr. Hardy, Mr. Barrett, and I attended. Four mobile teams of two persons each were trained to do the testing at 47 sites around the province. The provincial Premier, the Honorable Alex Campbell, and his wife opened the project by having their children tested in Summerside. This and other events provided for excellent media coverage. The response was nothing short of phenomenal, a tribute to the superb organizational skills and diligent work of Wiley Barrett, the 4 teams, and the enthusiasm of the many volunteers. Parents from the many rural communities throughout the length and breadth of the Island arrived at the testing sites with their children and gave the occasion a festive air.

The actual procedure took only 5 or 6 minutes per child. The volunteers arranged themselves in assembly line fashion so that the child went from person to person for each step in the process (registration, washing the forearm, applying a square of parafilm and the heated gel pack, and finally covering them with terry toweling fastened by Velcro straps). Each child's card was stamped with the time at the start. At the end of the line, when the time stamp matched the 5 minute delay time on the technician's clock, everything was quickly removed, the electrode applied, and the meter reading recorded. In the month long project, we tested 35,411 infants and children (over 90% of the childhood population of P.E.I.) from 3 weeks to 17 years of age with only a small number of equivocal tests.

The known cases were correctly identified and one additional case, a 2 year old girl with severe pulmonary disease, was found; she had a lung transplant in 1993 and still resides in P.E.I. While this was a successful mass screening operation, it was clear however that the test was not an "off the shelf" item, as it required the skill and expertise of trained individuals for its proper implementation and expert analysis of the results. Without the grant, the Minnesota support from Dr. Warwick and Ms. Koroshec, the fairly closed geography of the island, and the extensive cooperation of the island's physicians, the project simply would not have been possible.

This experience led us to a trial of neonatal screening using the same technique in newborn infants, knowing that newborns may not sweat adequately and it was possible that sufficient sweat might not be collected. This screening plan was predicated on the belief that early diagnosis in conjunction with early institution of treatment would go a long way in preventing or delaying the lung damage and malnutrition so characteristic of CF and ultimately would improve survival. In 1968, the CCFF approved my grant for a pilot study of newborn screening for CF at the Grace Maternity Hospital in Halifax, the principal obstetrical teaching hospital of the medical school conveniently located across the street from the pediatric hospital. With approval of the medical staff and parents, we screened all babies in the normal newborn nurseries between the 3rd and 5th day after delivery for a 6 week period in the summer of 1968. After 264 consecutive normal newborns were screened, a positive test was obtained on a 3 day old male infant. On the following day, the pilocarpine iontophoresis test confirmed the positive result with further confirmation at 9 and 14 days of age. In this patient, adequate amounts of sweat were obtained by iontophoresis without problem. This was an exciting development being the first time a neonate had been screened positive for CF with a sweat test and the result confirmed by the standard laboratory sweat test, pilocarpine iontophoresis. He continues to do well.

The screening program was repeated in the summer of 1969 but no new cases were found. In the summer of 1970, we used a new commercial unit consisting of a chloride electrode and a miniature iontophoresis device for screening, but this was unsatisfactory and we had to abandon the project. Later, with the advent of newer screening modalities, I sought to have a province-wide screening program introduced but, unfortunately, this was not supported by the Department of Health.

My fellowship experience had taught me that CF was indeed treatable and I came back with an attitude of hope and expectation of a better future for the children and families. In those two fellowship years, there were only 6 deaths among the more than 300 patients we followed. This very low mortality experience was in sharp contrast to my earlier two years of basic residency in Halifax with 5 deaths among the 6 children with CF whom I happened to see.

Rapid growth in patient numbers occurred over the decade ending July 1976. In addition to the increasing number of survivors as noted above and the newly diagnosed patients from N.S., there were 16 cases from N.B., 11 from P.E.I. and 1 from Newfoundland. The IWK Hospital was the only children's hospital in the Maritime Provinces so patients from the other two provinces and occasionally from Newfoundland were referred for evaluation and treatment.

Growth also included an increase in number of outpatient visits and hospital admissions (628 admissions in the 1966–1976 decade) and concomitant growth in a more positive attitude about CF, not only among the staff, but also in the involved families. These improvements were outgrowths of support provided by the CCFF, particularly in the form of annual clinic incentive grants. In the fall of 1967, we had our first site visit. Drs. Harry Shwachman, from Boston, and Douglas Crozier, from Toronto, visited the clinic on behalf of the CCFF and recommended that the clinic incentive grant be increased. They recommended more participation and involvement of house staff in the outpatient clinic and support for a clinical fellowship. Dr. Kenneth Wong was our first CF Fellow, followed by Drs. Vijaya Belgaumkar, Thomas Lee, Margaret Brown, and Irene O'Kane. In 1978, fellowship support was changed to support a CF Clinic Nurse Coordinator. We were fortunate in securing the services of Ms. Patricia Summers, R.N., an experienced Public Health Nurse, as the CF Nurse. Her work was primarily in the outpatient clinic and home visiting and, along with Marie Gallant our social worker, their visits to each CF family in the province twice yearly was invaluable in increasing the effectiveness of the comprehensive therapeutic program.

The Pulmonary Function Laboratory

Shortly after returning to Halifax, I submitted a proposal to the federal Department of National Health and Welfare and the Medical Research Council for funding for a pediatric pulmonary function laboratory. We needed this laboratory as a vital tool to monitor the disease processes and the effects of treatment in CF and a variety of other childhood pulmonary diseases. Thousands of children with chronic respiratory problems (especially asthmatic bronchitis) were living in the province but we had no means of directly measuring the extent of their disabilities and the impact of various therapies. This major but largely neglected area in child health required a laboratory to support much needed investigations and improvements in treatment.

Plans for the new hospital included space for a pulmonary function laboratory. My grant application for a technician was approved, and with funding from the new federal Health Resources Fund, pulmonary function equipment was ordered. Pending the opening of the new hospital in 1970, I obtained laboratory space in the Clinical Research Center located near the hospital. On the day in 1968 that the crates with the much anticipated new equipment were delivered to the laboratory, the Dean of Medicine also arrived and said very simply, "I'm sorry Dr. Gillespie, but you are going to have to move. The newly organized Family Medicine Division is going to need this space." There was only one problem, there was no place to go. As a result, the equipment went into storage in the basement of the newly opened Sir Charles Tupper Building where it remained for over two years until the new IWK Hospital opened in 1970.

Unfortunately, that wasn't the end of the matter; the provincial Hospital Services Commission delivered further bad news. It announced that when the new hospital opened, no monies would be available to pay technicians to perform the tests. Earlier, in preparation for the move to the new hospital, I arranged for each of our two inhalation therapists to obtain two weeks of training at Dr. Matthews' pediatric pulmonary function laboratory with Marvin Lough, and at Dr. Will Waring's laboratory at Tulane University Hospitals in New Orleans, Louisiana. Fortunately, when the new IWK Hospital did open, the Medical Director, Dr. A.S. Wenning approved a proposal to include pulmonary function testing in the job description of the inhalation therapists. At the same time, the CCFF agreed to provide a monthly stipend to pay for technical services. This arrangement continued for several years until the Hospital Services Commission agreed to a revised schedule of payments for pulmonary function testing. After these provisions were in place, we had a period of "dry runs" to insure that our techniques and procedures were satisfactory and reliable. Finally, on July 1, 1971, pulmonary function testing became available for children 5 years and older. All CF patients were tested periodically thereafter.

Satellite Clinics and Outreach Programs

From 1967 onward, there was rapid growth in the number of patients being followed and in the extent of clinic activities, including our outreach program. A satellite CF clinic in Charlottetown, P.E.I., was supported by the pediatricians and the Department of Health, and was underway in the fall of that year. It involved a 400 mile round trip including ferry travel across Northumberland Strait. Initially the clinic was a one day affair held on Saturdays 6 times a year. The active support and participation of the provincial Public Health Nurses provided enhanced support for the families and was a unique feature of these clinics. When pediatrician Dr. Parker left the Island in the early 1970s, Dr. Charlie Brown who, during his training had been a fellow with Dr. Cochrane in Halifax replaced him. Dr. Brown was familiar with CF so that it was not necessary to hold clinics as frequently. Later we were able to change to twice yearly clinics held over a two day period and attended by the full CF team from the IWK Hospital.

About the same time, Dr. Douglas Gibbon in Saint John, N.B. asked me to see the children with CF he was following and Dr. Claude Leighton, a Moncton, N.B. pediatrician, asked me to speak about CF at a public meeting. Nurses from the Moncton Hospital were in attendance and I was asked, in particular, to address the then current policy of isolating hospitalized CF children. Dr. Leighton felt that the only way to settle the matter was to have a public statement from a "visiting fireman" like me. After that meeting, the policy was changed to allow children with CF to be admitted to the open pediatric ward. During the late 1960s and early 1970s, whenever the schedule permitted, I included trips to Moncton and Saint John with the trip to Charlottetown to see patients with CF. Along with Dr. Lee Stickles, pediatrician in Fredericton, N.B., Drs. Gibbon and Leighton often referred their newly diagnosed patients to the IWK Hospital for initiation of treatment, as did physicians from a predominantly French speaking region of northeastern N.B.

In N.S. until 1971, I participated, along with other pediatric specialists, in the traveling clinics sponsored by the Rotary Clubs in N.S. Initially two orthopedic surgeons and two general pediatricians visited communities distant from Halifax to provide specialist care to the children in the area. Shortly after returning to Halifax, I was invited to participate in these biannual clinics. Later other pediatric sub-specialists joined in attending what were then called "the crippled children's clinics." On these trips, I saw mostly children with asthma and bronchitis, but also any children with CF living in the area. Local physicians found aerosol therapy used in CF very helpful in treating asthmatic children and its use spread widely throughout the province.

In 1973, Dr. Margaret Churchill (at that time the only pediatrician practicing outside Halifax) in Yarmouth, N.S. asked me to see selected children with chest problems. At the first such visit, I spoke briefly to the area physicians about preventive measures (such as daily aerosol treatments) for chronically ill asthmatic children. A Dr. Clark asked if I would visit his community also to see his patients with chest problems and thus began a unique experience that I like to call "The Pubnico Chronicles."

These trips provided a welcome respite from the hospital scene and we set up a twice yearly schedule. Similar to the P.E.I. clinic trips, they required a 450 mile round trip between Halifax and Yarmouth. Dr. Churchill was interested in bringing up to date care to her area so that children and families would not incur the difficulty and expense of travel to Halifax for consultation. I was interested in teaching physicians about daily preventive measures that could benefit many of their patients. After driving down the scenic southwestern shore of N.S., I saw Dr. Churchill's patients for 2 ½ days at the Yarmouth Regional Hospital. Then I drove some 35 miles up the shore to the village of Pubnico to see the pulmonary patients of Dr. Alexander "Sandy" Clark, the Pubnico physician who spoke to me after the luncheon meeting on my first trip to Yarmouth. Mariners and seafarers along the eastern coast of North America knew "The Pubnicos" as part of the rich fishing grounds and trade route for carrying goods and supplies between Canadian and American ports all along the coast. The main village, Pubnico, at the head of Pubnico Bay, a long inlet from the sea, is small with only a dozen or so homes, a general store, a gas station, and a garage. On the southwest side of the inlet were the bilingual Acadian communities and on the eastern side of Pubnico Bay, the population was much less homogeneous with a mixed background of English speaking folks. I usually arrived in Pubnico in mid afternoon Wednesday and saw Dr. Clark's patients from then until about 5 PM on Friday. Then I had a 3½ hour drive back to Halifax to prepare reports to Drs. Churchill and Clark. The welcome pleasures of these trips were the over night stays, especially with Dr. Clark in his beautiful old home that also served as the local Medical Centre. It held three offices, a small conference room, and a small dispensary (there was no pharmacy in the village). He had two associates and between the three of them covered a large section of the coastal area. Sandy was from the Lake District of England, a widower, and a first class physician who enjoyed his work. He was also a good cook, an avid gardener, and active in the local Lion's Club.

Apart from the opportunity of seeing patients closer to their homes and the medical challenges they presented, I have fond memories of the civility and pleasantries of those trips. In Yarmouth, Margaret Churchill exercised her hospitality and considerable culinary skills by treating us to evening dinner. In Pubnico, Sandy demonstrated his cooking skill with the evening meal (which he cooked) after which we had libations in front of a crackling fire in the fireplace.

From his predecessor Dr. Clark had inherited a patient with CF whom he seldom saw because the family made regular trips every six weeks to the CF clinic in Halifax. Like most physicians, he had no experience with CF. That changed in 1977 when he sent an infant with meconium ileus to Halifax for surgery. The father was a fisherman and could not be at the hospital. Since I was due in Pubnico soon after, I met with both parents there in Dr. Clark's conference room where we discussed CF for over two hours. Dr. Clark sat in on this session and became very interested. Later, seven more children with CF were diagnosed from his area and, after their initial treatment at the IWK Hospital, Sandy saw them regularly in follow-up. He and I kept in close touch, and the frequent trips to Halifax were no longer necessary for these children. Dr Clark provided first-class care for these children and their families in their own rural community. To me, this was a unique melding of the ivory tower and the front line physician in a rural medical practice. As a result, everyone benefited and no one lost. On the occasion of his retirement, Sandy received the "Breath of Life" award of the CCFF in recognition of his truly unique contribution to the care and well being of his CF patients.

Universal Drug Coverage

In N.S., as elsewhere in Canada, the provisions of the federal Canada Health Act govern health care. The five major provisions of this act assure a health care program that is universal, accessible, comprehensive, portable, and publicly administered through a series of agreements between the federal government and the ten provincial governments. While the details vary from one province to another, for families confronting the daily realities of dealing with all the problems presented by such a complex disease as CF, this program was a blessing. But this universal insurance program did not cover the cost of medications and for many years this was a deterrent and hindrance in the provision of care for the majority of patients and families.

In 1967, the CF Society of NS conducted a study of drug costs for outpatients and determined that the annual cost was $500 per patient. This was beyond the means of most families with CF children and the Society raised funds by every means possible to supplement the drug costs. As a result, no child went without necessary medications. But as more children survived and newer medicines were introduced, the costs required more substantial support. Each year, from 1959 onward, the CF Society submitted annual briefs to the Minister of Health requesting funds to assist in meeting the crippling drug costs. There was no support from government but in 1967, an addendum was attached to the annual brief. After a review of the results of comprehensive therapy, it ended with a statement that the outlook for children with CF was much better than generally believed providing the necessary medications and equipment were available to implement such treatment. There was no formal reply, but the Provincial Department of Health in the spring of 1968 provided a grant of $10,000. Subsequently annual increments were received so that by 1975-1976, the grant had reached $18,000. The drug costs the previous year were $36,000 and the CF Society continued its efforts to raise money to supplement the difference.

During the early 1970s, the Department of Pediatrics proposed to the provincial government the coverage of the cost of treatment of several chronic diseases, including CF. It was soon obvious that the Department of Health could not accept this proposal and we were advised to consider submitting proposals for individual conditions. Considering that children don't vote but their parents do, parents and families with CF submitted their concerns and complaints about the burden of drug costs directly to their political representatives in the provincial Legislative

Assembly. These complaints must have influenced the politicians. I was told that a letter to the provincial Minister of Health from a particularly vociferous mother of two children with CF (one of whom had died earlier) was shown to the members of the provincial cabinet with his comment, "Well gentlemen, what are we going to do about this?" By this time, in light of the annual briefs and the undeniable improvement in well being and survival that occurred after comprehensive care was introduced, the government was prepared to consider proposals for CF. A committee was formed with members from government, the Medical Society of Nova Scotia, the provincial pharmaceutical association, and other agencies. I was appointed as the representative of the Medical Society. We met for three sessions, during which the costs and details of such drug coverage were thoroughly considered and debated. The question of which medications would be covered was somewhat contentious. Despite one proposal that the plan cover only the major drugs then in use, I pushed for coverage of all drugs, both those currently in use and any new drugs that might be found in future to be beneficial. Fortunately the committee accepted this and submitted a report to the provincial Minister of Health who subsequently announced that, effective on October 1, 1976, all drugs and equipment used in the treatment of CF would be covered under a special plan as part of the provincial Medical Services Insurance program. Initially, $100,000 was earmarked for this program. There were two relatively minor exceptions, insulin (already covered under another provincial program) and oxygen. Oxygen was not considered to be a "drug" in the context of this plan. In later years, after the formation of the Adult CF Clinic in 1983-1984, arrangements were made to include coverage of home oxygen therapy. The institution of drug coverage for CF was the "jewel in the crown of Medicare" and stands as a tribute to the diligent and persistent work of the dedicated parents and volunteers who formed the Nova Scotia CF Society. I believe this program to be one of the best in the country and it remains fully in effect.

Two Special Families

The following two families stand out in my memory, especially the latter which helped in the search for the CF gene. Each family had five children with CF, taught me a great deal, and both serve to illustrate the wide and variable spectrum of disability and disease in this complex disorder. And of greater significance, the second family also showed how a clinical care oriented Center can assist in the research effort to conquer or cure CF.

In the first family, one infant died before the clinic opened in 1958 while four additional children were subsequently diagnosed, with two of them dying in infancy. When I succeeded Dr. Cochrane at the CF clinic, the two remaining children with CF in this family were among the 46 patients with CF living in the province. The older of these two children was 3 years old and was seriously ill with extensive lung disease when I first saw her on admission in August 1966. When diagnosed, she had been started on digestive enzymes, vitamins, and a low fat diet but because the chest x-ray was reported as "within normal limits," pulmonary therapy was not prescribed. By the time I saw her, her pulmonary disease was severe and progressive and she was the sickest of our patients. She died in 1967 before she was five years of age, having spent a total of 342 days of her short life in hospital. Her death from CF was the first I encountered after returning to Halifax a year earlier.

The fifth child with CF in this family was then two years of age. The family lived 275 miles from Halifax and trips to clinic were expensive and difficult as the father was on a disability pension and unable to travel. The mother developed serious health problems of her own, and, following the death of their fourth child with CF in 1967, the remaining CF child was seen only once in the following year. When I was unable to arrange local follow up, the family agreed to have their daughter admitted to the Children's Hospital in Halifax once or twice yearly for intensive treatment while continuing her daily home treatment as usual. This therapeutic compromise, in lieu of frequent and regular outpatient follow-up visits, did make a difference and she was able to finish primary school and enroll in high school. Unfortunately, she died in 1980, shortly before her 16th birthday. Despite the heartbreak endured by this courageous mother, she expressed her happiness in having at least one of the children with CF survive long enough to attend school successfully.

Somewhat later, the second family with five children (two girls and three boys ranging from 7 to 18 years of age at diagnosis) presented a pattern of symptoms that differed from the usual combination of recurrent respiratory trouble and growth failure usually seen in CF. This family played a significant part in the genetic studies by Dr. Lap-Chee Tsui and his colleagues in Toronto. The index case in the family was a 12 year old boy with a history of sinus trouble and intermittent wheezing who was referred to Dr. Lee Stickles, a Fredericton, N.B. pediatrician, for consultation. He ordered sweat tests because the boy had nasal polyps. Sweat testing (4 paired tests) gave "borderline" results ranging from 39 to 57 for chloride concentrations; all tests had adequate amounts of sweat. Additionally, the chest x-ray was reported as showing findings in keeping with allergic bronchopulmonary aspergillosis, a condition seen at our hospital only in children with CF. We discussed this boy's problem and jointly agreed to consider this as CF. Later in 1983 a series of sweat tests were performed on the other 4 children. A few results were in keeping with CF, but most were "borderline" or even within normal limits. Each child had nasal polyps and abnormal pulmonary function tests. When everything was considered, a diagnosis of CF in each of the children seemed justified. This serious diagnosis was discussed with the parents and Dr. Stickles and, after hospitalization at the IWK Hospital in January 1984 for further studies, the children were started on full CF therapy.

In 1984, in response to a request for blood samples from families with two or more children with CF from geneticists at the Hospital for Sick Children (HSC) in Toronto, we sent specimens from each child, the parents, the grandparents on one side, and an aunt. These blood specimens confirmed the diagnosis of CF in each of the 5 children and were used along with others from across Canada in the research that culminated in the exciting discovery of the location of the CF gene on chromosome 7 in 1989. Later, Dr. Manuel Buchwald, a geneticist from the HSC research team, told me that they might not have been able to complete their study without the samples obtained from this family. This was a very gratifying experience.

While the advent of genetic testing with DNA analysis has made diagnosis easier in situations where the sweat test gives equivocal or borderline results, neither method will produce infallible results. There is still a place for the exercise of common sense and good clinical judgment.

The Adult CF Clinic

Our first experience with transfer to adult care came in 1978 when I had to go on emergency medical leave. Since funding for a CF fellow had stopped in 1977, there was no other experienced pediatrician available and 12 adult patients had to be transferred to the adult teaching hospital. There was no time to make adequate arrangements at the adult hospital for allocation of beds and personnel necessary to accommodate the special CF needs. Additionally, when adult CF patients were admitted to the adult facility, the adult respirologist who had agreed to deal with their problems was not necessarily consulted, resulting in fragmentation and inconsistency of care. Soon after I returned to work, the adult respirologist left Halifax and the surviving 10 of the 12 patients who had been transferred returned to continue follow up at our clinic. Pending more satisfactory arrangements at the adult facility, subsequent hospital admissions were to the IWK Hospital. This unplanned transfer of care was an unhappy experience, both for the patients and the physicians. One example was that of a young woman in her early twenties with relatively little lung disease who had been diagnosed early in life. After the adult respirologist left Halifax, the medical resident staff, who had no prior exposure to CF, were managing the adult clinic. On her last visit there, despite a productive cough and marked weight loss, she was told by a resident to return for follow up in one year. She immediately returned to our IWK clinic where she was promptly admitted to hospital for a period of intensive treatment. While her clinical condition improved, she did not fully regain her former state of well being.

Five years later in 1983, there had been a considerable increase in the number of older patients, with 31 individuals now 18 years of age and older living in N.S. Another 35 young persons between 10 and 18 years of age would, in the near future, result in a further increase in the number of adults needing treatment. Except for the brief negative experience in 1978, patients of all ages with CF continued to be admitted to the IWK Hospital as there was simply nowhere else to go and most internists had not yet encountered CF adults.

In addition to our own adults with CF, we had additional adult patients from N.B. and P.E.I. who were referred for inpatient treatment. The lack of beds for adults at the IWK Hospital and the enlarging scope of the problems the adult patients had to contend with were beyond the purview of pediatrics and pediatricians. Issues about jobs, training and educational opportunities, marriage, and disability pensions required the expertise of health care workers experienced in these matters. Children's hospitals can be noisy and some of the adult CF patients found hospitalization there less tolerable because of that and the limitations that had to be imposed by the constraints of pediatrics.

Fortunately, Dr. Donald MacIntosh, the respirologist who established the first adult CF clinic in Canada at Montreal in 1969–1970, had recently relocated to Halifax. We discussed our situation with him and he supported Dr. Roger Michael, another adult respirologist, in the opening of an adult clinic at the Victoria General Hospital. Ms. Anna Freeman, a respiratory nurse specialist, assisted. The first patients were transferred in the fall and winter of 1983–1984. There were the inevitable growing pains but by the end of the first year, a specific number of beds had been allocated to CF on the respiratory ward at the Victoria General Hospital (VGH) and a cadre of allied health workers developed into a smoothly functioning team. Especially in the beginning, the transition process from a pediatric to an adult setting was not easy. Having been followed closely for years in a pediatric setting, patients and families were apprehensive about the change. It was the parents who perhaps had the most difficult time. Many years earlier, they had gone through the formative years of the CF clinic while coping with the stressful demands and needs of their CF children but now, much older, they had to face once again many of the same concerns experienced years before.

Individual circumstances determined the best time for transfer but we preferred to transfer after 19 years of age. This allowed time for completion of high school and for the turbulence of adolescence to settle. The respective CF clinic nurses were the key personnel in arranging the details of familiarization. After the adult clinic was firmly established in its own right, younger patients and their families were much less apprehensive about transfer and looked forward to the world beyond adolescence. This successful opening of the adult CF clinic was another major milepost in the CF story in the Maritimes.

Adult Respiratory Rounds: 1966 vs. 1999

Not long ago, I attended Grand Rounds at the new Halifax Infirmary site of the Queen Elizabeth Health Sciences Centre where the adult CF clinic is now located. CF was the topic for discussion and a number of specialists participated in a stimulating discussion of the many challenges they faced in coping with CF in adults. There are now 76 adults from 19 to 54 years of age registered in the clinic.

This experience took me back to 1966 and the VGH where I had my first encounter with adult medicine physicians. VGH was then the main adult teaching hospital. That summer, I was invited to attend the adult Respiratory Rounds when CF was the topic. The case for discussion was that of a 19 year old man admitted with pneumonia and a "presumed" diagnosis of CF. This patient happened to be the first person in N.S. that Dr. Cochrane had diagnosed in 1958 and subsequently cared for. Naturally, in preparation, I reviewed his file at diagnosis and follow up. At rounds, one of the medical residents presented the history of the present illness and physical and laboratory findings. Although the family doctor had referred the

Table 28.2 Patient Survival in Nova Scotia

Category	#Patients	Died (%)	Living (%)
Diagnosis pre–1958	75	62 (83%)	13 (17%)
Diagnosis 1958–66	67	23 (34%)	44 (65%)
Diagnosis 1966–74	38	0 (0%)	38 (100%)

patient to hospital with a diagnosis of "pneumonia," the resident said there was no evidence of "pneumonia" on the chest x-ray. The patient did have a productive cough and a culture report of *Staphylococcus pyogenes*, which were consistent with CF. The physician chairing the session, an adult respirologist, was very skeptical of the past diagnosis of CF and introduced me by saying, "And now Dr Gillespie will prove to us that this man has cystic fibrosis."

I began by reviewing Dr. Cochrane's findings at diagnosis in 1958 and subsequent follow up visits including a positive sweat test in 1959 and confirmed in 1964. On physical examination, I noted the small stature, an over inflated chest with harsh breath sounds on auscultation, and slight but definite enlargement of his liver, especially the left lobe (as observed in some patients with CF), and clubbing of the fingers, consistent with chronic lung disease. On questioning him, I learned that while working on his farm in warm weather, he would often have to wipe salt crystals away after sweating. My review of the chest x-rays clearly showed over inflation of the lungs and diffuse thickening of the bronchial walls.

This combination of history and physical findings in the presence of the two positive sweat tests could only mean a diagnosis of CF so I closed my remarks with "And now the chairman will prove to us that this patient does not have cystic fibrosis." When I sat down, no one disagreed and rounds were suddenly over. How things have changed in 30 years! CF is now a fact of life in adult medicine.

The Improved Outlook Since the 1950 Era

Dr. Cochrane diagnosed his first CF patient in N.S. in 1958. When CF was considered by most physicians to be a hopeless and fatal disease of early childhood. Most physicians had never encountered the disease and those few who did found that it was almost invariably fatal in infancy or very early childhood. Dr. Cochrane's investigations seeking a cause or causes of this severe disorder and his efforts in getting better care and a clinic underway provided a firm basis for the widespread improvement in well being and survival that followed in Nova Scotia and the Maritimes. Table 28.2 shows the improving survival in N.S. through 1974. Of the 75 patients with recognized and diagnosed CF in the province from 1950, only 13 patients survived to 1958 (83% mortality over the eight year span). To 1966, after

Table 28.3 Follow up of 67 Patients from the 1958-1966 Era

Period	# Patients	Deaths	Survivors	Age at Death (yrs) Range	Mean
1958-1966	67	23	44 (65%)	0.02-23.6	3.9
1966-1975	44	8	36 (81%)	4.7-25.2	12.8
1975-1984	36	10	26 (72%)	15.9-31.7	22.8

Table 28.4 Follow up of 38 Patients from the 1966-1974 Era

Period	# Patients	Deaths	Survivors	Age at Death (yrs) Range	Mean
1966–1974	38	0	38 (100%)	–	–
1974–1983	38	0	38 (100%)	–	–
1983–1992	38	8	30 (78%)	17.1–23.8	20.1

Dr. Cochrane's 1958 initiation of the special clinic dedicated to CF patients, mortality decreased to just 34% (4% per year) and no deaths occurred among the 38 patients diagnosed over the next 8 year period to 1974.

Table 28.3 shows the improved survival results in follow up of the 67 patients diagnosed from 1958 through 1966 (the years of Dr. Cochrane's clinic). In the first follow up period, survival increased to 81% and held at 72% through 1984 even though the patients were getting older. The mean age of death also increased markedly. Table 28.4 shows that, for the patients diagnosed in the 1966 to 1974 era, there was even further improvement in survival in the subsequent follow up periods (100% survival in 1983), and the 78% survival to 1992 was a further gain over the 72% observed in follow up among the 1958-1966 group (Table 28.3).

While the improvement in survival in N.S. has been gratifying, diagnosis of CF within the first few months of life, or at least by one year of age, has been disappointing. Table 28.5 shows the percent of patients diagnosed by one year of age was just 46% to 1966 with improvement to 63 % by 1974. Despite improved publicity, increasing numbers of pediatricians, and greater awareness of CF generally, this percentage did not increase beyond 68% by 1992. These data indicate that nearly one third of the patients continued to be diagnosed well after the possibility of irreversible lung damage, such as bronchiectasis, and/or significant nutritional deficit might occur. Universal newborn screening, now feasible, would eliminate

Table 28.5 Patients Diagnosed before 1 Year of Age

Period	Total Diagnosed	Less than Age 1 Year
1958-66	67	31 (46%)
1966-74	38	25 (63%)
1974-82	41	27 (65%)
1982-92	63	43 (68%)

most of the disability encountered in the more than 30% of cases still undiagnosed in the first year of life.

Looking back over the years to my first awareness of and involvement with CF, so much has changed. Far from a disease rarely encountered by most physicians, this almost universally fatal disease of infants and young children is now a major challenge in the world of adult medicine. CF stands at the forefront of major research in the basic sciences (genetics, immunology, etc.) and is in the center of clinical efforts to solve the pressing problems presented in adult life. I still recall the excitement generated when Danes and Bearne published their reports in the late 1960s about a possible marker, observed in certain skin cells, that seemed to enable detection not only of persons with CF but also carriers of the gene. Although hopes were dashed when it was found this characteristic was found in other situations, their work spurred renewed efforts to find a simple marker that would enable detection of patients or carriers. In the early 1970s, Dr. Alex Spock, a pediatric allergist at Duke University in North Carolina, reported a serum factor as another possible marker. While these studies and other researches were underway in many centers, at the clinical care level we had trials of newer antibiotics, new and better enzyme preparations, and other medications to enable our young patients to sustain normal growth and development. These efforts were in support of the daily unremitting treatment regimen at home carried out by the patients and their parents and siblings which was the backbone of treatment. None of this was easy, but, despite the inevitable setbacks and losses, it was so rewarding to witness the emergence into adulthood of so many vibrant and vigorous young men and women who continue to challenge all of us to do our utmost in conquering CF.

In the 26 years from 1966 to 1992, there were over 2400 admissions for CF to the IWK Hospital. Many sweat tests were performed every year. The introduction of DNA analysis, unheard of 20 years ago, now provides an additional diagnostic measure. Problems and unanswered questions remain but the struggle goes on. Thanks to the combined work of countless individuals and groups around the globe, the future is more promising than ever before.

Over 14 years ago, 17 year old Daniella with CF sent a poster for me to hang in my office. I still have that poster which depicts a rock strewn and bush covered valley with a shining mountain peak rising far beyond. The caption on the poster reads, "If there were no valleys, there would be no mountain to climb." Although we have not yet reached the summit, we are well out of the valley and the mountain peak is nearer and brighter still.

Can We Do Even Better?
Looking Ahead

29

The Advantages of Universal CF Neonatal Screening: Why We Need It

Philip M. Farrell, M.D., Ph.D.

The advantages and disadvantages of CF neonatal screening have been considered extensively [1-4] and may be summarized as follows. The most compelling argument to implement population-based screening is to provide each CF patient with an optimal opportunity for medical and psychosocial benefits. Diagnosis in early infancy combined with aggressive, effective nutritional management can prevent malnutrition in almost every child with CF [1,3,5]. With regard to preventing or ameliorating pulmonary disease, there is supportive evidence [3] and we should expect that many CF patients will benefit significantly from having their disease recognized before lung pathology becomes progressive. Stated another way, unless patients have been diagnosed before developing chronic obstructive, inflammatory lung disease, they cannot benefit fully from the advances in respiratory therapy of the past few decades. There is additional evidence to suggest that infection with *Pseudomonas aeruginosa* might be delayed by diagnosis in infancy and careful management.[6] The genetic counseling and psychosocial benefits of early diagnosis are obvious, and it is also possible that the cost of care will be reduced, particularly as fewer hospitalizations occur. Finally, early diagnosis through screening will undoubtedly prevent some deaths and alleviate parental suffering.

The major arguments against CF neonatal screening are the challenge and the start up costs of incorporating the trypsinogen/DNA test into the current battery of newborn screening tests available. All aspects of diagnosis and treatment must be addressed adequately during the planning and implementation processes. The comprehensive nature of newborn screening has been described [7] as "a population-based public health program applying preventive medicine in defined regions to reduce newborn morbidity and mortality from certain biochemical and genetic disorders by using pre-symptomatic detection/diagnosis with dried blood specimens analyzed in central laboratories employing automated procedures and linked to clinical follow up systems." Much can be learned from the Wisconsin and also the Massachusetts programs, each of which has devised its own program in consultation with its own professionals.

All of these components must be sustained with financial support to assure success. Many states recover newborn screening expenses through a variety of charge- back mechanisms, but others are dependent on governmental subsidy. In the latter situation, regions can implement CF neonatal screening by obtaining new financial allocations or by eliminating some existing newborn screening test(s) that can no longer be justified.[7] States that implement CF neonatal screening without assuring all of the follow up benefits and care enhancement strategies will be limiting the value of this diagnostic approach. Other challenges include the need for effective risk communication and genetic counseling sessions and accomplishing the goal of following pre-symptomatic patients at CF centers.

Because the intuitive and demonstrated advantages of CF neonatal screening are so compelling, many regions around the world have already implemented such testing. Entire countries such as Australia now screen and others such as France will soon follow. In the US as of 2000, eight states screen either their entire newborn population or at certain hospitals. Massachusetts is the most recent state to proceed and has more than a year of experience using a sixteen CFTR mutation kit.

CFTR multi-mutation analysis coupled to trypsinogen testing could eventually lead to actual diagnosis of most CF babies from the newborn dried blood specimen.[2] Ultimately, an IRT/CFTR multi-mutation testing strategy will become technically and financially feasible.[8] Rapidly emerging technology for expeditious inexpensive molecular genetics testing imparts a sense of optimism and confidence that neonatal diagnosis of CF will become the routine method. Although the optimum method among the various options for CFTR multi-mutation analysis remains to be determined, or even developed, one can be certain that the laboratory procedures will only improve as the Human Genome Project proceeds. It is already possible, however, to use the 12-16 CFTR mutation kits without prohibitive cost. Such a powerful technology that inexpensively converts a screening test to a quick and accurate diagnostic test will, in my judgment, be irresistible.

The question arises as to why more states in the US are not screening their newborn populations for CF. While explanations for the delay include a number of factors, perhaps the most important has been the lack of a "forcing factor." Many states want to see data that show a decrease in mortality, or a dramatic difference in pulmonary outcomes, or something else that brings pressure by organizations such as the CFF or Centers for Disease Control and Prevention. The position of the CFF has amounted to a "wait and see" attitude. During the long interval since the CFF Task Force report,[9] however, numerous articles have been written on the value of CF neonatal screening, while very little information has surfaced on risks. Data collected by the CFF Registry from 1983 through 1999 reveal that more than 15,000 children with CF have been born in the US and conservative estimates would suggest that 7,000 were severely malnourished at the time of diagnosis.[1,10] We lack good estimates of the amount of accompanying pulmonary disease. Therefore, the time has come when the CFF should take a new position, perhaps in association with the CDC. This will be facilitated by a growing national effort to

Table 29.1. Future Detection and Management of CF: Goals in a New Era

1. Routine neonatal genetic diagnosis through screening
    early detection before malnutrition and pulmonary involvement
    prompt referral to a certified CF Center
    genetic counseling provided to families

2. Prevention of macro- and micro-nutrient deficiencies
    support normal growth and development
    maximize genetic potential for growth and IQ

3. Monitor respiratory status reliably
    prompt identification of pulmonary involvement
    periodic pulmonary function test when age appropriate
    train parents and initiate pulmonary treatment as needed

4. Primary bronchopulmonary prophylactic interventions
    prevent the initiation and/or progression of disease
    maintain quality of life

5. Continue supportive management procedures
    educate and promote understanding and compliance
    improve quality of life

optimize and standardize newborn screening in general and to assure that all states have access to valuable tests.[11]

Looking ahead to the next decade, I envision a brighter prognosis for children with CF. This will occur in my judgment as an integral, and hopefully featured, component of the medical profession's ongoing transformation to a balanced combination of prevention and intervention. The latter strategy, of course, dominated the second half of the 20th century as the entire U.S. health care industry developed more and more interventions for diseased or injured individuals and assured that individualistic interventions predominated. On the other hand, population-oriented prevention of disease has become quite attractive recently and is more feasible now in the era of molecular medicine. I anticipate that this strategy will be increasingly preferred by both patients and third party payors.

With regard to the CF population, effective prevention of disease manifestations is only possible with early, presymptomatic diagnosis, and this can best be achieved through the screening of newborns. Table 29.1 describes my predictions for future diagnosis and treatment/prevention. If the expected transformation occurs nationally to implement such a preventive medicine strategy, I further predict that both the quality and quantity of life will be significantly increased for the next generation of patients with CF. Let's all rededicate ourselves to ensuring a more hopeful outlook for future children with this challenging disease. Prevention should be the passion and pride of Pediatrics.

References

1. Farrell PM, et al. "Improving the health of patients with cystic fibrosis through neonatal screening." *Adv Pediatr* 2000;47:79-115.
2. Wilcken B and Travert G. "Neonatal screening for cystic fibrosis: Present and future." *Acta Pediatr;* 1999;88 suppl 432:33-5
3. Water DL, Wilcken B, Irwig L, Van Asperen P, Mellis C, Simpson JM, et al. "Clinical outcomes of newborn screening for cystic fibrosis." *Arch Dis Child Fetal Neonatal Ed* 1999;80:F1-F7.
4. Centers for Disease Control and Prevention. "Newborn Screening for Cystic Fibrosis: A Paradigm for Public Health Genetics Policy Development." *Morbidity and Mortality Weekly Report.* U.S. Department of Health and Human Services, Vol. 46, No. RR-16, Dec. 1997.
5. Farrell PM, Aronson RA, Hoffman GL, et al. "Newborn screening for cystic fibrosis in Wisconsin: First application of population-based molecular genetics testing." *Wisc Med J* 1994;93:415-21.
6. Kosorok MR, Jalaluddin M, Farrell PM, Shen G, Colby CE, Laxova A, Rock MJ and Splaingard M. "Comprehensive analysis of risk factors for acquisition of *Pseudomonas aeruginosa* in young children with cystic fibrosis." *Pediatr Pulmonol* 26:81-88, 1998.
7. Allen DB, Farrell PM." Newborn screening." *Adv Pediatr* 1996;43:231-70.
8. McCabe ERB, McCabe LL. "State-of-the-art for DNA technology in newborn screening." *Acta Pediatr* 1999; 88 Suppl 432:58-60.
9. AD Hoc Committee Task Force on Neonatal Screening, Cystic Fibrosis Foundation. "Neonatal screening for cystic fibrosis: position paper." *Pediatrics* 1983; 72:741-5.
10. Lai HC, Kosorok MR, Sondel SA, et al." Growth status in children with cystic fibrosis based on the National Cystic Fibrosis Patient Registry data: evaluation of various criteria used to identify malnutrition." *J Pediatr* 1998;132:478-85.
11. A report from the newborn screening task force convened in Washington DC, May 10-11,1999. "Serving the family from birth to the medical home." *Pediatrics suppl* 2000;383-427.
12. Wagener JS, Farrell PM, and Corey M. "A Debate on Why My State (Province) Should or Should Not Conduct Newborn Screening for Cystic Fibrosis" (14th Annual North American Cystic Fibrosis Conference). *Pediatr Pulmon* 2001;32:385–396.

30

Emerging Biotechnologies

Mitchell L. Drumm, Ph.D.

Powerful computers, robotics and other emerging biotechnologies have provided new resources for understanding the complexities involved in normal biological functions, and how they are perturbed in disease. It is now possible to identify genes in a fraction of the time it took only a few years ago. We can now look at tens of thousands of genes simultaneously, whereas before we were limited to only a handful, to look at the interaction among many proteins, and to screen thousands of drugs in a matter of days. An idea of the future for these techniques is summarized below.

Human genome project

The human genome has been sequenced. But how will the knowledge of those 3 billion As, Ts, Cs and Gs benefit us? As we think back to 1989, the identification of the CFTR gene generated expectations of new CF treatments, and even cures, none of which have yet been realized. However, having CFTR in hand has tremendously increased our understanding of CF at the molecular and cellular levels, providing us with much better ideas of what actually needs to be corrected. Yet CFTR is but one gene of an estimated 75,000 to 100,000 found on our chromosomes, and about 10,000 of these genes are active in any one cell.† With thousands of other genes and their products around, it should come as no surprise that CFTR does not work all by itself. In fact, it is now clear that defective CFTR initiates a domino effect in the cells and tissues in which it is found, impacting on numerous enzymes and regulatory molecules encoded by other genes. Certainly much of the pathophysiology of CF is due to the effects CFTR has on these other proteins. CFTR has turned out to be a tough nut to crack, so while we continue to search for ways to correct the CFTR defect, an additional, rational therapeutic approach is to investigate these other proteins, which are all products of different genes. One might more easily think of this through an analogy with the Cleveland winters, in which the salt used to melt ice and snow slowly catalyzes the deterioration of our cars. We fight this battle by washing off the excess salt when possible, rust proofing the cars, replacing rusted parts, but not by ceasing to salt roads, which is the underlying cause. In CF, in which salt is also the underlying cause, we would like to find ways to restore the salt to a non disease status, just as washing the car attempts to do. We would also like to "rustproof" the airways against infection. We can already replace

---

†Since this chapter was prepared, a major finding is that completion of the human genome sequence suggests that we only have 30,000–40,000 genes, not 75,000 to 100,000 that we had thought.

damaged, or "rusted" parts by transplant, but this is not the first line of therapy, due to the availability of healthy, compatible organs. To develop better ways to resist and fight off infection and to find ways to restore salt transport requires identifying and understanding the proteins that carry out these processes. For diseases like CF, the identification step is the most immediate use of the human genome sequencing effort. Identifying the CF gene, a process that took nearly 4 years once its approximate location was determined, could now conceivably be done in days or weeks with a computer and the appropriate analysis software.

Microarray Technologies

The genome sequence will help in the identification of genes, but that information tells us relatively little about what the genes do. Microarrays have developed as a way to observe changes in gene expression of many genes at one time. Previously, one would analyze the level at which a single gene was expressed under a few conditions using radioactively labeled reagents and x-ray film and after a few days or more, one would have a notebook sized document showing the results for that gene. Now, using a couple of postage stamp sized chips and fluorescence technology, one can achieve nearly the same information on tens of thousands of genes and the results are fed directly into a computer. The power of these technologies is yet to be fully realized, as only a portion of the genes are currently known. As the genome project and related efforts identify more genes, the microarray studies will become even more comprehensive. This type of technology will allow comparison of small numbers of cells biopsied from CF and non-CF individuals for how different genes react to a CF environment. From that information, those genes that change their characteristics can be further studied for therapeutic purposes.

High Throughput Screening

Robotics and miniaturized biotechnologies are opening the door to faster screening for candidate drugs. Using culture dishes about the size of a recipe card, each with 384 wells, one can culture a few cells in each well and look for the effects of various drugs on those cells. A robot takes the rectangular culture dish and administers one of thousands of compounds to each well and then a computer, interfacing through an optic sensor, reads the response of the cells to the drugs. Dozens of culture plates can be screened in a day, allowing thousands of compounds to be screened very rapidly. Such studies are being carried out for CF currently, in which CF cells are cultured in these dishes, exposed to drugs and monitored for chloride channel activity. This type of technology also overlaps with the microarray technology, for as genes of interest are identified by the microarrays, compounds already known to act on those gene products, and derivatives of those compounds, can be tested for their effects on CF cells.

In summary, identification of the CF gene has not extended the life of a single CF patient. The gene has, however, provided us with immense amounts of information with which to devise new therapies. Combined with this genetic derived information and these available biotechnologies, a reasonable expectation should be that more effective treatments for CF should be realized.

31

Airway Epithelial Dysfunction and Lung Disease: Insights for Future Therapy

Michael R. Knowles, M.D. and Richard C. Boucher, M.D.

The study of normal airway epithelial cell function and the defective genetic and cell function in cystic fibrosis (CF) has been undertaken, in large part, to enable the development of better therapy. It has been a logical, albeit slower-than-desired, journey to understand key facets of the disease. A brief review of the sequential progress we have made in understanding the root cause (pathogenesis) of the lung disease will provide the basis for a rational approach to the development of new therapies, which we hope will occur in the near future.

Prior to identification of the CF gene, it was generally appreciated in the 1970s that CF was a disease of epithelial cells, but it was not clear whether the epithelial dysfunction was intrinsic to the epithelium, or reflected the effect of circulating factors on epithelial function. We developed a technique that measured a single parameter of epithelial function called the transepithelial potential difference (PD), and used this technique to define the salt (ion) transport properties of nasal and lower respiratory epithelium in normal humans *in vivo*, and subsequently in patients with respiratory disease. CF patients exhibited a striking finding that became the hallmark of CF airway epithelia; the transepithelial PD was markedly higher than normal. This higher transepithelial PD in CF was apparent within hours after birth, which pointed strongly to the likelihood that this reflected a primary genetic defect in CF airways epithelium, and was not a consequence of chronic infection or "circulating factors."

In further studies of the defective airway epithelial function in CF, instead of finding a single defect of Cl^- transport as seen in sweat ductal epithelium, we identified several defects in CF airways epithelium:[1,2,3]

A defect was identified in the ability of Cl^- to move across CF cells (transcellular Cl^- permeability).

The Cl^- permeability of CF airways epithelium was not activated by beta-agonists, as was seen in normal subjects.

The most striking defect in CF epithelia was the very rapid absorption of salt (NaCl,) and water, which was determined from the greater inhibition of the PD with a Na^+ channel blocker (amiloride) *in vivo*, and direct measurements of the absorption of Na^+ (and Cl^- ions *in vitro*, using open circuit flux techniques.

These observations led to the hypothesis that CF airways epithelium has an excessive rate of NaCl and water (volume) absorption, which would dehydrate airway secretions, and lead to reduced clearance of mucus from airways, and, ultimately, chronic airway infection. This hypothesis led to clinical studies with an aerosolized Na^+ channel blocker, e.g., amiloride that appeared to be effective in short-term studies of CF airways dysfunction, e.g., mucociliary clearance. However, amiloride was not effective as a therapeutic adjunct to the standard treatment of CF in the late 1980s.

Identification of the CF gene in 1989 led to better understanding of the role of the CFTR gene in healthy people, and the impact of defective function in CF. The following are four examples of how these studies advanced understanding and progress toward better therapy.

At the University of North Carolina at Chapel Hill, we were able to diagnose patients with very mild pulmonary disease, but normal sweat chloride values, and identified genetic mutations in CFTR. The disease in these patients reflected splicing defects in the CFTR gene, which resulted in relatively low levels of normal CFTR, so that 5-10% of the normal level of CFTR protected against "severe" CF, which was very useful in considering the degree of correction required for gene transfer or new drug therapy.

The availability of the CFTR gene made it possible to make a mouse model of CF, leading to the discovery that the CF mouse lungs had high levels of a Ca^{2+}-activated (or alternative) Cl^- channel. We recognized that the CF Cl^- channel defect could be bypassed, which, in some instances, would protect against disease. This observation contributed to the development of drugs that activate these alternative Cl^- channels via "purinergic" receptors (see below).

Studies established that CFTR is not only a cAMP-regulated Cl^- channel, but that it also inhibits the airway epithelial Na^+ channel.[4] In CF, where CFTR function is missing, the Na^+ channel is not inhibited, which provides a molecular understanding of the excessive salt (NaCl) and water absorption in CF airways *in vivo*. It also further reinforced the notion that therapy might be derived from drugs that effectively inhibit the Na^+ channel in CF airways, and thereby limit the excessive absorption of salt (and water) from airway surfaces.

Availability of the CFTR gene enabled the rapid testing of gene transfer as a potential therapeutic approach. The CF defect could be "corrected" by transfection of the normal CFTR gene, and preliminary studies suggested that only 3-10% of the cells might need to be corrected to be therapeutically important. It was shown both in animal models (including the CF mouse) and humans that major barriers exist to airway luminal delivery of gene transfer vectors containing the normal CFTR gene.[5] Recognition that new approaches are needed has set the stage for identifying receptors that bind and internalize gene transfer vectors into airway cells, and for ways to penetrate a "shield," i.e., the glycocalyx, on the luminal membrane of airway cells.[6]

After identifying cellular functions of CFTR, it was critical to define the pathogenesis of lung disease, i.e., to determine how the loss of CFTR function would affect airways and lead to disease. We, and others, measured the concentration of salt in airway surface liquid of normal subjects and CF infants prior to infectious lung disease, and found the concentration of salt to be similar in both normal and CF, and to be isotonic.[7,8] Further detailed studies identified dramatic differences in the rates of isotonic volume absorption between CF and normal. CF airways had very rapid (compared to normal) absorption of isotonic salt (and water), which abolished mucus transport after several hours.[9] The slowing of mucus transport included changes in the viscoelastic properties of the mucus layer, and also a depletion of the periciliary liquid layer. Thus, excessive absorption of salt (and water), and depletion of the periciliary liquid layer, not only abolishes the ciliary component of mucus clearance, but also allows the cell surface and mucus to come in contact, and "anneal" to one another. This combination of disease mechanisms provides a compelling scenario, whereby mucus plaques (and plugs) accumulate in airways, and become the site for infection on airway surfaces (biofilm infection). At a functional level, depletion of the periciliary liquid layer abolishes both major airway mucus clearance mechanisms, i.e., mucociliary clearance and cough-dependent clearance. This double hit on mucus clearance likely explains the severity of CF lung disease as compared to another lung disease with defects in only the ciliary-dependent component, i.e., primary ciliary dyskinesia.

Looking Ahead

Although there are many important scientific discoveries to be made in the context of CFTR function and the dysfunctions of the diseased tissues, much of the future work in CF will focus on developing novel therapies based on our current and emerging understanding of the functional problems encountering the CF patient. Three general strategies can be envisioned.

First, gene therapy represents perhaps the most elegant and simple form of therapy for this disease. As mentioned above, a single copy of the normal CFTR gene will correct the dysfunctions of CF cells. However, we greatly underestimated the difficulty of getting the normal CFTR gene into cells of the airways *in vivo*. Thus, major efforts are underway to identify molecules on the luminal membrane of airway cells, which will help mediate gene transfer. Future efforts will also require modifying the gene transfer vector so it can better interact with pertinent receptors on airway cells. This effort will also need to be coupled with methods to reduce the luminal membrane "shield" (glycocalyx) that confronts any vector. An ongoing challenge is getting the vector to the correct region of airways in humans *in vivo*, and the confounding effects of infection and inflammation in CF. Theoretically, the application of these vectors will be simplest in neonates with CF (no intrinsic airways/lung disease). However, there are real concerns about the safety/ advisability of initiating such forms of therapy in young children and how any measurements of "benefit" can be made in meaningful periods of time in this patient population.

Second, better definition of the "root cause" (pathogenesis) of the lung disease will identify potential therapeutic targets, and clearly expand the opportunities for better therapy. For example, patients homozygous for the $\Delta F508$ mutation have pulmonary disease ranging from very severe to very mild. This observation suggests that there are important interactions with the environment that affect the lung perhaps more than other organs, and that there are important modifier genes that modulate the severity (or mildness) of CFTR dysfunction in the lung. Therefore, we will search for these modifier genes using a series of hypothesis driven and screening (high-tech gene arrays) approaches. Identification of modifier genes and definition of their roles in the lung with respect to CFTR dysfunction will be important not only for understanding the pathogenesis in this disease, but also for identifying new targets for pharmacotherapy. Stated another way, if specific defects in cell function can be identified, then new drugs might be used to correct the defective functions. Some of these new drug targets are likely to be proteins that are normally regulated by CFTR, but dysregulated in CF patients. Currently, high throughput screening (see Drumm, Future Directions) is focused on identifying new drugs that can activate Cl⁻ channels. Future efforts will almost certainly include screening for drugs that target multiple other therapeutic targets. Now that the Pseudomonas aeruginosa genome has been sequenced, better understanding of this bacterium and new avenues of attack should likely identify new treatment approaches.

Third, it appears we are well poised to attack the initiating lesion in the CF airways, the mucus plaque/plug. Theoretically, we only have to replace 5–10 ml (1-2 tsp) of isotonic fluid on airway surfaces, which would not initially appear to be difficult. However, to achieve a persistent change of this magnitude will require new approaches. We are currently studying the use of inhaled "osmolites" based on the notion that small particles will draw water into the airways, and hydrate airway secretions. The challenge is to safely deliver sufficient quantities of osmolites that will stay on airway surfaces for therapeutically necessary intervals. New derivatives of Na⁺ channel blockers must be developed that will remain on airway surfaces and block salt (NaCl) and water absorption for longer intervals than the first generation drugs. These Na⁺ channel blockers may also potentially be used in conjunction with osmolites to rapidly restore liquid onto airway surfaces and maintain it. Finally, drugs to stimulate the airway surface, so-called "purinergic" receptors provides an attractive monotherapy of CF.[10] These purinergic receptor drugs (agonists) such as uridine triphosphate, or UTP,* not only activate alternative Cl⁻ channels to initiate Cl⁻ secretion, but also block Na⁺ absorption.[11] Thus, the development of long-acting purinergic receptor agonists that can be safely inhaled onto CF airway surfaces is moving rapidly, and clinical trials are anticipated in normal and CF subjects before long.

The unanswered question is whether other adjunctive therapies will be required to remove plaques. One might also need to think about additional strategies that would rehydrate mucus plaques more rapidly to augment the activity of specific drugs. Thus, it is hoped that these newer drugs will remove the mucus plaques that form the site of airways infection, and reduce the need for antimicrobial drugs.

Summary

The future is focused on developing better therapy for CF lung disease, based on a clearer understanding of the cause of the disease, and a rational approach to treat the defective cell functions. We already have well-defined pathophysiological targets, and several candidate approaches for therapy. Current high technology testing for additional therapeutic targets, and the application of high through-put screening to identify potential new therapeutic drugs, offer real opportunities to identify more effective pharmacological agents. Gene transfer of the normal CFTR gene is a realistic goal for treating CF lung disease in the new millenium, but it is likely to require more than five years to adequately develop gene transfer techniques for use in the clinic.

Note: R.C. Boucher and M.R. Knowles are founding scientists of Inspire Pharmaceuticals, which licensed the patent for aerosolized UTP from the University of North Carolina on March 10, 1995. R.C. Boucher, M.R. Knowles, and the University of North Carolina hold equity in Inspire Pharmaceuticals.

References

1. Boucher RC. "Human airway ion transport (Part 1)." *Am J Respir Crit Care Med.* 1994;150:271-281.
2. Boucher RC. "Human airway ion transport (Part 2)." *Am J Respir Crit Care Med.* 1994;150:581-593.
3. *Cystic Fibrosis in Adults.* Philadelphia, Knowles MR and Yankaskas JR ed. Lippincott-Raven, 1999.
4. Stutts MJ, Canessa CM, Olsen JC, Hamrick M, Cohn JA, Rossier BC, Boucher RC. "CFTR as a cAMP-dependent regulator of sodium channels." *Science* 1995;269:847-850.
5. Knowles MR, Hohneker KW, Zhou Z, Olsen JC, Noah TL, Hu PC, Leigh MW, Engelhardt JF, Edwards LJ, Jones KR, Grossman M, Wilson JM, Johnson LG, Boucher RC. "A controlled study of adenoviral vector-mediated gene transfer in the nasal epithelium of patients with cystic fibrosis." *N Engl J Med.* 1995;333:823-831.
6. Pickles RJ, Fahrner JA, Petrella JM, Boucher RC, Bergelson JM. "Retargeting the Coxsackivirus and adenovirus receptor to the apical surface of polarized epithelial cells reveals the glycocalyx as a barrier to adenovirus-mediated gene transfer." *J Virol* 2000;74:6050-6057.

7. Knowles MR, Robinson JM, Wood RE, Pue CA, Mentz WM, Wager GC, Gatzy JT, Boucher RC. "Ion composition of airway surface liquid of patients with cystic fibrosis as compared to normal and disease-control subjects." *J Clin Invest* 1997;100:2588-2595.

8. Hull J, Skinner W, Robertson C, Phelan P. "Elemental content of airway surface liquid from infants with cystic fibrosis." *Am J Respir Crit Care Med* 1998;157:10-14.

9. Matsui H, Grubb BR, Tarran R, Randell SH, Gatzy JT, Davis CW, Boucher RC." Evidence for periciliary liquid layer depletion, not abnormal ion composition, in the pathogenesis of cystic fibrosis airways disease." *Cell* 1998;95:1005-1015.

10. Bennett WD, Olivier KN, Zeman KL, Hohneker KW, Boucher RC, Knowles MR. "Effect of uridine 5'-triphosphate plus amiloride on mucociliary clearance in adult cystic fibrosis." *Am J Respir Crit Care Med* 1996;153:1796-1801.

11. Devor DC, Pilewski JM. "UTP inhibits Na^+ absorption in wild-type and DeltaF508 CFTR-expressing human bronchial epithelia." *Am J Physiol* 1999;276:C827-C837.

Patient Care and Research

Pamela B. Davis, M.D., Ph.D.

Where is the CF field going in the next five years? First of all, it will be vital to keep patients well enough to benefit from a cure when it comes, whether from gene therapy or from manipulation of ion transport. Maintenance of effective ongoing care is a critical part of the battle against CF. Almost as important as the drug development is the aggressive management of the patients now alive. The physicians on the front lines must defend aggressive therapy to insurers reluctant to spend money now for potential future gains. In addition, families must be encouraged to administer home treatments faithfully, and not to assume that modern medicine can rescue a lung badly damaged by neglect. We are in danger of being dazzled by our own accomplishments and caught up in the hope for the future because of the progress in the past, and behaving as if anything can be fixed with a new drug or a miracle cure. We cannot let patients pass some figurative "point of no return" because of insurance pressure or complacency. **Vigorous prosecution of conventional treatment should be the order of the day. Just as we cannot let up on the research to develop the cures of tomorrow, so too we cannot neglect the meticulous care of the patient today.**

In the meantime, there are many exciting areas of research that will teach us much about the basic science of the cystic fibrosis transmembrane conductance regulator protein (CFTR), epithelia, gene modifiers, and inflammation. However, the current excitement in the field is in the area of development of new therapeutics. Many drugs are under development that are relevant to CF. The CF Foundation is putting tens of millions of dollars into pursuing new opportunities for drug discovery and development. These include high throughput screening of compounds for their ability to activate chloride transport in epithelial cells, support for companies and laboratories to develop promising drugs and reagents, and organization of a network of clinical centers designed to test drugs in Phase I and Phase II testing. With all this activity, surely there will be some "hits," won't there?

Well, maybe. From my personal perspective, I worry that simply activating chloride transport in the apical membrane of airway epithelial cells (the goal for some of the high throughput screening assays) may not be sufficient to correct the pathophysiology of CF in the airways. It seems likely, at the very least, that to sustain chloride secretion, chloride entry at the basolateral membrane must be assured, as well as activation of a potassium channel. Some candidate drugs that activate CFTR may fail to activate epithelial chloride transport because they inhibit these other transporters (or even just fail to stimulate them). Moreover, in one model for

CF pathogenesis in the airway, excess sodium reabsorption occupies a central pathophysiologic position. If this model is correct, manipulating chloride transport without inhibiting sodium reabsorption will be insufficient. Thus, we may have to do more than activate chloride transport by any means to cure this disease. Developing agents for these additional interventions may become important as chloride transport activators come to clinical trial.

New antibiotics now under development will definitely help, as they have in the past, but we are not often hampered in CF care right now by "running out of antibiotics." Some of the high powered antibiotics are not convenient to use, but most bacteria can be treated. To me, the more pressing issues are:

1. how to best prevent establishment of chronic infection and

2. effective control of the ensuing inflammation.

New strategies of dealing with infection early in life need to be developed and validated in clinical testing. In addition, anti-inflammatory therapy is not in wide use for CF. Corticosteroids have limiting side effects. Despite very impressive results from high dose ibuprofen in younger patients with CF with few adverse effects, this drug has not gained wide acceptance, either. It may be that its profile of adverse effects is unacceptable (that is, gastrointestinal hemorrhage or renal insufficiency can be severe and life threatening), or it may be that no dramatic difference is noted by the patient (or physician) when it is taken compared to when it is not. The benefits of anti-inflammatory therapy are evident only with time and consistency of administration. This is a knotty problem for physicians. Prophylactic treatment is logical in CF, yet this effective drug goes unused. A better version of ibuprofen - one with a more favorable therapeutic index, or even one that some company will market vigorously - would be a great boon to CF patients.

To me, gene therapy still offers the best opportunity to "cure" patients with CF. Despite the false starts and the disappointments, the strategy in principle should work and should be fully corrective of all the defects in the disease. Devising a safe and effective gene therapy strategy is not trivial, however. There has been continuing progress by investigators who have not jumped immediately to clinical trials or who have used patient trials judiciously as tools to improve the current vectors. This progress should not be discounted, despite the evident failures in CF and other diseases. It seems to me likely in the next five years that nontoxic gene therapy approaches will come to clinical trial that will impact the electrophysiology of the airway epithelium, demonstrate gene transfer unequivocally, and correct some of the downstream manifestations of CF in the airways. It may require additional effort and time to produce high level, long lasting correction, but once the principle is established this reduces to a technical problem.

Glossary

ATP(T)	Association of Tennis Professionals
ATP	adenosine triphosphate
ATS	American Thoracic Society
B&C Hospital	Babies & Children's Hospital, Cleveland
CCFF	Canadian Cystic Fibrosis Foundation
CF	cystic fibrosis
CFF	Cystic Fibrosis Foundation
Cftr	the mouse counterpart to CFTR
CFTR	human cystic fibrosis transmembrane conductance regulator
CTR	Care Teaching and Research Center
CWRU	Case Western Reserve University, Cleveland
DNA	deoxyribonucleic acid
EC	Executive Committee of the International Association of Cystic Fibrosis Adults
ESCF	The European Society for Cystic Fibrosis (formerly the European Working Group)
FDA	Federal Drug Administration
GAP	Guidance, Action and Projection program
GMSAC	General Medical and Scientific Advisory Council
HCH	Halifax Children's Hospital
HSC	Hospital for Sick Children, Toronto
IACFA	The International Association of Cystic Fibrosis Adults
ICF[M]A	International Cystic Fibrosis [Mucoviscidosis] Foundation
IRT	immunoreactive trypsinogen
IV	intravenous
IWK	Isaac Walton Killam Hospital, Halifax
MAC	Medical Advisory Council
NCFRF	National Cystic Fibrosis Research Foundation
NEJM	New England Journal of Medicine
NHLBI	National Heart, Lung, and Blood Institute
NIAMD	National Institute for Arthritis and Metabolic Diseases
NIDDK	National Institute for Diabetes, Digestive, and Kidney Diseases

NIH	National Institutes of Health
PPC	Pediatric Pulmonary Center
RDP	Research Development Program
TDN	Therapeutics Development Network
UCLA	University of California Los Angeles
UT	University of Texas
VGH	Victoria General Hospital, Halifax

Name Index

Subject Index

Numerics

1,000 Years of Cystic Fibrosis 287, 329

A

A Plea for a Future 172, 233, 243
ABI Vest® 326, 341
adult 14, 69, 77, 101, 102, 113, 114, 118, 141, 170, 190, 237, 249, 259, 261, 264, 265, 266, 267, 270, 279, 287, 300, 303, 304, 307, 309, 310, 314, 332, 337, 338, 339, 345, 347, 350, 382, 383, 384, 386
Adult CF Clinic 380, 382
Adult Pulmonary Centers 224
aerosol 20, 68, 71, 72, 73, 143, 176, 177, 184, 198, 298, 305, 306, 307, 311, 336, 339, 340, 355, 364, 370, 371, 377
agar plate test 197
allele 297
alleles 132, 133, 146, 296
American Academy of Pediatrics 157, 353
American Association of Respiratory Care 345, 346
American College of Chest Physicians 353
American Thoracic Society 322, 353
amiloride 143, 398
anion gap 49, 50
antibiotic 7, 17, 19, 61, 66, 68, 69, 70, 72, 73, 98, 100, 101, 102, 117, 140, 143, 164, 176, 295, 297, 298, 299, 305, 306, 342, 348, 355, 366
aspergillosis 381
Associate Program 113
Association 263
   International Cystic Fibrosis Association 251, 253, 266, 330
Association of Tennis Professionals 168, 254, 255
asthma 5, 10, 63, 69, 224, 227, 309, 323, 324, 336, 339, 345, 361, 377

B

Babies and Children's Hospital 63, 75, 90, 93, 120, 138, 139, 154, 193, 200, 203, 220, 245, 247, 336, 346, 361, 367
Babies Hospital 18, 20, 23, 24, 25, 28, 30, 31, 68, 71, 138, 149, 152, 154, 164, 212
basic science advisory committee 207

Belgian CF Association 263
biotechnology 146, 266
Birth of the Foundation 152
Board of Trustees 153, 154, 161, 174, 180, 191, 195, 199, 201, 206, 210, 213, 214, 218, 219, 221, 225, 227, 228, 230, 234, 237, 240, 241, 243, 353
Boston Children's Hospital 57, 64, 138, 154, 169, 212, 361
Boylston Society 277
bronchiectasis 17, 39, 56, 66, 70, 116, 277, 284, 341, 385
bronchoscope 7, 113, 114, 115, 116, 117, 118, 307
bronchoscopy 7, 75, 113, 114, 115, 116, 117, 118, 119, 307, 341
Buckhill Falls 216
Burkholderia cepacia 140, 141, 265, 269, 306, 350

C

Canadian Cystic Fibrosis Foundation 363, 365
carbon dioxide 8, 28, 323, 347
Care Committee 221, 229
Care Teaching and Research Centers 138
Case Western Reserve University 90, 120, 145, 190, 191, 198, 225, 292
cause of death 3, 8, 9, 145, 322, 326
cDNA libraries 86, 87, 144
celiac disease 17, 18, 24, 30, 110, 194, 335, 362
Center Committee 74, 214, 221, 229, 275, 276, 317, 318, 327, 328, 329, 331, 332, 333, 348, 358
Center Director 60, 61, 120, 140, 142, 169, 281, 292, 310, 316, 318, 323, 326, 329, 358, 373
Center network 126, 139, 140, 142, 143, 144, 146, 340
Centers for Gene Therapy 145
Centers Program 77
Centers program 142, 240
central catheter 105
CF Center 7, 15, 60, 74, 90, 118, 120, 121, 124, 126, 127, 134, 136, 140, 141, 145, 204, 209, 215, 224, 247, 281, 282, 283, 289, 291, 292, 295, 304, 307, 308, 309, 310, 311, 316, 317, 318, 320, 322, 323,